Applications of Biomaterials
in
Facial Plastic Surgery

Editors

Alvin I. Glasgold, M.D.

Chairman, Department of Otolaryngology
Robert Wood Johnson University Hospital
and St. Peter's Medical Center
New Brunswick, New Jersey
and Attending Staff, Department of Otolaryngology
Manhattan Eye, Ear, and Throat Hospital
New York, New York

Frederick H. Silver, Ph.D.

Associate Professor, Department of Pathology
Robert Wood Johnson Medical School
and Director, Graduate Program
in Biomedical Engineering
Rutgers University
Piscataway, New Jersey

CRC Press
Boca Raton   Ann Arbor   Boston

Library of Congress Cataloging-in-Publication Data

Applications of biomaterials in facial plastic surgery/editors,
Alvin I. Glasgold, Frederick H. Silver.
   p. cm.
  Includes bibliographical references and index.
  ISBN 0-8493-5251-7
  1. Face--Surgery. 2. Biomedical materials. 3. Surgery, Plastic.
I. Glasgold, Alvin I. II. Silver, Frederick H., 1949-
  [DNLM: 1. Biocompatible Materials--therapeutic use. 2. Face-
-surgery. 3. Surgery, Plastic. WE 705 A652]
  RD523.A66 1991
  617.5′2′0592--dc20
  DNLM/DLC
  for Library of Congress

90-15144
CIP

Direct all inquiries to CRC Press, Inc., 2000 Corporate Blvd., N.W., Boca Raton, Florida 33431.

© 1991 by CRC Press, Inc.

International Standard Book Number 0-8493-5251-7

Library of Congress Card Number 90-15144
Printed in the United States

PREFACE

The use of autografts, homografts and off-the-shelf polymers was, in the past, sufficient to generate acceptable cosmetic results in facial surgery. However, during the last decade advances in surgical techniques, appreciation of the consequences of homograft resorption, as well as decreased use of homografts because of the increased risk of viral contamination, have led to an increased interest in the development of new implant materials.

The development of biological and synthetic implants has previously occurred via two almost independent pathways. Surgeons have traditionally pioneered the development of biological graft materials while engineers and scientists have been largely responsible for introduction of synthetic polymers in a variety of medical applications.

Increased sophistication of facial plastic surgeons has led to an increase in the number of cosmetic surgical procedures to correct genetic, traumatic, and cosmetic deformities as well as an increased expectation for positive results by the patient. The growing awareness of cosmetic procedures as well as the patient's expectation of positive results have led to a need for improved surgical techniques and "ideal" implants for each type of procedure. What was surgically acceptable ten years ago, falls short of being cosmetically acceptable by present standards.

Advances in research and surgical techniques have been a result of attracting greater talent to the field as well as development of an interdisciplinary approach to implant design. Integration of advances in surgical techniques with the design and evaluation of new biological and synthetic implants is an ongoing challenge that faces those who work in this interdisciplinary field. It is our hope that this book may expose those involved in this field to both the clinical and basic scientific principles and help to catalyze the assembly of strategic alliances between surgeons, engineers, and scientists to facilitate design and evaluation of new implant materials.

Alvin I. Glasgold, M.D.
Frederick H. Silver, Ph.D.

THE EDITORS

Alvin I. Glasgold, M.D., is Chairman of the Department of Otolaryngology—Head and Neck Surgery at Robert Wood Johnson University Hospital and St. Peter's Medical Center, New Brunswick, New Jersey. He is on the Attending Staff and is a Resident Instructor in Facial Plastic Surgery at Manhattan Eye, Ear, and Throat Hospital, New York, New York. He is also an Associate Clinical Professor of Surgery at the Robert Wood Johnson Medical School in New Jersey.

Dr. Glasgold graduated in 1957 from Alfred University, Alfred, New York with a B.A. degree (cum laude) and obtained his M.D. degree in 1961 from New York Medical College, New York. He was an intern at Beth Israel Hospital in New York and a resident physician at the Bronx Veteran's Hospital, New York (1961 to 1966).

Dr. Glasgold is a Fellow of the American College of Surgeons, the American Academy of Otolaryngology—Head and Neck Surgery, the American Society for Head and Neck Surgery, the American Academy of Facial Plastic and Reconstructive Surgery, the American Academy of Cosmetic Surgery and the American Society of Lipo-Suction Surgery. He is certified by the American Board of Otolaryngology—Head and Neck Surgery, and has served as a Board Examiner for the American Board of Facial Plastic and Reconstructive Surgery.

Dr. Glasgold has been a representative to the Board of Governors of the American Academy of Otolaryngology—Head and Neck Surgery. He was the first Chairman of the Facial Plastic Section of the New Jersey Academy of Ophthalmology and Otolaryngology and was the 1985 recipient of the Merit Award from the New Jersey Academy of Ophthalmology and Otolaryngology for his contributions to Facial Plastic Surgery. He is presently serving on the Credentials Committee of the American Academy of Facial Plastic and Reconstructive Surgery. He is President of the Facial Plastic Surgery Information Service.

Dr. Glasgold has been a guest lecturer throughout the United States in the field of Rhinoplasty, Facial Plastic Surgery, and the utilization of biomaterials in Facial Plastic Surgery and has published 20 scientific papers. He has chaired an annual course in External Rhinoplasty at Manhattan Eye, Ear, and Throat Hospital and served as chairman of the annual meetings of the Facial Plastic Section of the New Jersey Academy of Ophthalmology and Otolaryngology. His current research is in biomaterials and facial implants conducted at the Biomaterials Center of the Robert Wood Johnson Medical School.

Frederick H. Silver, Ph.D., is Associate Professor of Pathology at Robert Wood Johnson Medical School in Piscataway, New Jersey and Director of the Graduate Program in Biomedical Engineering jointly administered by the University of Medicine and Dentistry of New Jersey and Rutgers University.

Dr. Silver received his B.S. degree from Northeastern University, Boston, Massachusetts in 1972. He obtained his M.S. and Ph.D. degrees in 1975 and 1977, respectively, in polymer science from the Department of Mechanical Engineering at Massachusetts Institute of Technology. After doing postdoctoral work at Massachusetts General Hospital, Boston, Massachusetts, he was appointed an Assistant Professor of Pathology at Harvard Medical School in 1980. Concurrently, he was Adjunct Assistant Professor of Biomedical Engineering at Boston University, Boston, Massachusetts. He became an Associate Professor of Pathology in 1981 at Robert Wood Johnson Medical School (formerly Rutgers Medical School), Piscataway, New Jersey. In 1985, Dr. Silver was appointed Associate Director of the Biomedical Engineering Graduate Program and in 1990, became Director of the program.

Dr. Silver is a member of the American Association for the Advancement of Science, Biomedical Engineering Society, Society of Biomaterials, New York Academy of Sciences, and the honorary society, Sigma Xi.

Dr. Silver has been the recipient of research grants from the National Institutes of Health, the National Science Foundation, the Orthopedic Research and Education Foundation, the Veterans Administration, and from private industry. He has written 2 textbooks and published more than 80 scientific papers. His current research interests are in self assembly of macromolecules, physical properties of the extracellular matrix, biomaterials, and medical devices.

CONTRIBUTORS

Jeanne Adams, M.D., F.A.C.S.
McPherson Hospital
Duke University Medical Center
Durham, North Carolina

G. Jan Beekhuis, M.D., F.A.C.S.
Head and Neck Surgery
Wayne State University Medical Center
Detroit, Michigan

Richard A. Berg, Ph.D.
Department of Biochemistry
Robert Wood Johnson Medical School
Piscataway, New Jersey

Hilary Brodie, M.D., Ph.D.
Department of Otolaryngology—Head
  and Neck Surgery
University of California, Davis Medical
  Center
Sacramento, California

**Michael M. Churukian, M.D.,
  F.A.C.S.**
Otolaryngology—Head and Neck Surgery
University of Southern California
Los Angeles, California

Alfred Cohen, M.D., F.A.C.S.
Department of Otolaryngology
University of California in Los Angeles
Los Angeles, California

Jeffrey J. Colton, M.D.
Cosmetic Surgeons of Michigan
Birmingham, Michigan

Dale P. DeVore, Ph.D.
Autogenesis Technologies Inc.
Acton, Massachusetts

Paul J. Donald, M.D., F.R.C.S. (c)
Department of Otolaryngology—
  Head and Neck Surgery
University of California, Davis Medical
  Center
Sacramento, California

Michael G. Dunn, Ph.D.
Division of Orthopedic Surgery
University of Medicine and Dentistry
Brunswick, New Jersey

Jeffrey C. Geesin, Ph.D. Cand.
Johnson and Johnson Consumer Products,
  Inc.
Skillman, New Jersey

Alvin I. Glasgold, M.D.
Otolaryngology—Head and Neck Surgery
Robert Wood Johnson University Hospital
St. Peter's Medical Center
New Brunswick, New Jersey

Mark Glasold, M.D.
Otolaryngology—Head and Neck Surgery
Manhattan Eye, Ear and Throat Hospital
New York, New York

G. Richard Holt, M.D., M.S.E.
Otolaryngology—Head and Neck Surgery
University of Texas Health Science
  Center
San Antonio, Texas

Frank M. Kamer, M.D., F.A.C.S.
Lasky Clinic
Beverly Hills, California

Wayne F. Larrabee, M.D.
Department of Otolaryngology—
  Head and Neck Surgery
University of Washington
Seattle, Washington

Lawrence Lefkoff, M.D.
Lasky Clinic
Beverly Hills, California

**Lawrence J. Marentette, M.D.,
  F.A.C.S.**
Department of Otolaryngology
University Center for Craniofacial/Skull
  Base Surgery
University of Minnesota
Minneapolis, Minnesota

David S. Orentreich, M.D.
Orentreich Medical Group
New York, New York

Norman Orentreich, M.D.
Orentreich Medical Group
New York, New York

Francis R. Palmer III, M.D.
Lasky Clinic
Beverly Hills, California

J. Russell Parsons, Ph.D.
Department of Orthopedic Surgery
New Jersey Medical School
Newark, New Jersey

Carol A. Ross, R.N.
Lasky Clinic
Beverly Hills, California

Frederick H. Silver, Ph.D.
Department of Pathology
Robert Wood Johnson Medical School
Piscataway, New Jersey

Dean M. Toriumi, M.D.
Department of Otolaryngology—
  Head and Neck Surgery
University of Illinois College of Medicine
Chicago, Illinois

Claus Walter, M.D.
Plastische Chirurgie
Klinik am Rosenberg
Heiden, Switzerland

Arthur J. Wasserman, Ph.D.
Department of Medical Writing Division
Bio-Pharmaceutical Clinical Services
Blue Bell, Pennsylvania

TABLE OF CONTENTS

Part I—Basic Science

Chapter 1

OVERVIEW

Frederick H. Silver and Alvin I. Glasgold

In the 1950s, biomaterials were used as vascular grafts and wound dressings to avoid life-threatening complications of vascular disease and traumatic injury, respectively. Due to the life-threatening consequences of the illnesses, success of these implants was largely a result of trial and error modification of prototype medical devices.

Since, then, many advances have been made in the development of medical devices consisting of natural and synthetic polymers, and in the establishment of interdisciplinary research teams involving scientists, engineers, and clinicians. In addition, our understanding of what chemical components are present in facial tissues as well as the types of cells and the tissue architecture has expanded dramatically. In order to design biomaterials to be used in the face, it is necessary to understand (1) the chemical components and physical structure of facial tissues; (2) types of conditions that are seen in clinical medicine that require biomaterials; and (3) conventional implants and their biocompatibility.

All tissues are composed of cells, extracellular proteins in the form of fibers that form three-dimensional tissue scaffolds, factors that bind cells to extracellular tissue scaffolds, and other molecules required for nutrition and tissue homeostasis. Although the types of cells found in facial tissues differ for skin, cartilage, and bone, and the chemistry of the collagen types and attachment factors differ for each tissue, the generic nature of the building blocks of these tissues are similar.

It is of primary importance that biomaterials including polymers, metals, and ceramics used in medical devices not interfere with normal cellular processes, modify tissue architecture, nor result in abnormal cellular proliferation.

Biochemical components found in facial tissues are numerous (see Chapter 2), and the complexity of their molecular structures and interactions is only beginning to become apparent. Although the cell types found in facial tissues are less numerous, regulation of cell and tissue biochemistry continues to be somewhat of a challenge to the biochemist.

The structural complexity of skin, cartilage, and bone is a topic of intensive research interest (Chapter 3). As we learn more about development and maturation, we begin to better appreciate the complexity of living systems. Biomaterials used to augment facial structures must not affect dermal or epidermal structure, or create stress points that later will affect the mechanical properties of skin (Chapter 3).

The goal of the biomaterials scientist and engineer is to develop materials that maintain normal tissue architecture. In the case of biodegradable materials, restoration of normal tissue structure is promoted if the implant mimics the architecture of the tissue being replaced. For this reason a careful analysis of tissue structure and the introduction of appropriate pores required for cell ingrowth are essential aspects of the design of implants. Characterization of the mechanical properties of tissues is also important in order to develop implants with similar properties so that stress concentrations leading to failure do not occur at the interface between the implant and host tissues. Since skin, cartilage, and bone have widely varying properties, this presents a challenge to the development engineer to find the appropriate polymers, metals, and ceramics for implant design.

Trauma or surgical intervention to facial tissues sets into motion a series of events that lead to either wound healing and/or chronic inflammation (Chapter 4). The type of response observed depends on the type of tissue, degree of vascularity, type of implant used, contamination of implant with bacteria or wear particles, and motion of the implant relative to the surrounding tissues. Even in the presence of an inert implant, its functioning can be compromised by induction of chronic inflammation associated with implant movement and poor adhesion. In addition, release of biodegradation products or metal ions further complicates the wound healing response since these moieties may activate inflammatory cells to release enzymes that degrade tissue, prolonging inflammation.

Although scarring results from imperfect wound healing, the origin of wrinkles is somewhat more complex (Chapter 5). Even under optimum conditions, dermal wounds are repaired by scar tissue deposition and exhibit decreased tensile strengths and other physiochemical properties compared to normal skin. Excess collagen and increased rates of collagen synthesis or decreased levels of collagenolytic enzymes result in collagen accumulation and lead to more serious dermal scars. Wrinkles, in contrast, are normally observed with increased age and result from physical changes to the dermis and epidermis as well as decreased levels of soluble collagen, glycosaminoglycans, and elastic fibers. These decreases are associated with solar damages to skin and are corrected by injection of materials such as silicone, collagen, and fat (see Part III).

Before an implant can be used to correct a defect, it must be carefully characterized as discussed in Chapter 6. Metals, ceramics, and polymers are characterized prior to implantation for chemical and physical properties of the surface and bulk material. Surface characterization is achieved using a number of high resolution techniques before and after exposure to tissues to evaluate adsorption of proteins. Mechanical tests are conducted in an attempt to match the properties of the implant and the host tissue. *In vivo* studies focus on the nature of the interface between host tissue and the device in an attempt to select materials that minimize fibrous tissue encapsulation and induction of an inflammatory response. Selection of the appropriate material requires both short- and long-term animal studies before human use is even considered. Interdisciplinary cooperation between scientists, engineers, and physicians is required to facilitate implant development.

Parts II and III of this book deal with the use of tissue (Part II) and synthetic materials, also termed "alloplasts" (Part III). Although cartilage, bone, and fat are transplanted routinely into different areas of the face, the repair and biocompatibility responses to these tissues differ depending on the site and method of implantation. In addition, implant loss (resorption) and the degree of foreign body response due to breakdown by enzymes and biological fluids is also dependent on the site of implantation. Therefore, it is difficult to accurately characterize the biocompatibility of an implant without referencing the test model (animal species and site of implantation used). As discussed in the Consensus Development Conference on Clinical Applications of Biomaterials (Galletti and Boretos),[1] a balance between risk and benefit must be used in determining how biocompatible a material must be before it can be used clinically. In most instances, biocompatibility tests are conducted in the most appropriate animal model to establish that the material is likely to be safe in humans.

In instances where grafts are not available or are insufficient to fill the defect, manmade materials are used. Part III of this book covers clinical applications of polymeric materials including poly(ethylene), Medpor™, poly(ethylene terephthalate), Mersilene™, poly(siloxane), Silastic™, poly(tetrafluoroethylene), GORE-TEX® and Proplast™, poly(glycolic acid), Vicry™, and poly(amide), Supramid™. There is not only a variety of polymers with different chemistries available, but also a number of physical forms and textures that can be given to implant materials. For instance, injectable poly(siloxane) is an oil, while solid implants of Silastic™ are also available.

It is the hope of workers in the field that an interdisciplinary approach to studying the chemistry, physics, and biology of facial tissues will lead to advances in material development and clinical applications in facial plastic surgery.

REFERENCE

1. **Galetti, P. M. and Boretos, J. N.,** Consensus Development Conference on Clinical Applications of Biomaterials, *J. Biomed. Mater. Res.,* 5, 5, 1984.

Chapter 2

BIOCHEMISTRY OF SKIN, CARTILAGE, AND BONE

Jeffrey C. Geesin and Richard A. Berg

TABLE OF CONTENTS

I. INTRODUCTION

Skin, cartilage, and bone comprise the largest organ system of the body and provide a critical function; namely, protection from the environment and an articulated frame for the attachment of muscles. The protein components of this system comprise the building blocks of the extracellular matrix which is present not only in the skeletal system and skin but also in all other organ systems. In the face and head, the components are the collagens, proteoglycans, elastin, and a multitude of glycoproteins that are present as cell surface proteins, adhesion proteins, and specialized proteins that participate in mineralization, epithelium formation, and the formation of specialized structures like hair follicles and sebaceous glands. This review will focus on the chemical components of skin, cartilage, and bone, as these are all present in the face and are all tissues that are involved in facial plastic surgery.

II. SKIN

Human skin, measuring approximately 2 m^2, is functionally an organ, as opposed to a simple, inert covering. Consequently, it has activities which are not only critical for its own development, but also play essential roles in providing necessary factors for the function of other tissues. This tissue is involved in regulation of body temperature, repair of wounds, immunity from disease, removal of waste and synthesis of growth factors, vitamins, and other important molecules. In addition, the skin normally undergoes continual development and remodeling. Matrix proteins, responsible for maintaining the structure of skin, are constantly being degraded and replaced. Cells at the skin's surface flake off and are replaced by others which have migrated up from lower layers. These processes are essential in a tissue which is constantly being bombarded by external insults such as ultraviolet light, temperature, wind, and chemicals. The skin's role as defender of the body has necessitated the development of some novel methods of dealing with these insults which is represented by the presence of some unique structures and molecules designed for this function.

A. EPIDERMIS

The skin is composed of three distinct parts. The epidermis is the outermost layer of the skin and is predominantly cellular. The major cell type is the keratinocyte, which forms overlapping structures not unlike that of a brick wall (see Chapter 3). These are held together by desmosomes which serve as the mortar which binds the cells together. The innermost layer is the dermis, which, as opposed to the epidermis, is composed largely of matrix components, of which collagen is by far the most abundant. The collagen matrix gives skin its tensile strength and resistance to tearing, while fibers formed by elastin provide elasticity and flexibility. The cell type which is most prevalent and responsible for synthesizing and structuring the dermal matrix is the fibroblast. Its role is not only to synthesize the required proteins, but also to recognize and remove proteins that are damaged or no longer useful. In between the dermis and the epidermis lies the basement membrane, also known as the dermal-epidermal junction. This is a thin, acellular region which is important for adhesion between the dermis and the epidermis and probably plays a role in communication between the two layers. The molecules in this region may be synthesized by cells in either the dermis or epidermis.

1. Intracellular Matrix Components

There are a number of important molecules found in the epidermis which play important roles in providing the requirements for dealing with the environment. One major function of epithelial cells is to produce a protective cytoskeleton. The predominant molecules fall in a class of proteins called keratins which are important components of intermediate filaments that are found in all epithelial cells.[1-3] These molecules are produced by keratinocytes which attain various stages of differentiation as they migrate upwards through the epidermis. Keratinocytes near the basement membrane are called basal cells, and these cells synthesize a set of keratins which are necessary for their role in this area of the tissue. As keratinocytes migrate upwards toward the skin's surface, the set of keratins they produce is altered to meet the new requirements of this more exposed layer. This change in keratin expression involves the continued production of some keratins seen in the basal layer with the deletion of some and the addition of others. As epithelial cells approach the surface, they lose their metabolic functions and transform into an inert cytoskeleton and into cornified cells of the stratum corneum. This process continues until the keratinocytes completely denucleate, reach the surface, and flake off due to normal wear and tear on the skin. Altogether, there are four layers of the epidermis which represent different levels of differentiation and therefore have specific sets of ketatin molecules. The intermediate filaments are composed of a number of double helical keratin molecules. The molecules of each helix are different gene products with one subunit from a subclass of keratins known as type I (acidic), and the other from type II (basic). Any change in gene expression must still produce the necessary ratios of type I and type II keratins.[4]

The production of keratin fibers from these molecules is thought to be assisted by another protein known as filaggrin for its role as filament aggregating protein.[5-7] This protein is synthesized in the lower layers of the epidermis as a larger phosphorylated histidine-rich precursor of >350 kDa called profilaggrin which is processed in the intermediate layers to form several 37 kDa filaggrin molecules from each precursor.[8,9] As the cells migrate to the outermost layer of the epidermis (stratum corneum), filaggrin is reduced to its constituent amino acids, which are thought to play a role in water binding for skin moisture retention.[10] The fact that ichthyosis vulgaris, a genetic disorder involving the loss of keratohyaline granules with the presence of severe dry skin, has been associated with a defect in the synthesis of filaggrin, supports the proposed roles for this molecule.[11]

The previously mentioned desmosomes are structures which form at sites of contact between epithelial cells and are assumed to contribute to keratinocyte adhesion. Although the nature of assembly of proteins into this structure is unknown, the recent purification of two proteins from desmosomes, termed desmoplakin I and desmoplakin II, should provide a basis for further study.[12,199] These electron dense cytoplasmic plaques are composed of a number of proteins including desmoplakins I and II,[12,198,199] desmoglein I,[200-202] desmocollins,[202,203] plakoglobin,[204] and others.[205] The desmoplakins are found in regions of attachment of intermediate filaments,[198] while desmoglein I is transmembraneous[200-202] and desmocollins are found in the intracellular space of the desmosome.[202,203]

Another important structure of the epidermis is the cell envelope. As keratinocytes differentiate and migrate upwards through the epidermis towards the surface, they develop a rigid, alkali-resistant structure within the cytoplasm. This structure is composed of a number of proteins which, via the activity of a keratinocyte-specific transglutaminase, are joined through ϵ-(γ-glutamyl) lysine cross-links.[13-15] These proteins have not been completely defined, but they include both soluble and membrane bound constituents such as involucrin,[16,17] keratolinin,[18] loricrin,[206] and others.[19-22] The corneocyte envelope protects and gives form to cells in an environment (near the surface of the skin) in which a normal cell envelope would not be sufficient.

2. Other Matrix Components

Lipids are an integral part of the epidermis which also play important roles in water retention, stratum corneum cohesion, and prevention of invasion by external insults.[23,24] Their composition varies considerably depending on what layer of the epidermis is analyzed.[25] The predominant lipids in the lower layers are phosphatidylcholine, phosphatidylethanolamine, and sphingomyelin, while the major lipids in the stratum corneum are cholesteryl sulfate, ceramide, and fatty acids.[26,27]

TABLE 1
Specialized Collagens

Type IV	Basement membrane (blood vessels)
Type VI	Microfibrils (ubiquitous, cell binding, associated with type I)
Type VII	Dermal-epidermal junction skin (anchoring fibrils)
Type VIII	Endothelial cells (blood vessels)
Type X	Hypertrophic chondrocytes
Type XIII	Epidermis, bone, hair follicles, cartilage

The pigmentation of skin takes place just above the basement membrane in the epidermis. Melanocytes, cells which are located in the basal layer, produce and secrete melanosomes into receptive keratinocytes.[28] The pigment, called melanin, is composed of two similar molecules, eumelanin and phaeomelanin.[29] The predominant molecule in blacks is eumelanin with a larger proportion of phaeomelanin in individuals of Celtic origins. Skin color is also affected by the number, size, and distribution of melanosomes.[30] The secreted melanosomes collect just above the basal cells and are thought to protect the proliferative cells of the epidermis from sun exposure.

A recently described epidermal protein is also the most recently described collagen protein. Type XIII collagen is distributed throughout the epidermis and hair follicles, but its role in this tissue is not known.[31,32]

B. BASEMENT MEMBRANE

Directly below the epidermis, the basement membrane plays important roles in cell adhesion and cell growth regulation. Basement membrane forms an area of epidermal-dermal adherence, support for the epidermis, and a diffusion barrier for cells and large macromolecules. It is 70 to 100 nm thick and is composed of various components which are associated in an as yet undetermined fashion.[33-35] These components include type IV collagen,[36] BM-40 (also known as osteonectin or SPARC),[37-40] laminin,[41,42] nidogen,[43] and at least two heparan sulfate proteoglycans.[44-46] Type IV collagen is a member of a heterogeneous group of collagens that do not form fibers (see below) but appear to be more specialized in their function (Table 1). Interactions have been demonstrated between these molecules where type IV collagen self-associates to form a lattice that is coated with laminin, heparan sulfate proteoglycan, and fibronectin *in vitro* which are assumed to be reproduced *in vivo*.[43,47-49] Laminin and nidogen, not only possess cell-binding sequences Arg-Gly-Asp which bind cell surface receptors (see below) and are specific for certain cell types, but also bind to one another.[34,50-53] The function of these components in basement membranes is thought to regulate cell attachment, spreading, and selective growth of epithelial and endothelial cells.[54-57] Extending from the basement membrane into the dermis are anchoring fibrils composed of type VII collagen.[58-61] Their identification came from the observation that anchoring fibrils and type VII collagen are missing in epidermolysis bullosa,[62] a disease where the epidermis separates from the dermis to form blisters. The type VII molecule has been determined to exist as an antiparallel dimer of two triple helical subunits, each composed of three identical monomers.[63,64] In the proximity of the basement membrane, but apparently not in it, lies fibronectin, a dimer of two identical glycoprotein subunits. Fibronectin has both cell-binding and matrix-binding domains making it a potentially important molecule for cell-matrix interactions.[65] In cases of wound repair, both fibronectin and normally hidden portions of laminin and nidogen are made available to the keratinocytes, and these interactions have growth and migration stimulating effects on the keratinocytes.[54,66-68] This property is likely to prove important in wound healing. For example, laminin has been shown to have growth factor activity,[67] and nitogen/entactin contains several amino acid sequences that are shared by epidermal growth factor.[52,68] A recently described protein, called hexabrachion,

TABLE 2
Fibrillar Collagens

Fiber forming (skin, bone)	Type I, type III, type V
Fiber coating (skin, tendon)	Type XII
Fiber forming (cartilage)	Type II, type XI
Fiber coating (cartilage)	Type IX

tenascin, or cytoactin has distribution similar to fibronectin,[69] and also has growth factor activities.[70] Tenascin may interfere with cell binding to fibronectin.[71,72]

C. DERMIS
1. Extracellular Matrix
a. Collagen

The dermis is predominantly composed of collagen, elastin fibers, and a small amount of proteoglycan. The collagen fibers are composed largely of type I collagen[73,74] with a variable amount of type III collagen,[73-75] and lesser amounts of type V collagen fibers.[74,76] Type VI collagen forms a filamentous network in many connective tissues including the dermis.[78,79] All of these collagen types are composed of three α proteins with triple helical regions. Type III collagen is composed of three identical α chains, while type I is composed of two identical chains linked to a third different gene product.[79] Both type V and type VI are composed of proteins that are three different gene products (terms α_1, α_2 and α_3). Type I, III and V collagens are members of the fibrillar collagen group (Table 2), while type VI differs, in that it has two large noncollagenous domains and is not a predominant molecule of any fiber. The structure of type VI seems to play a role in anchoring large interstitial structures into connective tissue.[77] Type VI collagen also contains Arg-Gly-Asp sequences that suggest this type of collagen may bind to specific cell surface receptors.[78] The collagen fibers are known to interact with various other matrix molecules including proteoglycans,[80] heparan sulfate,[81] and a 59-kDa connective tissue matrix protein,[82] and also with the plasma proteins, vitronectin,[83] fibronectin,[84] von Willebrand factor,[85,86] and thrombospondin[87] (Table 3).

b. Elastin

While the collagen fibers are thought to give skin its ultimate structural rigidity and protection from tearing, the elastin fibers are thought to give the skin elasticity. The elastin network forms different types of structures depending upon how close they are to the basement membrane.[88] These fibers are fine structures which form candelabra type distribution in the upper regions of the dermis. Below this, are larger fibers running parallel to the surface. Recent sequencing of cDNAs have demonstrated that the elastin found in skin may be slightly different from that found in other tissues due to alternative splicing, and these differences may reflect its role in skin.[89-91]

The elastin fibers are generally associated with much smaller microfibrils.[92-94] These microfibrils are composed of a collection of several poorly defined molecules and may play a role in assembly of elastin fibers since their appearance precedes that of elastin in the development of these fibers. One of the more recently defined molecules present in microfibrils is fibrillin which is present in tissues containing types I, II and IV collagen, and is a component of microfibril fibers that contain elastin.[95]

c. Proteoglycans

The ground substance of the dermis is composed of various macromolecules including glycoproteins and glycosaminoglycans. The proteoglycans, formed through the linkage of glycosaminoglycans to their respective core proteins, have been most studied in cartilage,

TABLE 3
Skin Specific Proteins

	Function	**Refs.**
Epidermal		
Keratins	Intermediate filaments	1—3
Filaggrin	Filament aggregation	5—7
Desmoplakins	Cell adhesion	12
Involucrin	Corneocyte envelope formation	17
Keratolinin	Corneocyte envelope formation	18
Type XIII collagen	Unknown	31, 32
Lipids	Water retention, prevention of invasion	25
Basement membrane		
Collagens		
Type IV	Cell adhesion	36
Type VII	Anchoring fibrils	58—60
Laminin	Cell adhesion, growth and diff regulation (RGD)	41, 42
Nidogen, entactin	Cell adhesion (RGD)	43
Heparan sulfate proteoglycans	Cellular organization	44, 46
BM-40, SPARC, osteonectin	Unknown, cell binding	37, 38
Dermal		
Collagens		
Type I	Collagen fibers	73, 74
Type III	Reticulin and collagen fibers	73—75
Type V	Collagen fiber associated	76
Type VI	Filamentous network (RGD)	77, 78
Type XII	Coats type I fibers	197
Elastin	Elastin fibers	88, 92
Fibrillin	Microfibrils	95
Fibronectin	Cell adhesion, growth and diff regulation (RGD)	65
Hexabrachion, tenascin cytoactin	Cell adhesion, growth and diff regulation (RGD)	69—72
Proteoglycans	Matrix structure	96—99

Note: Abbreviation RGD, component contains an Arg-Gly-Asp sequence recognized by integrin family of receptors.

and skin proteoglycans are related to small proteoglycans of cartilage.[96,97] The four major glycosaminoglycans of the dermis are hyaluronate,[96] chondroitin 4-sulfate,[98] dermatan sulfate,[99] and heparin,[96] while heparan sulfate is found both in the basement membrane,[44,45,100,101] and is also a component of cell membranes.[102,103] Hyaluronate is found at its highest densities near thin collagen bundles of the papillary dermis, while dermatan sulfate, which can be found as two different species, is more evenly distributed throughout the dermis.[99,104-106] Dermatan sulfate associates with collagen fibers and may modulate fibrillogenesis. In general, proteoglycans of skin display a much higher ratio of protein to glycosaminoglycan when compared to cartilage.[96] Skin also contains small proteoglycans with side chains that differ from small proteoglycans found in other tissues.[98] Studies on cultured epithelial cells have shown that cell surface proteoglycans may consist of a single core to which both heparan sulfate and chondroitin sulfate glycosaminoglycans may be bound.[107,108]

2. Integrins

In addition to collagen, elastin, and proteoglycans in extracellular matrix are several adhesion proteins and their receptors. A recently described super family of receptors, the integrins, is present in the extracellular matrix of skin and other tissues.[109] The integrins are receptors that recognize Arg-Gly-Asp sequences in their ligands, also called RGD sequences using the single letter abbreviation for amino acids. The super family consists of one of three different β-subunits associated with one of several α-subunits. One subfamily of integrins, known as the VLA family, has a unique β-subunit combined with one of 6 different α subunits to produce a subfamily of 6 receptors that modulate cell binding to extracellular matrix components. Each member of the subfamily consists of an $\alpha_n\beta_1$ heterodimer that is a transmembrane protein. There are 6 αs in the VLA family where the αs confer ligand specificity for matrix components,[110] and these receptors bind to ligands having the Arg-Gly-Asp sequence.[111] The best characterized member of the family is VLA5 or $\alpha_5\beta_1$, the fibronectin receptor. The other members of this family of cell surface receptors bind to components of the extracellular matrix including several collagens (VLA2), fibronectin, laminin and collagen (VLA3), or laminin (VLA6).[109,110] These receptors also link these extracellular matrix components to the intracellular actin cytoskeleton.[112,113] The collagen-binding integrin, VLA2, binds to both extracellular collagen and the cell cytoskeleton.[112] Integrins are involved with attachment of cells to the extracellular matrix, the formation of focal adhesions between cells and their substrate, and cell mobility.

III. CARTILAGE

Cartilage is a specialized connective tissue that is composed of cells and extracellular matrix. It is exceptional in that it contains few vessels or nerves, and nutrition is accomplished through diffusion. Cartilage is divided into three types: hyaline, fibrous, and elastic (see Chapter 3). In the adult human head, hyaline cartilage is present in the nose, larynx, trachea, and bronchi. Elastic cartilage is also present in the larynx, the external ear, and the auditory tube. Fibrous cartilage is a transitional form between dense connective tissue and hyaline cartilage, and although it is found primarily in the meniscus and the annulus fibrosus of the intervertebral disk, it is often present in lacunae surrounded by hyaline cartilage.

A. COMPOSITION

Cartilage is a heterogeneous tissue depending on its location and how closely it is juxtaposed to bone.[114] Cartilage consists of cells surrounded by a metachromatic substance composed of aggregates of large proteoglycans,[115] interspersed with thin collagen fibers and various noncollagen proteins.[116] Cartilage nearest to bone contains many cells that are proliferating in a transition zone from cartilage to bone where the matrix is undergoing calcification.

1. Collagen

Cartilage is composed of several types of collagen,[79,117] proteoglycans,[115] glycoproteins,[116,118] and other proteins including cleaved COOH-terminal propeptides of type II collagen,[119] and anchorin,[120] a cell attachment factor (Table 4). Although type II collagen predominates, the collagens found in cartilage are more heterogeneous than those found in other tissues. Type II collagen is a homotrimer containing only $\alpha_1(II)$ chains.[79] Type XI collagen is more complex in that it is predominantly a heterotrimer containing three different α chains $\alpha_1(XI)$, $\alpha_2(XI)$, and $\alpha_3(XI)$ in a single helical molecule.[121] Type IX collagen is also composed of three different α chains, $\alpha_1(IX)$, $\alpha_2(IX)$, and $\alpha_3(IX)$.[122,123] Type IX collagen is covalently bound to type II collagen fibrils and also contains a glycosaminoglycan side chains.[123] Type II collagen is distributed in few tissues other than cartilage. An exception is the cornea which contains type II collagen, and also type IX collagen,[124] although the type IX found in the cornea differs slightly from that found in cartilage in one domain only.[124] The association between types IX, XI, and II collagen appears to be important as they are expressed together and form mixed fibrils.[117]

The function of the types IX and XI in cartilage collagen fibril is not completely known. Type XI collagen has been reported to interact with proteoglycans but not hyaluronic acid[125] and, therefore, may play a role in matrix assembly. Since type IX collagen is distributed on the surface of type II fibrils, the type IX collagen may play a role in limiting fiber

TABLE 4
Cartilage Specific Proteins

	Function	Refs.
Collagens		
Type II collagen	Structure, tensile strength	79, 117
Type V collagen	Unknown	129
Type VI collagen	Unknown	77, 78
Type IX collagen	Coats type II fibers	117, 122, 124
Type X collagen	Mineralization?	126—128
Type XI collagen	Matrix assembly, binds proteoglycans	121
Proteoglycans		
Large proteoglycan	Hydration of matrix	115, 132, 131
Core protein	Organizes gycosaminoglycans	131
Link protein	Stabilizes proteoglycan aggregate	133
Small proteoglycan (PGI)	Unknown	136, 139
Small proteoglycan (PGII)	Collagen binding, fibrillogenesis	136, 139
Other matrix proteins		
Fibromodulin, 59K protein	Collagen binding, fibrillogenesis	83
Anchorin	Cell attachment factor, binds type II collagen	121, 143
Chondrocalcin, C-propeptide	Mineralization?	115, 149
Collagen-binding protein	Orients collagen fibrils	140
Cartilage matrix protein	Unknown	141
CH 21	Mineralization?	148

diameter or modulating the interaction of cartilage collagen fibrils with other components of the extracellular matrix. In addition to these collagen types, cartilage also contains specialized collagen types such as type X collagen which is associated with hypertrophic chondrocytes.[126-128] Other types of collagen present in cartilage include type V which may form cross hybrids with type XI.[129] Cartilage also contains type VI collagen that is not covalently cross-linked and can be extracted with guanidine hydrochloride.[77] It forms a filamentous network in cartilage as it does in other connective tissues.[78] Type VI collagen is also composed of $\alpha_1(VI)$, $\alpha_2(VI)$ and $\alpha_3(VI)$ in a heterotrimer.[78]

The cartilage forming cell is the chondrocyte which synthesizes the collagens that are unique to cartilage as well as the proteoglycans that are found in cartilage. The chondrocyte is unstable genetically and can be altered in its transcription of collagen. Depending on the culture condition, chondrocytes may stop synthesizing type II collagen and begin synthesizing type I collagen.[130] This transition in collagen types is especially important where cartilage is being replaced by bone because bone contains only type I collagen, whereas cartilage does not contain type I.

2. Proteoglycans

The most prevalent proteoglycan, comprising 5 to 10% of cartilage tissue by weight, is a high molecular weight aggregate that contains a single type of core protein having a molecular weight of 210 kDa.[115,131] Large proteoglycan was first purified from bovine nasal cartilage,[132] and has been well characterized.[115,131] Various glycosaminoglycans are covalently attached to the core protein through a linkage that includes *o*-glycosidic linkages to xylose and serine or threonine amino residues.[115] Glycosaminoglycan side chains are also linked to the core protein by *N*-glycosidic linkages to asparagine to produce proteoglycan monomers. The most abundant glycosaminoglycan found on monomers of large aggregating proteoglycan is chondroitin sulfate; however, it also contains a region rich in keratin sulfate. The large proteoglycan found in cartilage forms an aggregate involving proteoglycan monomers, link protein, and hyaluronic acid.[115,132,133] Its major physical property is that it contains a large number of fixed negative charges on approximately 100 chondroitin sulfate chains each having approximately 100 negatively charged carboxyl or sulfate groups. This poly-anionic matrix molecule associates with water and ions and, therefore, serves to hydrate cartilage. Expansion is limited by the tensile forces carried by the collagen fibers to cause the tissue to behave as a viscoelastic substance that can withstand limited deformation. Besides the large aggregating proteoglycan, another large proteoglycan is present in cartilage but does not aggregate with hyaluronic acid.[115,134] This proteoglycan is also found in nasal cartilage,[134] and has a higher protein content than large aggregating proteoglycan.

The second type of proteoglycan includes lower molecular weight forms that have a more limited number of glycosaminoglycans including chondroitin sulfate or dermatan sulfate. These together comprise less than 2% of nasal cartilage by weight.[135] The protein cores of the two bone small proteoglycans, PG-I and PG-II, are homologous but nonidentical,[136] and although similar to the core proteins isolated from cartilage, small proteoglycans are apparently identical.[137] The PG-II from bone was shown to be similar to PG-II from cartilage but contains chondroitin sulfate,[138] instead of either chondroitin sulfate or dermatan sulfate found in cartilage.[135,139] Although the function of small PG-I is not known, small PG-II binds collagen types I and II.[83] The first of the small proteoglycans to be purified from nasal cartilage contained predominantly chondroitin sulfate. The molecular weight of the proteo-glycan itself is less than 100,000 with the molecular weight of the core protein less than 50,000.[135] Two species of similar sized proteoglycans were isolated from articular cartilage by Rosenberg et al.,[139] and were found to contain dermatan sulfate. The core proteins had 45-kDa mol wt, but sequencing showed them to be nonidentical proteins.[139] They were named DS-PGI and DS-PGII. These proteoglycans are called biglycan and decorin, respectively.[118]

Cartilage tissue is rich in proteoglycan and collagen; however, the association between the two may be complex. Various proteoglycans have been tested for their interaction with collagen and recently, it was found that proteoglycan monomers, derived from large aggregating cartilage proteoglycans, bound to type XI collagen in solution.[125] Heparan, but not hyaluronic acid, could compete with the interaction. As referred to above, the small pro-teoglycan PG-II from tendon having dermatan sulfate side chains binds to type I and II collagen.[83] Another protein isolated from cartilage named 54K protein or cartilage matrix protein was shown to bind to type II collagen and decrease the rate of fibril formation.[140] Several proteins including small proteoglycans and a 59-kDa protein and a 54-kDa protein may, therefore, influence collagen matrix assembly in cartilage tissues.

B. INTERACTIONS BETWEEN COMPONENTS

Several cartilage specific proteins are present in cartilage, including cartilage matrix protein, which consists of three subunits of 54-kDa mol wt.[141] This protein is present in tracheal cartilage. Another protein called 59-kDa protein,[83] or fibromodulin,[142] which may be related to the core protein of PG-II, does not contain glycosaminoglycan but does bind collagen types I and II.[83] Anchorin is a protein that specifically binds type II collagen.[121,143] The protein has a 34-kDa mol wt, and is found associated with chondrocytes and may function as a cell attachment factor.[144] Cartilage also contains residual amounts of C-pro-peptide that was cleaved from the type II collagen after its biosynthesis.[119] This protein is also called chondrocalcin.[145,146] Chondrocalcin was originally found associated with miner-alizing cartilage.[145] Although it may merely represent the propeptide released during bio-synthesis of type II collagen, it also binds to hydroxyapatite and may play a role in mineralization.

Hypertrophic cartilage present in the transition zone between cartilage and bone contains an unusual type of collagen named type X,[126,128,147] which is also associated with other marker molecules like CH 21,[148] and occurs in the same location where mineralization is proceeding. Cartilage that is undergoing mineralization has been shown to contain both type X collagen and chondrocalcin in close association.[147,149] CH 21 is a low molecular weight protein that has been isolated from chick chondrocytes and may be associated with the hypertrophy of the cells prior to mineralization.[148]

Cartilage contains adhesion molecules that are thought to mediate cell attachment to the extracellular matrix. The first such molecule that was characterized was chondronectin.[150] As indicated above, another such molecule to be characterized was anchorin CII which was purified from chick chondrocytes plasma membranes.[121,144] Since anchorin is associated with the chondrocyte plasma membrane, and chondrocytes were shown to be able to use anchorin CII to bind to type II collagen substrates,[144] anchorin may be a major adhesion molecule in cartilage.

IV. BONE

Several types of bone exist in the body which are differentiated one from the other by the way it is produced during growth and development. Bones are organized as either cancellous or spongy bone that consists of trabeculae which branch and interact to form a sponge-like network, or as compact bone that is macroscopically a dense mass devoid of spaces. Long bones have both an epiphyseal region of spongy bone at the ends adjacent to the cartilage and a diaphysial region of compact bone in the middle. Mature compact bone, also called Haversion bone, contains concentrically arranged laminae that are organized to accommodate small arteries, arterioles, capillaries, and vesicles of a microcirculatory system. Bones are distinguished from other tissues in the body by consisting of a collagenous matrix that contains the mineral hydroxyapatite which gives this tissue the ability to withstand compressive and torsional stresses. Bone differs from cartilage not only in stiffness but also in being a highly vascularized tissue compared with cartilage.

The collagens of bone consist primarily of type I collagen with only very small amounts of type V and other minor collagens, including type X. Bone contains lesser amounts of small proteoglycans as well as noncollagen proteins such as osteonectin, osteocalcin, phosphoproteins, glycoproteins, and other proteins that are involved in regulating the mineralization process.

A. COMPOSITION

Bone is often composed of both compact and spongy bone. Flat bones of the skull consist of two thick layers of compact bone called the trabecula externa and trabecula interna. Other bones such as the maxillary bones contain both compact and spongy bone. Except for the cartilage covered epiphyseal surface where joints articulate, bone is covered by a dense layer of connective tissue called the periosteum. A thin layer of connective tissue also coats the marrow cavity of bones. These two surfaces of long bones possess osteogenic capacity to form new bone. The periosteum is a vascular connective tissue that contains osteoblasts in direct contact with bone. The outer layer of the periosteum consists of denser tissue with larger blood vessels and is stitched onto the underlying bone with collagenase fibers called Sharpey's fibers that hold the periosteum firmly onto the bone.

Compact bone is produced primarily from cartilage which is transformed into bony tissue by proliferation of osteoblasts and fibroblasts that replace chondrocytes, and which are genetically programmed so that proteins specific to bone are synthesized and secreted into the extracellular matrix. Chondrocytes produce a proportionately larger amount of proteoglycan than osteoblasts and also produce primarily type II collagen as well as chondronectin and anchorin which are cell adhesion proteins found in cartilage. This process of the conversion of cartilage into bone is termed endochondral ossification. Certain bones are formed directly from mesenchymal cells. This process is termed intermembranous ossification. The flat bones of the skull and portions of the mandible are formed by this mechanism.

TABLE 5
Bone Specific Proteins

	Function	Refs.
Collagens		
Type I collagen	Fibril formation, matrix structure	115
Type V collagen	Fibril organization	129
Type X collagen	Mineralization?	124, 127
Proteoglycans		
Glycosaminoglycans		
Bone small proteoglycan I, biglycan	Matrix organization	136, 141, 153
Bone small proteoglycan II, decorin	Matrix organization, collagen binding	152, 153
Other matrix proteins		
Bone acidic glycoprotein	Cell attachment, mineralization	196
Osteonectin, SPARC, BM-40	Regulation of mineralization	37, 38, 40, 48, 169
Osteopontin, bone sialoprotein I (BSP)	Cell adhesion (RGD) binds hydroxyapatite	155, 179
Bone sialoprotein II	Matrix organization	153, 155, 156
Osteocalcin, bone Gla protein	Regulation of mineralization Ca^{++} homeostasis	159
Matrix Gla protein	Regulation of mineralization Ca^{++} homeostasis	162
Chondrocalcin, carboxy-terminal propeptide	Mineralization	145
Phosphoproteins	Mineralization	171, 172
Phosphoryn (dentin only)	Mineralization	167
BP2	Mineralization	166
BMP	Differentiation	175
Osteogenin	Differentiation	176
Thrombospondin	Cell adhesion (RGD)	178

1. Collagen

Bone contains almost exclusively type I collagen which forms a cross-linked matrix that is associated with noncollagen proteins and mineral. Many bones are derived from cartilage that undergoes calcification and upon conversion into bone the type of collagen is switched from type II to type I. Chondrocytes that make type II collagen are known to be able to switch to type I collagen in culture, but it is unknown whether this process occurs *in vivo* where osteoblast proliferation may be the predominate method to increase type I collagen synthesis. Bone formation involves the expression of a specific set of matrix molecules that include not only type I collagen but numerous small molecules that regulate mineralization and differentiation of bone cells (Table 5).

2. Proteoglycans

The proteoglycans are a small but significant component of mineralized matrix. Two low molecular weight proteoglycans isolated from bone were shown to be similar to but not identical with two small proteoglycans from cartilage.[136,151-153] A second proteoglycan has a higher molecular weight similar to cartilage aggregating proteoglycan; however, this proteoglycan is not present in fully mineralized bone, and may represent a molecule persisting after development of bone from cartilage.[151] There has been shown to be two small proteoglycans from bone having different core proteins of similar size.[136] One of the small proteoglycans, PS-1,PGI (biglycan), has a core protein with 38,000 mol wt, and 2 chondroitin sulfate side chains of about 40,000.[151] The smaller proteoglycan, PS-2,PGII (decorin), has a similar but structurally distinct core protein[136,153] from that of PGI, and has only one glycosaminoglycan chain which is also chondroitin sulfate.[138] Although the function of the proteoglycans is not known, it has been suggested that they orient collagen and fill the hole region in nonmineralized collagen fibrils.[154]

3. Other Matrix Molecules

Bone sialoproteins containing phosphate and sialic acid have also been isolated from mineralized bone.[155] Bone sialoprotein II was shown to be a proteoglycan containing keratan sulfate.[156] The relationship between mineralization and proteoglycan in bone has been examined, and both hydroxyapatite size and bone density was found to be inversely proportional to glycosaminoglycan content.[157] Other matrix proteins include the γ carboxyglutamic acid (Gla) containing protein or Gla protein, which is a small molecular weight protein also termed osteocalcin.[158,159] This protein has a 5.8 kDa mol wt, and is found only in bone and teeth and, owing to the presence of Gla, is thought to be involved in the mineralization process.[158] Its synthesis is stimulated by vitamin D.[159] The protein binds to hydroxyapatite[160] and may be an inhibitor of hydroxyapatite crystal growth.[160] Since vitamin D stimulates osteocalcin and matrix Gla protein synthesis, these proteins may also be involved in calcium homeostasis.[161,162]

B. MINERALIZATION

The regulation of the mineralization process is not well understood. The noncollagen anionic proteins seem to be required for mineralization; however, their exact functions are not understood.[163] They may serve as nucleators, provide a surface for mineralization, help organize and inhibit crystal growth, or serve as a reservoir for calcium.[164] In endochondral bone formation where chondrocytes are replaced by bone cells, a transition zone occurs where chondrocytes become hyperplastic, larger and metabolically more active. Such chondrocytes synthesize a unique type of collagen, type X, whose precise function in mineralizing cartilage is presently unknown.[126-128] Osteoblasts that produce type I collagen and are involved in the mineralization of bone produce substantial amounts of alkaline phosphatase and in many cases matrix vesicles, which are thought to be involved in initial minerlization or crystallization of hydroxyapatite. As the osteoblasts are surrounded by bone matrix, they become less metabolically active and are transformed into osteocytes which have only limited function, serving primarily to break down bone matrix in their immediate vicinity in response to several mediators. The process is stimulated by parathyroid hormone and inhibited by calcitonin and is part of the mechanism for calcium homeostasis in the body.[165] Several proteins found in bone are capable of binding calcium.[163] Additional proteins have been isolated from bone including several uncharacterized proteins such as BP2.[163,166] Phosphoryn isolated from dentin that may also be involved in mineralization.[167] Another widely studied bone protein called SPARC is a major calcium binding protein,[168] also named osteonectin.[138,48,169] Although it is widely distributed in connective tissues, including endoderm and dermis, its function in bone may be in part to either bind calcium[172] or to poison the mineralization surface, thereby limiting mineralization.[170] Several additional phosphoproteins are found in bone such as the amino terminal propeptide of type I[171] and other phosphoproteins[172] which may regulate mineralization.[163]

C. REMODELING

Bones undergo continual growth and remodeling with the growth phase taking place during the enlargement of the animal and the remodeling phase taking place after the bones have reached maximal size. Remodeling is influenced by mechanical stress as well as internal and external electrical properties of the bone and its environment.[163,173] Remodeling is performed by a cell type called the osteoclast which is derived from a different precursor cell than the osteoblast and which secretes collagenase for the specific degradation of the collagen extracellular matrix, and which also lowers the pH of the extracellular environment promoting the dissolution of hydroxyapatite crystals. The actions of osteoclasts and osteoblasts are coupled. Collagenase is a member of the metalloproteinase family which itself is a highly regulated family of proteases that are synthesized as latent enzymes and are activated by enzymatic and other processes.[174] Osteoclasts have properties similar to macrophages or monocytes derived from the bone stem cells. A second phase of remodeling is the synthesis of new bone which is brought about by the osteoblast that is regulated by a number of both systemic and local growth factors.[173,175] Intramembranous ossification may be similar to the bone formation that is induced by bone morphogenic protein[173] and osteogenin.[175,176] The relationship of peripheral bone formation to the developmentally significant mechanisms of bone formation is not completely understood.

Adhesion molecules that are present in bone mediate cell attachment. Thrombospondin has been shown to mediate cell-matrix interaction.[177,178] Bone sialoprotein also called osteopontin[179] was purified from bovine bone,[153] has 59-kDa mol wt, and shows some homology to a newly isolated bone acidic glycoprotein.[196] It contains sialic acid and recent studies demonstrate that the protein contains an RGD sequence that is present on many proteins that bind to cell surface receptors.[179] The protein also binds hydroxyapatite and contains acidic amino acids.

V. MODULATION OF CONNECTIVE TISSUE CELLS BY EXTRACELLULAR MATRIX

The role of the extracellular matrix in the regulation of cell function has received much recent attention. In soft tissues and cell culture where it has been most studied, binding of extracellular matrix through integrin receptors can produce alterations in both the differentiation state and growth rate of the affected cells. For example, fibronectin promotes spreading and migration of cultured cells,[179-182] and has been reported to inhibit the terminal differentiation of keratinocytes,[30] whereas tenascin[71] may inhibit fibronectin mediated cell migration. Since the expression of two proteinases involved in the degradation of the extracellular matrix can be regulated through the cellular fibronectin receptor, this is one mechanism by which the matrix can control its own synthesis and degradation.[183] The occupation of the fibronectin receptor has also been identified as a control point for myogenic differentiation.[184] Laminin is also involved in the regulation of differentiation of various cell types.[50,184,185] In addition, these receptors have been implicated in the chemoattractant ability of peptides released upon proteolytic degradation of extracellular matrix molecules such as fibronectin.[186] Some extracellular matrix molecules, such as laminin, hexabrachion, and entactin, have been shown to possess sequences with considerable homology to epidermal growth factor.[67,69,79] This domain of these molecules has been shown to be associated with growth regulation activity similar to that exhibited by epidermal growth factor itself.[67] The role these activities play in native tissues is not yet clear, but a picture of how these receptors for extracellular matrix molecules might affect tissue development and wound repair is emerging. The extracellular matrix itself may provide a reservoir to which growth factors or angiogenic factors such as FGF may be bound through interaction with proteoglycans present.[187] The state of the extracellular matrix or the presence or absence of various matrix molecules can alter the response of cells to soluble growth factors such as EGF,[188] FGF,[189] and TGF-B.[190,191] How these receptors mediate the vast array of effects on cells they control is not clear. However, the recent findings that receptor phosphorylation and other changes in receptor structures appears to be involved in cell differentiation and transformation,[192-194] and that these receptors can form bridges between the cytoskeleton and the extracellular matrix[195] will provide testable hypotheses for future study.

REFERENCES

1. **Moll, R., Franke, W. W., Schiller, D. L., Geiger, B., and Krepler, R.,** The catalog of human cytokeratins: patterns of expression in normal epithelia, tumors and cultural cells, *Cell,* 31, 11, 1982.
2. **Sun, T-T., Eichner, R., Nelson, W. G., Tseng, S. C. G., Weiss, R. A., Jarvinen, M., and Woodcock-Mitchell, J.,** Keratin classes: molecular markers for different types of epithelial differentiation, *J. Invest. Dermatol.,* 81, 109s, 1983.
3. **Eichner, R., Bonitz, P., and Sun, T-T.,** Classification of epidermal keratins according to their immunoreactivity, isoelectric point, and mode of expression, *J. Cell Biol.,* 98, 1388, 1984.
4. **Fuchs, E., Tyner, A. L., Giudice, G. J., Marchuk, D., RayChaudhury, A., and Rosenberg, M.,** The human keratin genes and their differential expression, in *Current Topics in Development Biology,* Vol. 22, Sawyer, R. H., Ed., Academic Press, Orlando, FL, 1987, 5.
5. **Sibrack, L. A., Gray, R. H., and Bernstein, I. A.,** Localization of the histidine-rich protein in keratohyalin: a morphologic and macromolecular marker in epidermal differentiation, *J. Invest. Dermatol.,* 62, 394, 1974.
6. **Dale, B. A., Holbrook, K. A., and Steinert, P. M.,** Assembly of stratum corneum basic protein and keratin filaments in macrofibrils, *Nature,* 276, 729, 1978.
7. **Lynley, A. M. and Dale, B. A.,** The characterization of human epidermal filaggrin, a histidine-rich, keratin filament-aggregating protein, *Biochim. Biophys. Acta,* 744, 28, 1983.
8. **Fleckman, P., Dale, B. A., and Holbrook, K. A.,** Profilaggrin, a high-molecular-weight precursor of filaggrin in human epidermis and cultured keratinocytes, *J. Invest. Dermatol.,* 85, 507, 1985.
9. **Resing, K. A., Walsh, K. A., Haugen-Scofield, J., and Dale, B. A.,** Identification of proteolytic cleavage sites in the conversion of profilaggrin to filaggrin in mammalian epidermis, *J. Biol. Chem.,* 264, 1837, 1989.
10. **Scott, I. R., Harding, C. R., and Barrett, J. G.,** Histidine-rich protein of the keratohyaline granules. Source of the free amino acids, urocanic acid and pyrrolidone carboxylic acid in the stratum corneum, *Biochim. Biophys. Acta,* 719, 110, 1982.
11. **Sybert, V. P., Dale, B. A., and Holbrook, K. A.,** Ichthyosis vulgaris: identification of a defect in synthesis of filaggrin correlated with an absence of keratohyaline granules, *J. Invest. Dermatol.,* 84, 191, 1985.
12. **O'Keefe, E. J., Erickson, H. P., and Bennett, V.,** Desmoplakin I and desmoplakin II: purification and characterization, *J. Biol. Chem.,* 264, 8310, 1989.
13. **Rice, R. H. and Green, H.,** The cornified envelope of terminally differentiated human epidermal keratinocytes consists of cross-linked protein, *Cell,* 11, 417, 1977.
14. **Buxman, M. M. and Wuepper, K. D.,** Cellular localization of epidermal transglutaminase: a histochemical and immunochemical study, *J. Histochem. Cytochem.,* 26, 340, 1978.
15. **Thacher, S. M. and Rice, R. H.,** Keratinocyte-specific transglutaminase of cultured human epidermal cells: relation to cross-linked envelope formation and terminal differentiation, *Cell,* 40, 685, 1985.
16. **Rice, R. H. and Green, H.,** Presence in human epidermal cells of a soluble protein precursor of the cross-linked envelope: activation of the cross-linking by calcium ions, *Cell,* 18, 681, 1979.
17. **Simon, M. and Green, H.,** The glutamine residues reactive in transglutaminase-catalyzed cross-linking of involucrin, *J. Biol. Chem.,* 263, 18093, 1988.
18. **Zettergren, J. G., Peterson, L. L., and Wuepper, K. D.,** Keratolinin: the soluble substrate of epidermal transglutaminase from human and bovine tissue, *Proc. Natl. Acad. Sci. U.S.A.,* 81, 238, 1984.
19. **Simon, M. and Green, H.,** Participation of membrane-associated proteins in the formation of the cross-linked envelope of the keratinocyte, *Cell,* 36, 827, 1984.
20. **Ma, A. S-P. and Sun, T-T.,** Differentiation-dependent changes in the solubility of a 195 kD protein in human epidermal keratinocytes, *J. Cell Biol.,* 103, 41, 1986.
21. **Kubilus, J. and Baden, H. P.,** Isolation of two immunologically related transglutaminase substrates from cultured human keratinocytes, *In Vitro,* 18, 447, 1982.
22. **Baden, H. P., Kubilus, J., and Phillips, S. B.,** Characterization of monoclonal antibodies generated to the cornified envelope of human cultured keratinocytes, *J. Invest. Dermatol.,* 89, 454, 1987.
23. **Imokawa, G. and Hattori, M.,** A possible function of structural lipids in the water-holding properties of the stratum corneum, *J. Invest. Dermatol.,* 84, 282, 1985.
24. **Wertz, P. W., Swartzendruber, D. C., Kitko, D. J., Madison, K. C., and Downing, D. T.,** The role of the corneocyte lipid envelopes in cohesion of the stratum corneum, *J. Invest. Dermatol.,* 93, 169, 1989.
25. **Lampe, M. A., Williams, M. L., and Elias, P. M.,** Human epidermal lipids: characterization and modulations during differentiation, *J. Lipid Res.,* 24, 131, 1983.
26. **Elias, P. M.,** Epidermal lipids, membranes, and keratinization, *Int. J. Dermatol.,* 20, 1, 1981.
27. **Lampe, M. A., Burlingame, A. L., Whitney, J., Williams, M. L., Brown, B. E., Roitman, E., and Elias, P. M.,** Human stratum corneum lipids: characterization and regional variations, *J. Lipid Res.,* 24, 120, 1983.

28. **Prota, G.,** Recent advances in the chemistry of melanogenesis in mammals, *J. Invest. Dermatol.,* 75, 122, 1980.

29. **Szabo, G., Gerald, A. B., Pathak, M. A., and Fitzpatrick, T. B.,** Racial differences in the fate of melanosomes in human epidermis, *Nature,* 222, 1081, 1969.

30. **Mosher, D. B., Fitzpatrick, T. B., and Ortonne, J. P.,** Abnormalities of pigmentation, in *Dermatology in General Medicine,* 2nd ed., Fitzpatrick, T. B., Eisen, A. Z., Wolff, K., Freedberg, I. M., and Austen, K. F., Eds., McGraw-Hill, New York, 1979, 568.

31. **Tikka, L., Pihlajaniemi, T., Henttu, P., Prockop, D. J., and Tryggvason, K.,** Gene structure for the α1 chain of a human short-chain collagen (type XIII) with alternatively spliced transcripts and translation termination codon at the 5' end of the last exon, *Proc. Natl. Acad. Sci. U.S.A.,* 85, 7491, 1988.

32. **Pihlajaniemi, T. and Tamminen, M.,** The α1 chain of type XIII collagen: polypeptide structure, alternative splicing and tissue distribution in *Structure, Mol. Biol. and Pathol. of Collagen,* Vol. 580, Fleischmajer, R., Olsen, B. R., and Kahn, K., Eds., New York Academy of Science, New York, 1990, 440.

33. **Briggaman, R. A. and Wheeler, C. E.,** The epidermal-dermal junction, *J. Invest. Dermatol.,* 65, 71, 1975.

34. **Timpl, R. and Aumailley, M.,** Biochemistry of basement membranes, *Adv. Nephrol.,* 18, 59, 1989.

35. **Timpl, R.,** Structure and biological activity of basement membrane proteins, *Eur. J. Biochem.,* 180, 487, 1989.

36. **Yurchenco, P. D. and Ruben, G. C.,** Basement membrane structure in situ: evidence for lateral associations in the type IV collagen network, *J. Cell Biol.,* 105, 2559, 1987.

37. **Lankat-Buttgereit, B., Mann, K., Deutzmann, R., Timpl, R., and Krieg, T.,** Cloning and complete amino acid sequences of human and murine basement membrane protein BM-40 (SPARC, osteonectin), *FEBS Lett.,* 236, 352, 1988.

38. **Engel, J., Taylor, W., Paulsson, M., Sage, H., and Hogan, B.,** Calcium binding domains and calcium-induced conformational transition of SPARC/BM-40/osteonectin, an extracellular glycoprotein expressed in mineralized and nonmineralized tissues, *Biochemistry,* 26, 6958, 1987.

39. **Timpl, R. and Dziadek, M.,** Structure, development and molecular pathology of basement membranes, *Int. Rev. Exp. Pathol.,* 29, 1, 1986.

40. **Malaval, L., Fournier, B., and Delmas, P. D.,** Radioimmunoassay for osteonectin. Concentrations in bone, nonmineralized tissues, and blood, *J. Bone Miner. Res.,* 2, 457, 1987.

41. **Timpl, R. and Rohde, H.,** Laminin—a glycoprotein from basement membranes, *J. Biol. Chem.,* 254, 9933, 1979.

42. **Sasaki, M., Kleinman, H. K., Huber, H., Deutzmann, R., and Yamada, Y.,** Laminin, a multidomain protein: the A chain has a unique globular domain and homology with the basement membrane proteoglycan and the laminin B chains, *J. Biol. Chem.,* 263, 16536, 1988.

43. **Paulsson, M.,** The role of Ca^{2+} binding in the self-aggregation of laminin-nidogen complexes, *J. Biol. Chem.,* 263, 5425, 1988.

44. **Hassel, J. R., Leyshon, W. C., Ledbetter, S. R., Tyree, B., Suzuki, S., Kato, M., Kimata, K., and Kleinman, H. K.,** Isolation of two forms of basement membrane proteoglycans, *J. Biol. Chem.,* 260, 8098, 1985.

45. **Fujiwara, S., Wiedemann, H., Timpl, R., Lustig, A., and Engel, J.,** Structure and interactions of heparan sulfate proteoglycans from a mouse basement membrane, *Eur. J. Biochem.,* 143, 145, 1984.

46. **Noonan, D. M., Horigan, E. A., Ledbetter, S. R., Vogeli, G., Sasaki, M., Yamada, Y., and Hassell, J. R.,** Identification of cDNA clones encoding different domains of the basement membrane heparan sulfate proteoglycan, *J. Biol. Chem.,* 263, 16379, 1988.

47. **Laurie, G. W., Bing, J. T., Kleinman, H. K., Hassell, J. R., Aumailley, M., Martin, G. R., and Feldmann, R. J.,** Localization of binding sites for laminin, heparan sulfate proteoglycan and fibronectin on basement membrane (type IV) collagen, *J. Mol. Biol.,* 189, 205, 1986.

48. **Bolander, M. E., Young, M. F., Fisher, L. W., Yamada, Y., and Termine, J. D.,** Osteonectin cDNA sequence reveals potential binding regions for calcium and hydroxyapatite and shows homologies with both a basement membrane protein (SPARC) and a serine proteinase inhibitor (ovomucoid), *Proc. Natl. Acad. Sci. U.S.A.,* 85, 2919, 1988.

49. **Tsilibary, E. C. and Charonis, A. S.,** The role of the main noncollagenous domain (NCI) in type IV collagen self-assembly, *J. Cell Biol.,* 103, 2467, 1986.

50. **Goodman, S. L., Deutzmann, R., and von der Mark, K.,** Two distinct cell-binding domains in laminin can independently promote nonneuronal cell adhesion and spreading, *J. Cell Biol.,* 105, 589, 1987.

51. **Aumailley, M. and Timpl, R.,** Attachment of cells to basement membrane collagen type IV, *J. Cell Biol.,* 103, 1569, 1986.

52. **Mann, K., Deutzmann, R., Aumailley, M., Timpl, R., Raimondi, L., Yamada, Y., Pan, T., Conway, D., and Chu, M-L.,** Amino acid sequence of mouse nidogen, a multidomain basement membrane protein with binding activity for laminin, collagen IV and cells, *EMBO J.,* 8, 65, 1989.

53. **Engvall, E., Davis, G. E., Dickerson, K., Ruoslahti, E., Varon, S., and Manthorpe, M.,** Mapping of domains in human laminin using monoclonal antibodies: localization of the neurite-promoting site, *J. Cell Biol.,* 103, 2457, 1986.

54. **Herbst, T. J., McCarthy, J. B., Tsilibary, E. C., and Furcht, L. T.,** Differential effects of laminin, intact type IV collagen, and specific domains of type IV collagen on endothelial cell adhesion and migration, *J. Cell Biol.,* 106, 1365, 1988.

55. **Terranova, V. P., Aumailley, M., Sultan, L. H., Martin, G. R., and Kleinman, H. K.,** Regulation of cell attachment and cell number by fibronectin and laminin, *J. Cell Physiol.,* 127, 473, 1986.

56. **Tomaselli, K. J., Damsky, C. H., and Reichardt, L. F.,** Interactions of a neuronal cell line (PC12) with laminin, collagen IV, and fibronectin: identification of integrin-related glycoproteins involved in attachment and process outgrowth, *J. Cell Biol.,* 105, 2347, 1987.

57. **Aumailley, M., Nurcombe, V., Edgar, D., Paulsson, M., and Timpl, R.,** The cellular interactions of laminin fragments. Cell adhesion correlates with two fragment-specific high affinity binding sites, *J. Biol. Chem.,* 262, 11532, 1987.

58. **Lunstrum, G. P., Sakai, L. Y., Keene, D. R., Morris, N. P., and Burgeson, R. E.,** Large complex globular domains of type VII procollagen contribute to the structure of anchoring fibrils, *J. Biol. Chem.,* 261, 9042, 1986.

59. **Sakai, L. Y., Keene, D. R., Morris, N. P., and Burgeson, R. E.,** Type VII collagen is a major structural component of anchoring fibrils, *J. Cell Biol.,* 103, 1577, 1986.

60. **Keene, D. R., Sakai, L. Y., Lunstrum, G. P., Morris, N. P., and Burgeson, R. E.,** Type VII collagen forms an extended network of anchoring fibrils, *J. Cell Biol.,* 104, 611, 1987.

61. **Leigh, I. M., Purkis, P. E., and Bruckner-Tuderman, L.,** LH7.2 monoclonal antibody detects type VII collagen in the sublamina densa zone of ectodermally-derived epithelia, including skin, *Epithelia,* 1, 17, 1987.

62. **Bruckner-Tuderman, L., Mitsuhashi, Y., Schnyder, U. W., and Bruckner, P.,** Anchoring fibrils and type VII collagen are absent from skin in severe recessive dystrophic epidermolysis bullosa, *J. Invest. Dermatol.,* 93, 3, 1989.

63. **Bruckner-Tuderman, L., Schnyder, U. W., Winterhalter, K. H., and Bruckner, P.,** Tissue form of type VII collagen from human skin and dermal fibroblasts in culture, *Eur. J. Biochm.,* 165, 607, 1987.

64. **Morris, N. P., Keene, D. R., Glanville, R. W., Bentz, H., and Burgeson, R. E.,** The tissue form of type VII collagen is an antiparallel dimer, *J. Biol. Chem.,* 261, 5638, 1986.

65. **Clark, R. A. F.,** Fibronectin in the skin, *J. Invest. Dermatol.,* 81, 475, 1983.

66. **Adams, J. C. and Watt, F. M.,** Fibronectin inhibits the terminal differentiation of human keratinocytes, *Nature,* 340, 307, 1989.

67. **Panayotou, G., End, P., Aumailley, M., Timpl, R., and Engel, J.,** Domains of laminin with growth-factor activity, *Cell,* 56, 93, 1989.

68. **Durkin, M. E., Chakravarti, S., Bartos, B. B., Liu, S.-H., Friedman, R. L., and Chung, A. E.,** Amino acid sequence and domain structure of entactin. Homology with epidermal growth factor precursor and low density lipoprotein receptor, *J. Cell Biol.,* 107, 2749, 1988.

69. **Lightner, V. A., Gumkowski, F., Bigner, D. D., and Erickson, H. P.,** Tenascin/Hexabrachion in human skin: biochemical identification and localization by light and electron microscopy, *J. Cell Biol.,* 108, 2483, 1989.

70. **Jones, F. S., Burgoon, M. P., Hoffman, S., Crossin, K. L., Cunningham, B. A., and Edelman, G. M.,** A cDNA clone for cytotactin contains sequences similar to epidermal growth factor-like repeats and segments of fibronectin and fibrinogen, *Proc. Natl. Acad. Sci. U.S.A.,* 85, 2186, 1988.

71. **Chiquet-Ehrismann, R., Kalla, P., Pearson, C. A., Beck, K., and Chiquet, M.,** Tenascin interferes with fibronectin action, *Cell,* 53, 383, 1988.

72. **Bourdon, M. A. and Rouslahti, E.,** Tenascin mediates cell attachment through an RGD-dependent receptor, *J. Cell Biol.,* 108, 1149, 1989.

73. **Fukai, K., Ishii, M., Chanoki, M., Kobayashi, H., Hamada, T., Muragaki, Y., and Ooshima, A.,** Immunofluorescent localization of type I and III collagens in normal human skin with polyclonal and monoclonal antibodies, *Acta Derm. Venereol.,* 68, 196, 1988.

74. **Smith, L. T., Holbrook, K. A., and Madri, J. A.,** Collagen types I, III, and V in human embryonic and fetal skin, *Am. J. Anat.,* 175, 507, 1986.

75. **Keene, D. R., Sakai, L. Y., Bachinger, H. P., and Burgeson, R. E.,** Type III collagen can be present on banded collagen fibrils regardless of fibril diameter, *J. Cell Biol.,* 105, 2393, 1987.

76. **Woodley, D. T., Scheidt, V. J., Reese, M. J., Paller, A. S., Manning, T. O., Yoshiike, T., and Briggaman, R. A.,** Localization of the alpha 3(V) chain of type V collagen in human skin, *J. Invest. Dermatol.,* 88, 246, 1987.

77. **Keene, D. R., Engvall, E., and Glanville, R. W.,** Ultrastructure of type VI collagen in human skin and cartilage suggests an anchoring function for this filamentous network, *J. Cell Biol.,* 107, 1995, 1988.

78. **Chu, M-L., Conway, D., Pan, T., Baldwin, C., Mann, K., Deutzmann, R., and Timpl, R.,** Amino acid sequence of the triple-helical domain of human collagen type VI, *J. Biol. Chem.,* 263, 18601, 1988.
79. **Miller, E. J. and Gay, S.,** Collagen; an overview, *Methods Enzymol.,* 82, 3, 1982.
80. **Scott, J. E. and Haigh, M.,** Proteoglycan-type I collagen fibril interactions in bone and non-calcifying connective tissues, *Biosci. Rep.,* 5, 71, 1985.
81. **LeBaron, R. G., Hook, A., Esko, J. D., Gay, S., and Hook, M.,** Binding of heparan sulfate to type V collagen: a mechanism of cell-substrate adhesion, *J. Biol. Chem.,* 264, 7950, 1989.
82. **Hedbom, E. and Heinegard, D.,** Interaction of a 59-kDa connective tissue matrix protein with collagen I and collagen II, *J. Biol. Chem.,* 264, 6898, 1989.
83. **Gebb, C., Hayman, E. G., Engvall, E., and Rouslahti, E.,** Interaction of vitronectin with collagen, *J. Biol. Chem.,* 261, 16698, 1986.
84. **Ingham, K. C., Brew, S. A., and Isaacs, B. S.,** Interaction of fibronectin and its gelatin-binding domains with fluorescent-labeled chains of type I collagen, *J. Biol. Chem.,* 263, 4624, 1988.
85. **Roth, G. J., Titani, K., Hoyer, L. W., and Hickey, M. J.,** Localization of binding sites within human von Willebrand factor for monomeric type III collagen, *Biochemistry,* 25, 8357, 1986.
86. **Takagi, J., Kasahara, K., Sekiya, F., Inada, Y., and Saito, Y.,** A collagen-binding glycoprotein from bovine platelets is identical to propolypeptide of von Willebrand factor, *J. Biol. Chem.,* 264, 10425, 1989.
87. **Galvin, N. J., Vance, P. M., Dixit, V. M., Fink, B., and Frazier, W. A.,** Interaction of human thrombospondin with types I-V collagen: direct binding and electron microscopy, *J. Cell Biol.,* 104, 1413, 1987.
88. **Jarrett, A.,** The elastic tissue of the dermis, in *The Physiology and Pathophysiology of the Skin,* Vol. 3, Jarrett, A., Ed., Academic Press, New York, 1974, 847.
89. **Fazio, M. J., Olsen, D. R., Kauh, E. A., Baldwin, C. T., Indik, Z., Ornstein-Goldstein, N., Yeh, H., Rosenbloom, J., and Uitto, J.,** Cloning of full-length elastin cDNAs from a human skin fibroblast recombinant cDNA library: further elucidation of alternative splicing utilizing exon-specific oligonucleotides, *J. Invest. Dermatol.,* 91, 458, 1988.
90. **Bashir, M. M., Indik, Z., Yeh, H., Ornstein-Goldstein, N., Rosenbloom, J. C., Abrams, W., Fazio, M., Uitto, J., and Rosenbloom, J.,** Characterization of the complete human elastin gene. Delineation of unusual features in the 5'-flanking region, *J. Biol. Chem.,* 264, 8887, 1989.
91. **Fazio, M. J., Olsen, D. R., Kuivaniemi, H., Chu, M.-L., Davidson, J. M., Rosenbloom, J., and Uitto, J.,** Isolation and characterization of human elastin cDNAs and age-associated variation in elastin gene expression in cultured skin fibroblasts, *Lab. Invest.,* 58, 270, 1988.
92. **Ross, R. and Bornstein, P.,** The elastic fiber. I. The separation and partial characterization of its macromolecular components, *J. Cell Biol.,* 40, 366, 1969.
93. **Uitto, J.,** Biochemistry of the elastic fibers in normal connective tissues and its alterations in diseases, *J. Invest. Dermatol.,* 72, 1, 1979.
94. **Varadi, D. P.,** Studies on the chemistry and fine structure of elastic fibers from normal adult skin, *J. Invest. Dermatol.,* 59, 238, 1972.
95. **Sakai, L. Y., Keene, D. R., and Engvall, E.,** Fibrillin, a new 350-kD glycoprotein, is a component of extracellular microfibrils, *J. Cell Biol.,* 103, 2499, 1986.
96. **Lapiere, C. M. and Nusgens, B. V.,** Fibroblasts, collagen, elastin, proteoglycans and glycoproteins, in *Pharmacology of the Skin I.,* Greaves, M. W. and Shuster, S., Eds., Springer-Verlag, Berlin, 1989, 69.
97. **Heinegard, D., Bjorne-Persson, A., Coster, L., Franzen, A., Gardell, S., Malmstrom, A., Sandfalk, R., and Vogel, K.,** The core proteins of large and small interstitial proteoglycans from various connective tissues form distinct subgroups, *Biochem. J.,* 230, 181, 1985.
98. **Damle, S. P., Kieras, F. J., Tzeng, W. K., Gregory, J. D.,** Isolation and characterization of proteochondroitan sulfate from pig skin, *J. Biol. Chem.,* 254, 1614, 1979.
99. **Matsunaga, E. and Shinkai, H.,** Two species of dermatan sulfate proteoglycans with different molecular sizes from newborn calf skin, *J. Invest. Dermatol.,* 87, 221, 1986.
100. **Hassel, J. F., Robey, P. G., Barrach, H.-J., Wilczek, J., Rennard, S. I., and Martin, G. R.,** Isolation of a heparan sulfate-containing proteoglycan from basement membrane, *Proc. Natl. Acad. Sci. U.S.A.,* 77, 4494, 1980.
101. **Kanwar, Y. S., Veis, A., Kimura, J. H., and Jakubowski, M. L.,** Characterization of heparan sulfate-proteoglycan of glomerular basement membrane, *Proc. Natl. Acad. Sci. U.S.A.,* 81, 762, 1984.
102. **Fransson, L. A., Coster, L., Carlstedt, I., and Malmstrom, A.,** Domain structure of proteoheparan sulphate from confluent cultures of human embryonic skin fibroblasts, *Biochem. J.,* 231, 683, 1985.
103. **Stow, J. L. and Farquhar, M. G.,** Distinctive populations of basement membrane and cell membrane heparan sulfate proteoglycans are produced by cultured cells, *J. Cell Biol.,* 105, 529, 1987.
104. **Tajima, S. and Nagai, Y.,** Distribution of macromolecular components in calf dermal connective tissue, *Connect. Tissue Res.,* 7, 65, 1980.

105. **Habuchi, H., Kimata, K., and Suzuki, S.,** Changes in proteoglycan composition during development of rat skin: the occurrence in fetal skin of a chondroitin sulfate proteoglycan with high turnover rate, *J. Biol. Chem.,* 261, 1031, 1986.

106. **Choi, H. U., Johnson, T. L., Pal, S., Tang, L.-H., Rosenberg, L., and Neame, P. J.,** Characterization of the dermatan sulfate proteoglycans, DS-PGI and DS-PGII, from bovine articular cartilage and skin isolated by octyl-sepharose chromotography, *J. Biol. Chem.,* 264, 2876, 1989.

107. **Rapraeger, A., Jalkanen, M., Endo, E., Koda, J., and Bernfield, M.,** The cell surface proteoglycan from mouse mammary epithelial cells bears chondroitin sulfate and heparan sulfate glycosaminoglycans, *J. Biol. Chem.,* 260, 11046, 1985.

108. **David, G. and Van den Berghe, H.,** Heparan sulfate-chondroitin sulfate hybrid proteoglycan of the cell surface and basement membrane of mouse mammary epithelial cells, *J. Biol. Chem.,* 260, 11067, 1985.

109. **Hynes, R. O.,** Integrins: a family of cell surface receptors, *Cell,* 48, 549, 1987.

110. **Wayner, E. A. and Carter, W. G.,** Identification of multiple cell adhesion receptors for collagen and fibronectin in human fibrosarcoma cells possessing unique α and common β subunits, *J. Cell Biol.,* 105, 1873, 1987.

111. **Ruoslahti, E. and Piershbacher, M. D.,** New perspectives in cell adhesion: RGD and integrins, *Science,* 238, 491, 1987.

112. **Carter, W. G. and Wayner, E. A.,** Characterization of the class III collagen receptor, a phosphorylated, transmembrane glycoprotein expressed in nucleated human cells, *J. Biol. Chem.,* 263, 4193, 1988.

113. **Chen, W. T., Hasegawa, E., Hasegawa, T., Weinstock, C., and Yamada, K. M.,** Development of cell surface linkage complexes in cultivated fibroblasts, *J. Cell Biol.,* 100, 1103, 1985.

114. **Stockwell, R. A.,** *Biology of Cartilage Cells,* Cambridge University Press, London, 1979.

115. **Heinegard, D. and Paulsson, M.,** Structure and metabolism of proteoglycans, in *Extracellular Matrix Biochemistry,* Piez, K. A. and Reddi, A. H., Eds., Elsevier, New York, 1984.

116. **Paulsson, M. and Heingard, D.,** Noncollagenous cartilage proteins, current status of an emerging research field, *Collagen Related Res.,* 4, 219, 1984.

117. **Mendler, M., Eich-Bender, S. G., Vaughan, L., Winterhalter, K. H., and Bruckner, P.,** Cartilage contains mixed fibrils of collagen types II, IX, and XI, *J. Cell Biol.,* 108, 191, 1989.

118. **Heinegard, D. and Oldberg, A.,** Structure and biology of cartilage and bone matrix non-collagenous macromolecules, *FASEB J.,* 3, 2042, 1989.

119. **Niyibizi, C., Wu, J.-J., and Eyre, D. R.,** The carboxypropeptide trimer of type II collagen is a prominent component of immature cartilages and intervertebral-disc tissue, *Biochim. Biophys. Acta,* 916, 493, 1987.

120. **Fernandez, M. P., Selmin, O., Martin, G. R., Yamada, Y., Pfaffle, M., Deutzmann, R., Mollenhauer, J., and von der Mark, K.,** The structure of anchorin CII, a collagen binding protein isolated from chondrocyte membrane, *J. Biol. Chem.,* 263, 5921, 1988.

121. **Morris, N. P. and Bachinger, H. P.,** Type XI collagen is a heterotrimer with the composition ($1\alpha,2\alpha,3\alpha$) retaining non-triple-helical domains, *J. Biol. Chem.,* 262, 11345, 1987.

122. **Bruckner, P., Mendler, M., Steinman, B., Huber, S., and Winterhalter, K. H.,** The structure of human collagen type IX and its organization in fetal and infant cartilage fibrils, *J. Biol. Chem.,* 263, 16911, 1988.

123. **Vasios, G., Nishimura, I., Konomi, H., van der Rest, M., Ninomiya, Y., and Olsen, B. R.,** Cartilage type IX collagen-proteoglycan contains a large amino-terminal globular domain encoded by multiple exons, *J. Biol. Chem.,* 263, 2324, 1988.

124. **Svoboda, K. K., Nishimura, I., Sugrue, S. P., Ninomiya, Y., and Olsen, B. R.,** Embryonic chicken cornea and cartilage synthesize type IX collagen molecules with different amino-terminal domains, *Proc. Natl. Acad. Sci. U.S.A.,* 85, 7496, 1988.

125. **Smith, G. N., Williams, J. M., and Brandt, K. D.,** Interaction of proteoglycans with the pericellular ($1\alpha,2\alpha,3\alpha$) collagens of cartilage, *J. Biol. Chem.,* 260, 10761, 1985.

126. **Schmidt, T. M. and Conrad, H. E.,** A unique low molecular weight collagen secreted by cultured chick embryo chondrocytes, *J. Biol. Chem.,* 257, 12444, 1982.

127. **LeBoy, P. S., Shapiro, I. M., Uschmann, B. D., Oshima, O., and Lin, D.,** Gene expression in mineralizing chick epiphyseal cartilage, *J. Biol. Chem.,* 263, 8515, 1988.

128. **Gibson, G. J. and Flint, M. H.,** Type X collagen syntheses by chick sternal cartilage and its relationship to endochondral development, *J. Cell Biol.,* 101, 277, 1985.

129. **Niyibizi, C. and Eyre, D. R.,** Identification of the cartilage $\alpha1$(XI) chain in type V collagen from bovine bone, *FEBS Lett.,* 242, 314, 1989.

130. **Benya, P. D. and Brown, P. D.,** Modulation of the chondrocyte phenotype *in vitro,* in *Articular Cartilage Biochemistry,* Kuettner, K., Ed., Raven Press, New York, 1986.

131. **Doege, K., Sasaki, M., Horigan, E., Hassell, J. R., and Yamada, Y.,** Complete primary structure of the rat cartilage proteoglycan core protein deduced from cDNA clones, *J. Biol. Chem.,* 262, 17757, 1987.

132. **Hascall, V. C. and Sajdera, S. W.,** Proteinpolysaccharide complex from bovine nasal cartilage. The function of glycoprotein in the formation of aggregates, *J. Biol. Chem.,* 244, 2384, 1969.

133. **Goetinck, P. F., Stirpe, N. S., Tsonis, P. A., and Carlone, D.,** The tandemly repeated sequences of cartilage link protein contain the sites for interaction with hyaluronic acid, *J. Cell Biol.,* 105, 2403, 1987.

134. **Heinegard, D. K. and Hascall, V. C.,** Characteristics of the nonaggregating proteoglycans isolated from bovine nasal cartilage, *J. Biol. Chem.,* 254, 927, 1979.

135. **Heinegard, D., Paulsson, M., Inerot, S., and Carlstrom, C.,** A novel low-molecular-weight chondroitin sulphate proteoglycan isolated from cartilage, *Biochem. J.,* 197, 355, 1981.

136. **Fisher, L. W., Termine, J. D., and Young, M. F.,** Deduced protein sequence of bone small proteoglycan I (biglycan) shows homology with proteoglycan II (decorin) and several nonconnective tissue proteins in a variety of species, *J. Biol. Chem.,* 264, 4571, 1989.

137. **Vogel, K. G. and Fisher, L. W.,** Comparisons of antibody reactivity and enzyme sensitivity between small proteoglycans from bovine tendon, bone and cartilage, *J. Biol. Chem.,* 261, 11334, 1986.

138. **Fisher, L. W.,** The nature of the proteoglycans of bone, in *The Chemistry and Biology of Mineralized Tissues,* Butler, W. T., Ed., Ebsco Media, Birmingham, AL, 186, 1985.

139. **Rosenberg, L. C., Choi, H. U., Tang, L.-H., Johnson, T. L., Pal, S., Webber, C., Reiner, A., and Poole, A. R.,** Isolation of dermatan sulfate proteoglycans from mature bovine articular cartilage, *J. Biol. Chem.,* 260, 6304, 1985.

140. **Chandrasekhar, S., Laurie, G. W., Cannon, F. B., Martin, G. R., and Kleinman, H. K.,** *In vitro* regulation of cartilage matrix assembly by a GMW 54,000 collagen binding protein, *Proc. Natl. Acad. Sci. U.S.A.,* 83, 5126, 1986.

141. **Argraves, W. S., Deak, F., Sparks, K. J., Kiss, I., and Goetinck, P. F.,** Structural features of cartilage matrix protein deduced from cDNA, *Proc. Natl. Acad. Sci. U.S.A.,* 84, 464, 1987.

142. **Heinegard, D., Larsson, T., Sommarin, Y., Franzen, A., Paulsson, M., and Hedbom, E.,** Two novel matrix proteins isolated from articular cartilage show wide distributions among connective tissues, *J. Biol. Chem.,* 261, 13866, 1986.

143. **Pfaffle, M., Ruggiero, F., Hofmann, H., Fernandez, M. P., Selmin, O., Yamada, Y., Garrone, R., and von der Mark, K.,** Biosynthesis, secretion and extracellular localization of anchorin CII, a collagen-binding protein of the calpactin family, *EMBO J.,* 7, 2335, 1988.

144. **Mollenhauer, J., Bee, J. A., Lizarbe, M. A., and von der Mark, K.,** Role of anchorin C11, a 31,000-mol-wt membrane protein in the interaction of chondrocytes with type II collagen, *J. Cell Biol.,* 98, 1572, 1984.

145. **Poole, A. R., Pidoux, I., Reiner, A., Choi, H., and Rosenberg, L. C.,** Association of an extracellular protein (chondrocalcin) and with the calcification of cartilage in endochondral bone formation, *J. Cell Biol.,* 98, 54, 1984.

146. **Van der Rest, M., Rosenberg, L. C., Olsen, B. R., and Poole, A. R.,** Chondrocalcin is identical to the C-propeptide of type II procollagen, *Biochem. J.,* 273, 923, 1986.

147. **Poole, A. R., Pidoux, I., Linsenmayer, T. F., and Schmidt, T. M.,** Type X collagen and the calcification of cartilage matrix: an immunoelectron microscopic study, *Trans. ORS,* 13, 155, 1988.

148. **Cancedda, F. D., Manduca, P., Tacchetti, C., Fossa, P., Quarto, R., and Cancedda, R.,** Developmentally regulated synthesis of a low molecular weight protein (Ch 21) by differentiating chondrocytes, *J. Cell Biol.,* 107, 2455, 1988.

149. **Hinek, A., Reiner, A., and Poole, A. R.,** The calcification of cartilage matrix in chondrocyte culture: studies of the C-propeptide of type II collagen (chondrocalcin), *J. Cell Biol.,* 104, 1435, 1987.

150. **Hewitt, A. T., Varner, H. H., Silver, M. H., Dessau, W., Wilkes, C. M., and Martin, G. R.,** The isolation and partial characterization of chondronectin, an attachment factor for chondrocytes, *J. Biol. Chem.,* 257, 2330, 1982.

151. **Fisher, L. W., Termine, J. D., Dejter, S. W., Whitson, S. W., Yanagishita, M., Kimura, J. H., Hascall, V. C., Kleinmann, H. K., Hassell, J. R., and Nilsson, B.,** Proteoglycans of developing bone, *J. Biol. Chem.,* 258, 6588, 1983.

152. **Franzen, A. and Heinegard, D.,** Characterization of proteoglycans from the calcified matrix of bovine bone, *Biochem. J.,* 224, 59, 1984.

153. **Fischer, L. W., Hawkins, G. R., Tuross, N., and Termine, J. D.,** Purification and partial characterization of small proteoglycans I and II, bone sialoproteins I and II, and osteonectin from the mineral compartment of developing human bone, *J. Biol. Chem.,* 262, 9702, 1987.

154. **Scott, J. E. and Haigh, M.,** Proteoglycan-type I collagen fibril interactions in calcifying and non-calcifying connective tissues, *Biochem. Soc.,* 13, 933, 1985.

155. **Franzen, A. and Heinegard, D.,** Isolation and characterization of two sialoproteins present only in bone calcified matrix, *Biochem. J.,* 232, 715, 1985.

156. **Kinne, R. W. and Fisher, L. W.,** Keratine sulfate proteoglycan in rabbit compact bone is bone sialoprotein II, *J. Biol. Chem.,* 262, 10206, 1987.

157. **Grynpas, M. D. and Hunter, G. K.,** Bone mineral and glycosaminoglycans in newborn and mature rabbits, *J. Bone Miner. Res.,* 3, 159, 1988.

158. **Price, P. A.,** Vitamin K-dependent bone proteins, in *Calcium Regulation and Bone Metabolism: Basic and Clinical Aspects,* Vol. 9, Cohn, D. V. et al., Eds., Elsevier, Amsterdam, 1987, 419.
159. **Price, P. A.,** Role of vitamin K-dependent proteins in bone metabolism, *Ann. Rev. Nutr.,* 8, 565, 1988.
160. **Romberg, R. W., Werness, P. G., Riggs, B. L., and Mann, K. G.,** Inhibition of hydroxyapatite crystal growth by bone-specific and other calcium binding proteins, *Biochemistry,* 25, 1176, 1986.
161. **Fraser, J. D., Otawara, Y., and Price, P. A.,** 1,25-Dihydroxyvitamin D_3 stimulates the synthesis of matrix γ-carboxyglutamic acid protein by osteosarcoma cells. Mutually exclusive expression of vitamin K-dependent bone proteins by clonal osteoblastic cell lines, *J. Biol. Chem.,* 263, 911, 1988.
162. **Otawara, Y. and Price, P. A.,** Developmental appearance of matrix GLA protein during calcification in the rat, *J. Biol. Chem.,* 261, 10828, 1986.
163. **Boskey, A. L.,** Noncollagenous matrix proteins and their role in mineralization, *Bone Miner.,* 6, 111, 1989.
164. **Elliott, J. C.,** Controlled crystallization, *Nature,* 317, 387, 1985.
165. **Bronner, F.,** Calcium homeostasis, in *Disorders of Mineral Metabolism,* Bronner, F. and Coburn, J. W., Eds., Academic Press, New York, 1982, 43.
166. **Mardon, H. and Triffit, J. T.,** A tissue-specific protein in rat osteogenetic tissues, *J. Bone Miner. Res.,* 3, 191, 1987.
167. **DiMuzio, M. T. and Veis, A.,** Phosphoryn: major noncollagenous proteins of rat incisor dentin, *Calcif. Tissue Int.,* 25, 169, 1978.
168. **Mason, I. J., Taylor, A., Williams, J. G., Sage, H., and Hogan, B. L. M.,** Evidence from molecular cloning that SPARC, a major product of mouse embryo parietal endoderm, is related to an endothelial cell "culture shock" glycoprotein of M_r 43,000, *Eur. J. Biochem.,* 161, 455, 1986.
169. **Termine, J. D., Kleinman, H. D., Whitson, S. W., Conn, K. M., McGarvey, M. L., and Martin, G. R.,** Osteonectin, a bone-specific protein linking mineral to collagen, *Cell,* 26, 99, 1981.
170. **Doi, Y., Okuda, R., Takezawa, Y., Shibata, S., Moriwaki, Y., Wakamatsu, N., Shimizu, N., Moriyama, K., and Shimokawa, H.,** Osteonectin inhibiting de novo formation of apatite in the presence of collagen, *Calcif. Tissue Int.,* 44, 200, 1989.
171. **Fisher, L. W., Robey, P. G., Tuross, N., Otsuka, A. S., Tepen, D. A., Esch, F. S., Shimasaki, S., and Termine, J. D.,** The M_r 24,000 phosphoprotein from developing bone is the NH_2-terminal propeptide of the α-1 chain of type I collagen, *J. Biol. Chem.,* 262, 13457, 1987.
172. **Uchiyama, A., Suzuki, M., Lefteriou, B., and Glimcher, M.,** Isolation and chemical characterization of the phosphoproteins of chicken bone matrix: heterogeneity in molecular weight and composition, *Biochemistry,* 25, 7572, 1986.
173. **Urist, M. R., Delange, R. J., and Finerman, G. A. M.,** Bone cell differentiation and growth factors, *Science,* 220, 680, 1983.
174. **Jeffrey, J. J.,** The biological regulation of collagenase activity, in *Regulation of Matrix Accumulation,* Median, R. P., Ed., Academic Press, New York, 1986, 53.
175. **Canalis, E.,** Effect of growth factors on bone cell replication and differentiation, *Clin. Orthop.,* 193, 246, 1985.
176. **Sampath, T. K., Muthukumaran, N., and Reddi, A. H.,** Isolation of osteogenin and extracellular matrix-associated bone inductive protein by heparin affinity, *Chromotography,* 84, 7109, 1987.
177. **Tuszynski, G. P., Rothman, V., Murphy, A., Siegler, K., Smith, L., Karczewski, J., Knudsen, K. A.,** Thrombospondin promotes cell-substratum adhesion, *Science,* 236, 1570, 1987.
178. **Gehron-Robey, P., Young, M. F., Fischer, L., and McClain, T.,** Thrombospondin is an osteoblast-derived component of mineralized extracellular matrix, *J. Cell Biol.,* 108, 719, 1989.
179. **Oldberg, A., Franzen, A., and Heinegard, D.,** Cloning and sequence analysis of rat bone sialoprotein (osteopontin) cDNA reveals an Arg-Gly-Asp cell-binding sequence, *Proc. Natl. Acad. Sci. U.S.A.,* 83, 8819, 1986.
180. **Lewandowska, K., Choi, H. V., Rosenberg, L. C., Zardi, L.,and Culp, L. A.,** Fibronectin-mediated adhesion of fibroblasts: inhibition by dermatan sulfate proteoglycan and evidence for a cryptic glycosaminoglycan-binding domain, *J. Cell Biol.,* 105, 1443, 1987.
181. **Jones, G. E., Arumugham, R. G., and Tanzer, M. L.,** Fibronectin glycosylation modulates fibroblast adhesion and spreading, *J. Cell Biol.,* 103, 1663, 1986.
182. **Pierschbacher, M. D., Hayman, E. G., and Ruoslahti, E.,** Location of the cell attachment site in fibronectin with monoclonal antibodies and proteolytic fragments of the molecule, *Cell,* 26, 259, 1981.
183. **Werb, Z., Tremble, P. M., Behrendtsen, O., Crowley, E., and Damsky, C. H.,** Signal transduction through the fibronectin receptor induces collagenase and stromelysin gene expression, *J. Cell Biol.,* 109, 877, 1989.
184. **Menko, A. S. and Boettiger, D.,** Occupation of the extracellular matrix receptor integrin, is a control point for myogenic differentiation, *Cell,* 51, 51, 1987.

185. **Grant, D. S., Tashiro, K.-I., Segui-Real, B., Yamada, Y., Martin, G., and Kleinman, H. K.,** Two different laminin domains mediate the differentiation of human endothelial cells into capillary-like structures, *in vitro, Cell,* 58, 933, 1989.

186. **Albini, A., Allavena, G., Melchiori, A., Giancotti, F., Richter, H., Comoglio, P. M., Parodi, S., Martin, G. R., and Tarone, G.,** Chemotaxis of 3T3 and SV3T3 cells to fibronectin is mediated through the cell-attachment site in fibronectin and a fibronectin cell surface receptor, *J. Cell Biol.,* 105, 1867, 1987.

187. **Bashkin, P., Doctrow, S., Klagsbrun, M., Svahn, C. M., Folkman, J., and Vlodavsky, I.,** Basic fibroblast growth factor binds to subendothelial extracellular matrix and is released by heparitinase and heparin-like molecules, *Biochemistry,* 28, 1737, 1989.

188. **Colige, A., Nusgens, B., and Lapiere, C. M.,** Effect of EGF on human skin fibroblasts is modulated by the extracellular matrix, *Arch. Dermatol. Res.,* 280, S42, 1988.

189. **Ingber, D. E. and Folkman, J.,** Mechanochemical switching between growth and differentiation during fibroblast growth factor-stimulated angiogenesis *in vitro:* role of extracellular matrix, *J. Cell Biol.,* 109, 317, 1989.

190. **Madri, J. A., Pratt, B. M., and Tucker, A. M.,** Phenotypic modulation of endothelial cells by transforming growth factor-β depends upon the composition and organization of the extracellular matrix, *J. Cell Biol.,* 106, 1375, 1988.

191. **Nakagawa, S., Pawelek, P., and Grinnell, F.,** Extracellular matrix organization modulates fibroblast growth and growth factor responsiveness, *Exp. Cell Res.,* 182, 572, 1989.

192. **Nagata, K. and Yamada, K. M.,** Phosphorylation and transformation sensitivity of a major collagen-binding protein of fibroblasts, *J. Biol. Chem.,* 261, 7531, 1986.

193. **Dahl, S. C. and Grabel, L. B.,** Integrin phosphorylation is modulated during the differentiation of F-9 teratocarcinoma stem cells, *J. Cell Biol.,* 108, 183, 1989.

194. **Plantefaber, L. C. and Hynes, R. O.,** Changes in integrin receptors on oncogenically transformed cells, *Cell,* 56, 281, 1989.

195. **Horwitz, A., Duggan, K., Buck, C., Beckerle, M. C., and Burridge, K.,** Interaction of plasma membrane fibronectin receptor with talin-a transmembrane linkage, *Nature,* 320, 531, 1986.

196. **Gorski, J. P. and Shimizu, K.,** Isolation of a new phosphorylated glycoprotein from mineralized phase of bone that exhibits limited homology to adhesive protein osteopontin, *J. Biol. Chem.,* 263, 15938, 1988.

197. **Olsen, B. R., Gerecke, D., Gordon, M., Green, G., Kimura, T., Konomi, H., Muragaki, Y., Ninomiya, Y., Nishimura, I., and Sugrue, S.,** A new dimension in the extracellular matrix, in *Collagen,* Vol. 4, Molecular Biology, Olsen, B. R. and Nimni, M. E., Eds., CRC Press, Boca Raton, FL, 1989, 1.

198. **Jones, J. C. R. and Goldman, R. D.,** Intermediate filaments and the initiation of desmosome assembly, *J. Cell Biol.,* 101, 506, 1985.

199. **Green, K. J., Parry, D. A. D., Steinert, P. M., Virata, M. L. A., Wagner, R. M., Angst, B. D., and Nilles, L. A.,** Structure of the human desmoplakins: implications for function in the desmosomal plaque, *J. Biol. Chem.,* 265, 2603, 1990.

200. **Schmelz, M., Duden, R., Cowin, P., and Franke, W. W.,** A constitutive transmembrane glycoprotein of M_r 165,000 (desmoglein) in epidermal and non-epidermal desmosomes. I. Biochemical identification of the polypeptide, *Eur. J. Cell Biol.,* 42, 177, 1986.

201. **Schmelz, M., Duden, R., Cowin, P., and Franke, W. W.,** A constitutive transmembrane glycoprotein of M_r 165,000 (desmoglein) in epidermal and non-epidermal desmosomes. II. Immunolocalization and microinjection studies, *Eur. J. Cell Biol.,* 42, 184, 1986.

202. **Jones, J. C. R.,** Characterization of a 125K glycoprotein associated with bovine epithelial desmosomes, *J. Cell Sci.,* 89, 207, 1988.

203. **Miller, K., Mattey, D., Measures, H., Hopkins, C., and Garrod, D.,** Localization of the protein and glycoprotein components of bovine nasal epithelial desmosomes by immunoelectron microscopy, *EMBO J.,* 6, 885, 1987.

204. **Cowin, P., Kapprell, H.-P., Franke, W. W., Tamkun, J., and Hynes, R. O.,** Plakoglobin: a protein common to different kinds of intercellular adhering junctions, *Cell,* 46, 1063, 1986.

205. **Green, K. J. and Jones, J. C. R.,** Interaction of intermediate filaments with the cell surface, in *Intermediate Filaments,* Goldman, R. D. and Steinert, P. M., Eds., Alan R. Liss, New York, 1989, 147.

206. **Mehrel, T., Hohl, D., Rothnagel, J. A., Longley, M. A., Bundman, D., Cheng, C., Lichti, U., Bisher, M. E., Steven, A. C., Steinert, P. M., Yuspa, S. H., and Roop, D. R.,** Identification of a major keratinocyte cell envelope protein, loricrin, *Cell,* 61, 1103, 1990.

Chapter 3

MORPHOLOGY AND MECHANICS OF SKIN, CARTILAGE, AND BONE

Arthur J. Wasserman and Michael G. Dunn

TABLE OF CONTENTS

I. INTRODUCTION

Understanding the structure of skin, bone, and cartilage is important to the biomaterial specialist as well as the surgeon. For the biomedical engineer, a prosthesis should be a likeness of the tissue to be replaced, and it is therefore imperative to understand its morphology. For the surgeon, an understanding of the morphology and biology of diseased, damaged, or malformed tissues is required to optimize a method for their repair, replacement, and return to normal function.

In this chapter, skin, cartilage, and bone will be discussed in the context of their basic development and structure. This will provide the framework for a further discussion on the biomechanical properties of these tissues. In addition, this chapter will provide a foundation for future applications, dealing with afflictions to these tissues, which require an understanding of their structure and function.

II. MORPHOLOGY OF THE SKIN

Management of facial skin disfigurement, resulting from disease, congenital defects or trauma, and the development of biomaterials for tissue augmentation, requires a working knowledge of skin biology and morphology. For example, scar revision and congenital nonprogressive defects of facial skin, can be treated with dermal grafts. Incisions made in facial skin during graft transfer should be made after carefully considering the numerous folds and clefts of the skin. This is of critical importance, since facial skin is vulnerable to scarring, and a cosmetic blemish to the face can adversely effect the quality of a patient's life. In the case of burn management, depending upon the category of a burn, a split thickness or full-thickness graft may be applied. Before these clinical problems can be addressed, a strong understanding of skin morphology is required. In the following section, the basic development and morphology of skin is reviewed.

A. THE EPIDERMIS

The skin is divided into two anatomically distinct regions. The outermost layer is the *epidermis*. Embryologically (Figure 1), this epithelial layer is derived from ectoderm,[1] and its layers are established by the end of the second trimester.[2] When fully differentiated, the epidermis contains other cells originating from bone marrow mesenchyme and neural crest.[2] The subjacent *dermis* is derived from mesenchymal cells,[1,3] and is established during the first 2 months.[2] This section of the skin differentiates into a fibrous connective tissue layer which contains nerve endings, blood vessels, and numerous wandering cells of various origins. The hypodermis is a superficial fascia which interfaces the dermis to underlying deeper structures and/or fascia. It is composed of fat and loose connective tissue.

The *epidermal layer* of the skin (Figures 2 and 3) varies in thickness depending upon its location on the body. The epidermis is composed of several divisions each of which has a unique structure and function. The *stratum basal* is the bottom or lowest layer of the epidermis (Figure 3). It is usually a one-cell thick layer of cuboidal or low columnar shaped basal cells. It is responsible for maintaining the progeny of cells which differentiate into the upper layers of the epidermis (described below). Because of its keratin synthesizing capability, cells of the stratum basal (and their progeny) are called keratinocytes. The cells adhere to each other through the formation of junctional specializations called desmosomes.[4] A basement membrane is secreted by keratinocytes and they attach to the membrane by hemidesmosomes. Beneath this basement membrane is the dermis, which will be discussed below.

Immediately above the basal layer is the *stratum spinosum* (Figure 3). More extensive keratinization and an increase in the number of desmosomes between spinous cells is a prominent feature of this layer. A transition from cuboidal shaped cells near the basal layer

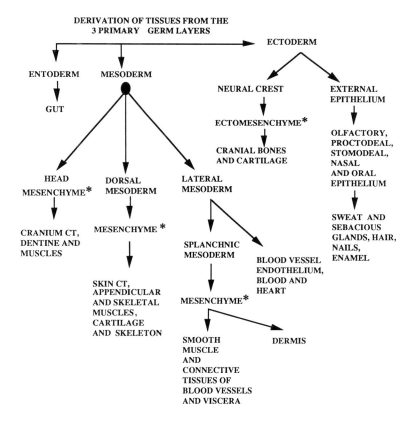

DERIVATION OF TISSUES FROM THE 3 PRIMARY GERM LAYERS

FIGURE 1. Flow chart showing the differentiation of tissue from the three primary germ layers. CT, connective tissue; *, mesenchyme—this is tissue of mesodermal origin which has broken away and migrated through the matrix of the embryo, destined to differentiate into structures unrelated to the original mesodermal mass.

to flattened squamous type cells near the surface layer occurs. The spinosal layer is several cells thick. The uppermost cells contain cytoplasmic inclusions composed of sterols and glycolipids.[4] These bodies are called lamellar granules. Their function is manifested in layers above the stratum spinosum (discussed below) where they create a lipidous barrier which establishes a water seal against the external milieu.[5]

The *stratum granulosum* is a transitional zone between the viable epidermal cells below and the devitalized cells of the outermost surface layer above (Figure 3). It is characterized by dense irregular shaped protein granules composed of keratohyaline. It is possible that these structures represent a concentration of enzymatically digested cellular debris and are not related to the keratinization process.[4,6,7] These cells do not contain nuclei and it is likely that acid nucleases and other cytoplasmic enzymes digest the nucleus as well as other cell organelles.[8] Failure of the cell contents to undergo autolytic digestion results in skin pathologies of keratin.[9] The lamellar granules are more abundant and cluster near the plasma membrane of the granule cells. Within the fully differentiated top layer of the stratum granulosum the granules are released by exocytosis into the extracellular space. Shortly thereafter, enzymatically degraded subcellular organelles also pass through the cell membrane.[7] This process of devitalization ultimately leads to a transformation of the granulosum cells into the cells which compose the superficial stratum corneum.

In the *stratum corneum,* a dense nonkeratinous material is deposited on the plasma membrane of the flattened cells (Figures 2, 3). The cells contain mostly keratin filaments, and keratohyaline along with vestiges of cellular debris. There are no cell nuclei, and

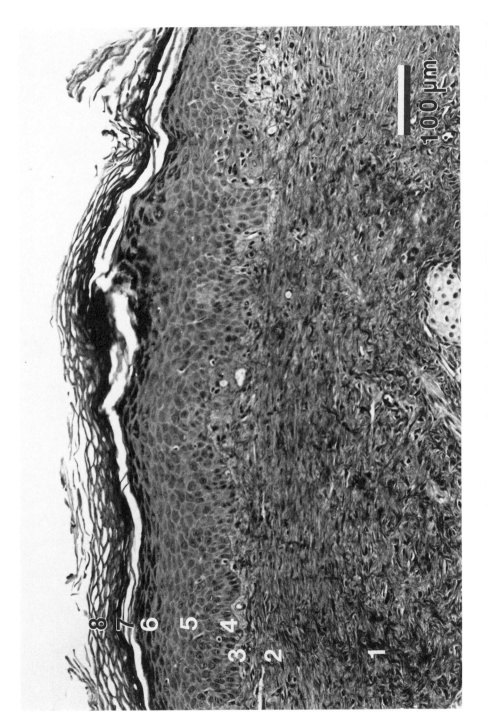

FIGURE 2. Light photomicrograph of the skin. Seen here are the epidermis and dermis. The subdivisions of these two layers are numbered 1 to 8 and identified as follows: (1) reticular dermis; (2) papillary dermis; (3) dermo-epidermal junction; (4) stratum basal of epidermis; (5) stratum spinosum of epidermis; (6) stratum granulosum of epidermis; (7) stratum lucidum of corneum (epidermis); (8) stratum disjunctum of corneum (epidermis).

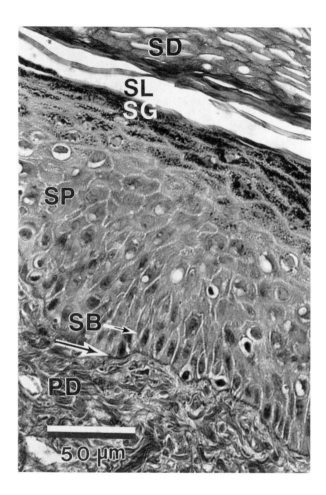

FIGURE 3. Light photomicrograph of the skin. Seen here is the upper portion of the dermis called the papillary dermis (PD); the dermo-epidermal junction (arrow); the stratum basal (SB); the stratum spinosum (SP); the stratum granulosum (SG); the stratum lucidum (SL); and the stratum disjunctum (SD).

desmosomes do not hold the cells together although they can be detected. Exfoliation of these devitalized cells occurs at the surface of the cornified layer.

Thickness variations of the stratum corneum and the development of pathologic states is related to hydrolytic activities which occur in the stratum granulosum. When the hydrolysis of cytoplasmic contents is at a minimum or absent, the nucleus and cellular contents become keratinized resulting in a parakeratotic keratin layer having psoriatic scales (characteristic of psoriasis). If the nucleus only is enzymatically degraded but the cell contents are only minimally affected, a palmar or plantar like corneum will result. Finally, if the extent of hydrolysis is great, only the cytoplasmic keratin filaments of the granule cells are incorporated into the stratum corneum resulting in a thin keratin layer.[8,9] These differences in epidermal cell physiology are expressed phenotypically as differences in skin morphology. Facial and ear skin is pliable and supple whereas plantar and palmar epithelium is coarse and tough.[8]

Two subdivisions of the corneum are sometimes referred to by histologists. The *stratum lucidum* is a translucent layer of tightly packed cells located between the corneum and granulosum. The *stratum disjunctum* is the fully mature outermost layer of the corneum where exfoliation of the devitalized squamous cells is constantly taking place (Figure 2).

TABLE 1
Epidermal Cell Types, Location, and Function

Cell type	Location	Function	Origin
Keratinocyte	Epidermis-stratum basal	Synthesizes keratin; gives rise to cells in upper epidermis	Ectoderm
Merkel cells	Epidermis	Transmit sensory tactile information	Neural crest or mesenchyme
Dendritic cells	Epidermis	Group of cells characterized by long thin dendritic processes	Varied
Melanocyte (dendritic cell)	Epidermis-basal cell layer	Protect skin from radiation damage	Neural crest ectoderm
Langerhans cells (dendritic cell)	Epidermis-stratum spinosum	Contact mediated allergic reactions	Bone marrow mesenchyme
Schwann cells (dendritic cell)	Epidermis	Accompanies sensory nerves which end in the epidermis	Neural crest
Mast cells (dendritic cell)	Epidermis	Induce localized inflammatory responses	Pleuripotential mesenchyme
Macrophage (dendritic cell)	Epidermis	Phagocytic cells; active during inflammation	Monocytes and pleuripotential mesenchyme

Note: Cells found in the epidermis. Described are the locations of the cells, their function, and cell line from which they are derived.

Within the corneum, several specialized cells can be found which are integral components of this layer. These cells are listed below and in Table 1.

1. *Keratinocytes* are an integral cell of the epidermis. They originate in the stratum basal. These cells differentiate into cells of the upper epidermal layers.
2. *Merkel cells* are the last cells to appear in the epidermis. They may be derived from neural crest or mesenchyme. It is believed these cells transmit sensory tactile information in the epidermis.[10] Merkel cells are characterized by the presence of intracellular dense cored vesicles similar to monoamine containing neurons and cells of the adrenal medulla.[11]
3. Another population of cells in the epidermis have a stellate shape with long thin dendritic processes. Because of their characteristic morphology, this group is called *dendritic cells*. Dendritic cells include Langerhans cells and melanocytes. Schwann cells, mast cells, and macrophages have been included in this category.[6]

    a. *Melanocytes* are a specialized cell of the skin that are derived from the neural crest ectoderm. They initially reside in the basal cell layer of the epidermis and appear at about the second month.[12] Because of their long branching, cell processes are referred to as dendritic type cells. The pigment melanin is produced in these cells and stored in pigment granules called melanosomes.[13] Through a process known as cytocrine secretion, the pigment can be transferred to adjacent keratinocytes. However, only melanocytes produce melanin. Their primary function is to protect the epidermis and underlying dermis from radiation damage induced by the environment. It is not surprising to find nearly twice as many melanocytes in the face as in the arms, legs and trunk.[14]

    b. *Langerhans cells* originate from bone marrow mesenchyme and have their greatest density in the stratum spinosum at about the third month of fetal development.[2,15,16] Ultrastructural observations of these cells show that they contain rod-shaped vermiform or Langerhans cell granules. These cells are found in apposition to lymphocytes during allergic reactions possibly causing antigen induced responses of the latter. Furthermore, their migration to lymph nodes has implicated them as triggers of immunoproliferative mechanisms.[4,17] Because of their location in the epidermis, it is thought these cells play a role in contact mediated allergic reactions.[18]

    c.   *Schwann cells* are derived from neural crest and may find their way to the epidermis by migrating along sensory nerves which end in the epidermis.[6]

    d.   *Mast cells* are mobile cells which are responsible for initiating localized inflammatory responses associated with allergic responses. Mast cells contain 3 cytoplasmic granules which are released extracellularly. These granules contain serotonin which causes vasoconstriction, heparin which is an anticoagulant, and histamine which causes increased vascular permeability.[4,6]

    e.   *Macrophages* are phagocytic cells of the connective tissue. They will internalize and enzymatically digest bacteria, cellular debris, and other invading foreign body material. The origin of these cells is from monocytes of the blood. They are recruited during times of inflammation. Monocytes penetrate the endothelial layer of the blood vessels where they transform into macrophages with long lamellapodia and lysosomes. A second source of macrophages is from pluripotential mesenchymal cells which are dormant in the connective tissues. These sessile cells are called histiocytes, and upon activation by external stimulation they will differentiate into activated macrophages. During chronic inflammation, macrophages will merge to form multinucleated *giant cells.*

B. THE DERMIS

The *dermis* differs from the epidermis not only in its genesis but in its morphology and composition. The dermis has an endogenous population of fibroblasts but a more complex system of migratory cells including: monocytes, lymphocytes, granulocytes, eosinophils, mast cells, plasma cells, macrophages, blood vessels, sensory nerves and organs, hair follicles, and glands.

The dermis is divided into two layers. That surface in contact with the epidermis is the *papillary layer* (Figures 2, 3, 4). There is a greater density of fibroblasts and other cells in this layer. It contains fiber bundles of small diameter collagen fibrils (Figure 4) which are composed of a higher ratio of type III to type I collagen.[19,20] Immature elastic fibers of oxytalan are a second structural element found in the papillary dermis.[21] The line of demarcation between the papillary and the *reticular dermis* is not clearly distinguishable (Figure 2). However, a major structural feature which distinguishes the reticular from the papillary dermis is the larger diameter collagen fibrils,[22,23] and thicker fiber bundles (Figure 5). These fibers are composed of a higher ratio of type I to type III collagen.[2] Elastic fibers of various stages of maturity and elastin matrix are also present throughout the reticular dermis.[21] These fibers form a tracery, entwining the various glands and hair follicles. There are fewer cells in this layer.

The dermo-epidermal junction is a region where the epidermis and dermis interface (Figure 3). Basal cells of the epidermis and fibroblasts of the dermis are thought to share the function of synthesizing the basal lamina which separates the 2 layers.[6] Hemidesmosomes between basal cells of the epidermis and the basal lamina form a tenacious connection. Anchoring filaments and fibrils pass through the basal lamina adding additional strength to the connection.[2] Anchoring fibrils and fibers, called oxytalin, also extend from the basal lamina into the dermal collagen.[24] These physical structures provide the mechanism of epidermal-dermal adhesion. This interface region is a highly plastic zone which undergoes constant alterations in response to environmental pressures.

The biomechanical properties of skin are dependent upon three variables: first, the types and ratios of collagen and the fibril diameters, second, the elastin/elastic fiber content, and third, the type and quantity of proteoglycans present. In a thorough report of the structure of the dermal matrix, Smith[24] indicates that the glycosaminoglycans dermatan sulfate, chon-

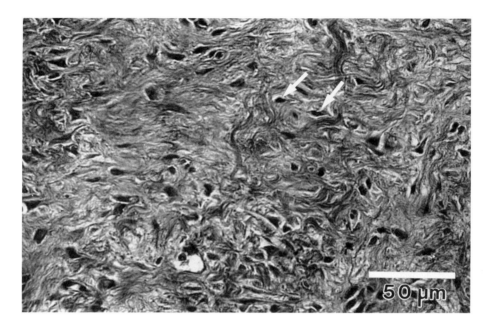

FIGURE 4.   Light photomicrograph of the papillary dermis. Collagen fibrils are thin and the fibril bundles are not tightly packed. Note the numerous cells of this layer (arrows).

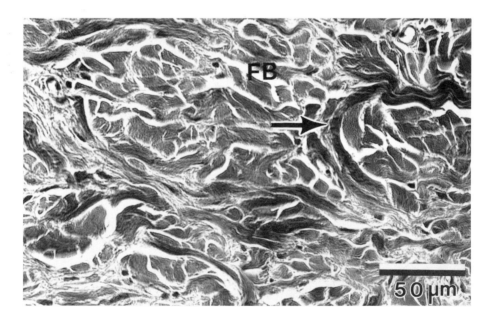

FIGURE 5.   Light photomicrograph of the reticular layer of the dermis. The collagen fibrils of this layer are coarse and form fibril bundles that are tightly packed (FB). Note that some collagen fibril bundles run perpendicular (arrow) to the predominantly parallel orientation.

droitin 4 and 6-sulfate and hyaluronic acid influence the kinetics and morphology of collagen fibril synthesis and elastic fibril structure. Dermatan sulfate is also implicated in controlling collagen fibril diameter. Larger diameter fibrils have a higher dermatan sulfate content and smaller fibrils have a lower content.[24-27] Scott[28] proposes that dermatan sulfate binds to both thick and thin collagen fibrils, but that the lower concentration of chondroitin sulfate in the coarse fibrils causes the dermatan sulfate content to appear greater. Changes in the chondroitin sulfate content of connective tissues has also been implicated in controlling collagen fibril diameter. In this case, increasing collagen fibril diameters are associated with a lower chondroitin sulfate content.[26,28] Developmentally, the diameter of collagen fibrils in the skin increases over time and range from about 25 nm at 14 weeks to 75 nm at 70 years.[27] Furthermore, tissues requiring a high tensile strength and serving an active mechanical role will have larger diameter fibrils.[23,27,29-31]

It is appropriate to point out at this point that facial skin contains many natural lines of expression, flexion creases and folds. The elastic fibers and collagen bundles of the dermis maintain the skin in a state of constant tension. Langer[32] in 1861 described lines of tension which may actually represent skin extensibility.[33] Creases and folds of the skin are frequently referred to as relaxed skin tension lines, lines of minimal tension, or lines of maximal tension. Their definition and role in selecting a site for surgical incisions is reviewed by Converse.[34] It is at these lines that elastic and collagen fibers are oriented parallel relative to the lines or creases. These collagen and elastic fibers are perpendicular to the underlying muscles. It is important to note that an incision made perpendicular to a line of tension will result in the deposition of large amounts of collagen due to the constant tension changes produced during underlying muscle activity. Such a hypertrophic scar can be avoided if incisions are made parallel to facial folds creases and lines since tension in this direction is minimal.

In many animals a thin layer of subcutaneous muscle attaches to the dermis which allows voluntary skin movement. This layer is called the *panniculus carnosus*. A less sophisticated arrangement of muscle is present in man. These muscles located in the face allow for frowning, smiling, and movement of the ears and scalp. There is also a plexus of loose smooth muscle cells located in the lower reticular layer of the penis, areolae, perineum, and scrotum which allow contraction and expansion of these structures upon thermal and tactile stimulation. Smooth muscles connected to hairs of the dermis allow for hair erection upon thermal stimulation and are called arrector pili.

Hairs develop from dermal mesenchyme at about 9 weeks.[35] They are supported and held in place by elastin and collagen fibers. As previously mentioned, hairs can be raised and lowered by a network of smooth muscle, called arrector pili. These smooth muscles extend from the connective tissue encasement around the hair to the papillary layer of the dermis.

Sebaceous glands associated with each hair can be identified as early as 15 weeks of fetal development. They secrete sebum through a duct and onto the epidermal surface. Some glands are very large and open directly onto the epidermal surface. There are no sebaceous glands on the palms of the hands and the soles of the feet. The glands are greatest in density and largest on the forehead, auditory meatus, anogenital surfaces and face (cheeks, chin, and alae of the nose).[36] To distinguish the larger glands from normal sized glands they are referred to as follicles.[37] Sebaceous glands contribute endogenous lipids to the epidermal surface and increase the impermeability of the epidermal layer.[38]

Sweat glands are of two types. *Eccrine glands* secrete a watery fluid directly onto the epidermis. These glands function to dissipate heat during periods of raised body temperature. They originate from epithelial cells which grow down into the dermis. The distribution of eccrine sweat glands is variable. There are many more glands in the face than the legs, trunk, or arms.[39] Activation of sweating is governed by a thermostatic center in the hypothalamus. Thermal stimulation of hypothalamic neurons results in activation of autonomic pathways to unmyelinated sympathetic fibers that innervate the eccrine sweat glands.[4] This reflex usually is initiated by stimulation of thermal receptors located in the deep muscles of the body, veins, and in the skin.[40] Reflex arcs triggered by emotional stimulation can also stimulate the eccrine glands to sweat. This latter response may be due to innervation by adrenergic neurons whereas the thermal responses may be due to cholinergic innervation.

Apocrine sweat glands located in the mons pubis, the mammary gland, and the peripheral-anal area are much larger in size than the eccrine glands. These glands arise as outpouchings from the base of the hair follicles. They receive adrenergic innervation and produce a thick secretion which is initiated at puberty.

Blood vessels supply the dermis in great abundance. Their function is not in nutrition alone but also in thermal and pressure regulation. The rete cutaneum network located below the dermis supplies blood to the lower portions of hair follicles, and sweat glands. This network also branches off to form the subpapillary plexis (rete subpapillare) which is a blood vessel layer located between the papillary and reticular dermis. From this network of vessels a capillary bed forms in the papilla of the papillary dermis. The subpapillary plexus supplies nutrition to the avascular epidermis.[41] A dense network of capillaries derived from this layer surrounds the sebaceous and sweat glands. *Lymphatic vessels* are dense in the papillary layer of the dermis but they are not associated with the hair, sweat glands, and sebaceous glands.

Several types of *sensory nerve endings* are embedded in the epidermis and dermis. These convey sensory information about touch, temperature, and pain. *Free nerve endings* located in the epidermis provide a sensitive reference for tactile discrimination or acuity.[42] Free nerve endings also envelop hair follicles forming a plexus or fusiform termination. This mechanoreceptor is activated upon deformation of the hair. A second group of nerve endings form organs, corpuscles, bulbs or capsules. *Meissner's* and *Merkel's* corpuscles are located in the upper dermis and epidermis, respectively, and are tactile endings. *Pacinian corpuscles* are pressure and vibratory sensors located in the dermis. *Ruffini's corpuscles* and *Krause's end-bulbs* are thermoreceptors and are also located in the dermis.

III. MORPHOLOGY OF CARTILAGE

Facial reconstruction involves the use of biomaterials for maintenance of contour restoration. Cartilage grafts are one material used to augment soft tissues. A working knowledge of the composition and morphology of cartilage is important to understanding this material when it is used as an autograft or allograft. Repopulation of cartilagenous graft materials by host chondrocytes is prerequisite to their viability and integration with host tissue. It is necessary to examine the basic development and morphology of cartilage in order to understand the structural changes that take place when it is used as a graft.

It is difficult to describe the development and structure of cartilage and bone since embryologically many bones start out as cartilage. The formation of cartilage and bone in the adult head, neck, axial skeleton, and limbs involves a prescribed sequence of events known as chondrogenesis and osteogenesis. In the following sections, cartilage and bone genesis, composition, and structure will be discussed.

The development of chondrification centers is initiated in specific regions where cartilage formation is to occur. Cartilage development is established by a transient phenomenon called cell condensation.[43,44] This involves a clustering, or an increase in cell packing or density of mesodermal cells, called mesenchyme.[43,45-48] During condensation, cell-to-cell contacts are established between mesenchymal cells which eventually differentiate into chondrocytes.[48,49] Mesenchymal cells give rise to identical cartilages but are thought to be distinctly different from one and other.[50] It is likely that these cells are pluripotential in that they can develop into nonchondrogenic cell types.

At the edges of the condensed protochondral tissue, mesenchymal cells form a membrane called the perichondrium. The inner surface of the perichondrium is a chondrogenic layer of tissue which continually produces chondrocytes throughout embryonic life. The chondrocytes produce new matrix and the cartilage enlarges from the surface. Cartilage growth which results from chondrogenesis of perichondrial chondrocytes is called *appositional growth*.[4,51] This process occurs primarily during embryonic development. Cells on the outer surface of the perichondrium differentiate into fibroblasts. These cells synthesize the fibrous

TABLE 2
Structural Components of Cartilage: Their Location and Function

Structure	Location	Function
Territorial matrix (TM)	Surrounds the lacuna; forms a capsule around the chondrocyte	Fine CF and small PG form a fibril basket that provides support for C; provides an ideal chemical environment for C
Interterritorial matrix (ITM)	Area between chondrocytes; begins outside of the TM	Coarse CF and PG aggregates provide compressive stiffness to cartilage
Matrix vesicles (MV)	Form clusters in the TM and ITM; bud off of C cell membrane	Provide a seeding site for mineralization
Lacuna	The cavity which contains a chondrocyte	Provides a compartment and ideal environment
Proteoglycan (PG)	Exist as monomers and aggregates; distributed throughout cartilage	Holds CF together and to C cell membrane; cements all components of cartilage together
Chondrocyte (C)	Cells of cartilage; sit within a lacuna; are surrounded by the territorial matrix	Produce CF, PG, and MV; maintain cartilage viability
Collagen fibrils (CF)	Compose the TM and ITM; fibrils are held together by PG	Forms a basket which holds C; forms cartilage suprastructure

Note: Listed are the components of cartilage. The location and function of these components are described.

layer of the perichondrium which contains extensive collagen fibers. Within the mass of protochondral tissue, mesenchymal cells continue to differentiate into chondrocytes which produce new malleable matrix. The chondrocytes divide several times resulting in cartilage expansion. This type of cartilage enlargement from within is termed *interstitial growth*.[4,51] Blood vessels are located in the perichondrium.[52] These vessels supply oxygen and metabolites by diffusion through the extracellular spaces. Blood vessels do not penetrate cartilage sufficiently to deliver metabolic substrates as occurs in other tissues of the body. However, in cartilage that will become bone, the blood vessels will penetrate into the cartilage. This heralds the transition from a cartilagenous state to a mineralizing state.

There are 3 different types of cartilage. The basic cartilage is termed *hyaline cartilage*. The components of hyaline cartilage are listed and described in Table 2. It has a glassy translucent appearance due to the amount of intercellular substance or matrix present. Included in this category are, cartilagenous tissues which differentiate into the articular surfaces of joints and growth plates of bones,[53,54] the cartilagenous precursor of bone, the costal cartilages, nasal septal cartilage, tracheal, bronchial cartilages, and alar cartilage.[55]

Hyaline cartilage contains chondrocytes, proteoglycans, and loose fibrils of type II collagen. The chondrocytes elaborate collagen fibrils and proteoglycans and eventually become surrounded by the extracellular matrix they produce (Figures 6, 7, 8). The cells reside within a space or compartment called a lacunae.[56-58] The morphology of the chondrocytes and lacunae are variable since their architecture is vulnerable to the effects of fixation. An excellent review of cartilage ultrastructure is provided by Sheldon.[57]

Chemical fixation will result in a loss of soluble organic constituents including proteoglycans,[59-61] causing detachment of chondrocytes from the extracellular matrix. There is also shrinkage of the chondrocytes,[62] and cartilage matrix.[63] Chondrocytes will appear to have long cytoplasmic fingers, and the lacuna will include a pericellular space (Figures 7, 8, 9). Following cryofixation, the chondrocytes appear oval or round and fill the entire lacuna.[64] The chondrocyte plasma membrane is intimately associated with the collagenous matrix they secrete.[65,66]

The proteoglycans of cartilage matrix are composed of chondroitin sulfate, dermatan sulfate, and keratin sulfate glycosaminoglycans.[60,67-71] Proteoglycan monomers attach to hyal-

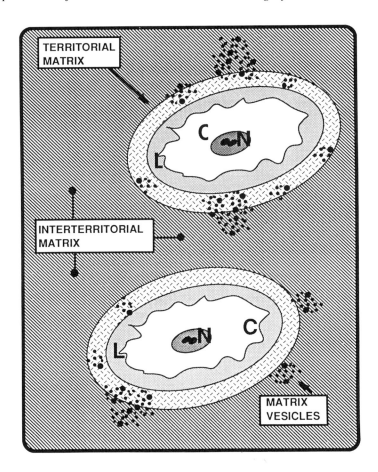

FIGURE 6.   Diagram of hyaline cartilage showing typical components. Compare this drawing
to the actual photograph of cartilage shown in Figures 7 to 9. Abbreviations: C, chondrocyte;
N, nucleus; L, lacuna.

uronic acid, via a link protein to form a proteoglycan aggregate or matrix granule.[53,69,71-76]
When cartilage is fixed with aldehydes for electron microscopy, the proteoglycans appear
as condensed granules (Figure 9), however, when cartilage is rapidly frozen, proteoglycans
appear filamentous and form a trabecular network.[64] Proteoglycans attach to collagen fibers
in the matrix and proteins in the plasma membrane of the chondrocytes. As a result, a
collagen fibril basket is created which suspends the chondrocytes. All of the components of
cartilage are held in place by the proteoglycans. Water reversibly binds to the proteoglycans
creating a viscous gel which is thought to provide compressive stiffness to this tissue.[77] Any
perturbation of proteoglycan homeostasis results in an inability to maintain the normal
collagen matrix suprastructure.[78,79]

The collagenous network immediately surrounding the chondrocyte forms a capsule
referred to as the territorial matrix (Figures 6, 7, 8, 9).[58,60] The matrix immediately surrounding chondrocytes may provide a biochemical environment responsible for inducing and
maintaining the differentiated phenotype of chondrocytes.[50] Several chondrocytes at once
may be found within the territorial matrix,[58,61] and cytoplasmic processes from the chondrocytes terminate here. Small vesicles bud off from the ends of these processes and remain
circumferentially situated in the matrix around the cells (Figures 6, 8, 9). They are very
abundant and frequently form large pools. These structures are known as matrix vesicles
and may play a role in the mineralization of cartilage[53,57,58,60] (see bone section for further
discussion on mineralization). Outside of the territorial matrix, fewer vesicles are found.

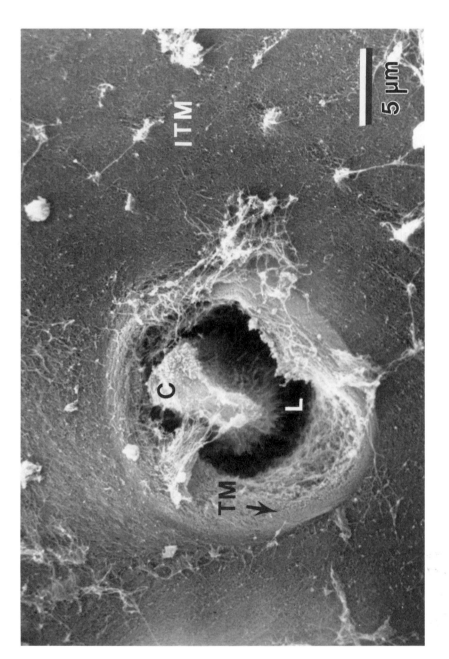

FIGURE 7. Scanning electron micrograph of typical chondrocyte from human nasal septum. Shown is a chondrocyte (C) in a lacuna (L). The lacuna is artifactually enlarged as a result of the fixation process. Surrounding the lacuna is a territorial matrix (TM). Outside of the territorial matrix and between the chondrocytes is the interterritorial matrix (ITM).

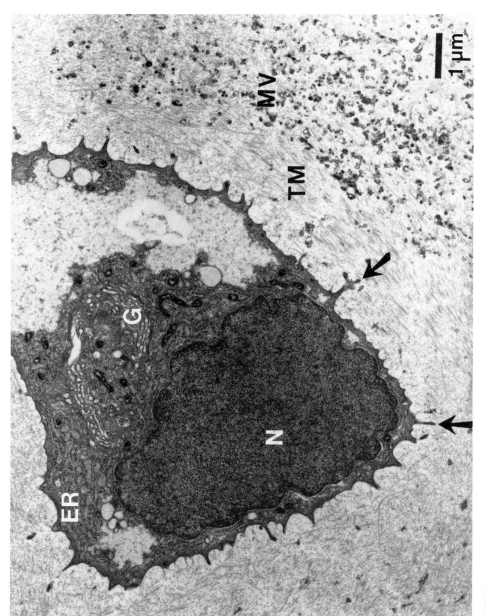

FIGURE 8.   Transmission electron micrograph of typical nasal septal chondrocyte (same tissue shown in Figure 7). The chondrocyte is surrounded by the territorial matrix (TM). Long thin cytoplasmic fingers from the chondrocyte project into the territorial matrix (arrow). Numerous matrix vesicles can be seen (MV). Inside the chondrocyte is a large nucleus (N), endoplasmic reticulum (ER), and Golgi (G). (From *Scanning Microscopy*, Johari, O., Ed., AMF O'Hare, 1988, 1641. With permission.)

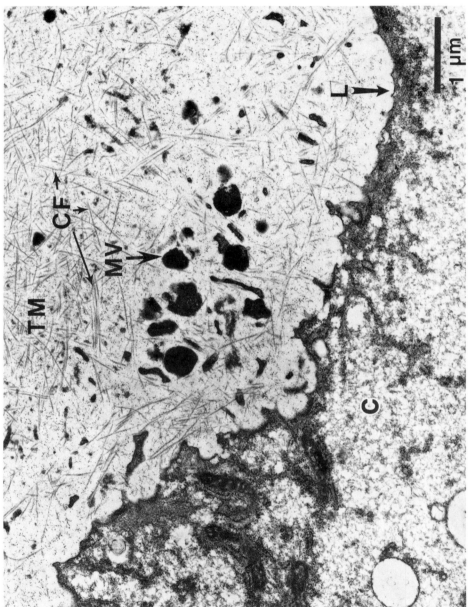

FIGURE 9. Transmission electron micrograph. Depicted here are numerous matrix vesicles (MV) embedded in the collagen fibers (CF) of the territorial matrix (TM) which surrounds the chondrocyte (C). Collagen fibers can be seen projecting from the plasma membrane of the cell (arrows). Proteoglycan aggregates are dispersed throughout the matrix and appear as fine specks or dots in the background. Proteoglycans function by holding the matrix suprastructure together. A thin lacuna (L) exists between the chondrocyte and the matrix, and is seen here as a thin space.

The collagen fibrils become coarser and more widely spaced. This region is called the interterritorial matrix (Figures 6, 7).[56,73,81] It is reported that proteoglycan structure is variable and that larger aggregates are found in the interterritorial matrix and smaller ones in the pericellular and territorial areas.[73] Because of this heterogeneity in proteoglycan ultrastructure, it is possible that the interterritorial matrix is less vulnerable to physical stresses, and therefore provides cartilage with its compressive stiffness.

The nose is a facial structure composed primarily of hyaline cartilage. It is frequently reconstructed as a result of injuries or inherited deformities. Nasal cartilage is also frequently used as a source of graft material. Bones of the nose include the maxillae (frontal process), the frontal bone (nasa spine), and the ethmoid (which forms part of the bony septum). Cartilages of the nose include the upper lateral cartilages, the nasal septum, and the lower cartilages. The attachment of the cartilages to the bones of the face and the overall structure of the nose, associated bones, and cartilages is provided in an excellent review of upper airway anatomy by Morris.[82]

The second type of cartilage is called *elastic cartilage*. This type differs from hyaline cartilage because it contains elastic fibers in addition to the normal contents of hyaline cartilage.[53,54] A characteristic of elastic cartilage is its relative flexibility. The auricle of the external ear, areas of the larynx, epiglottis, eustachian tube, and the external auditory canal are made of elastic cartilage. Embryologically, prechondrogenic mesenchyme differentiates into fibroblasts,[83] which may initially synthesize microfibrillar fibrils along with collagen fibrils. These may be the formative stages of elastin development. Eventually chondrocytes are recognizable, and at maturity, a matrix of collagen and elastin surround the cells. A perichondrium forms and appositional growth takes place. Sulfated glycosaminoglycans such as proteoglycan complexes are located within the interstices of the reticulum of fibers making up the matrix.

The third type of cartilage is *fibrocartilage* which is tough and resilient. Fibrocartilage is a mixture of connective tissue, fibroblasts, hyaline cartilage, and chondrocytes. It surrounds many organs as a capsular membrane. It also constitutes the cartilage of the symphysis pubis, lateral and medial meniscus, and intervertebral disks.[54] Tendon insertions into bone and cartilage are also composed of fibrocartilage.[84] As with elastic cartilage, prechondrogenic tissue gives rise to fibroblast like cells which produce extensive amounts of collagen fibrils. These fibrils become organized into collagen fibers. The fibroblasts may transform into chondrocytes which secrete a matrix of glycosaminoglycans. This matrix is limited in quantity compared to the other cartilage types.[53] It is the extensive collagen content which endows fibrocartilage with its superior biomechanical properties. For example, fibrocartilage at the ends of tendons coalesces with the collagen fibers of the tendon on the one end and the bone on the other. This provides a very strong link between the tendon and the bone. Microscopically, the collagen fibers of the tendon transform into a denser more compact region of collagen fibers. The fibroblasts of the tendon undergo a diminution and are gradually replaced by chondrocytes which are surrounded by a paucity of ground substance. It is this region of dense collagen and chondrocytes which constitutes the fibrocartilage.

IV. MORPHOLOGY OF BONE

Understanding bone development, physiology, and morphology is a necessary part of engineering bone alternatives (substitutes), and utilizing the dynamic responses of bone to develop new methods for facial reconstruction and treating bone diseases. The success of bone grafts for the replacement of diseased or damaged bones depends on several factors, including the source and structure of the original transplant. Cancellous bone autografts are quite desirable since their porous nature facilitates serum permeation through the open channels and maximizes osteoblast survival. These graft materials become integrated with new host bone. Bone allografts and xenografts if untreated (made deantigenic) are isolated

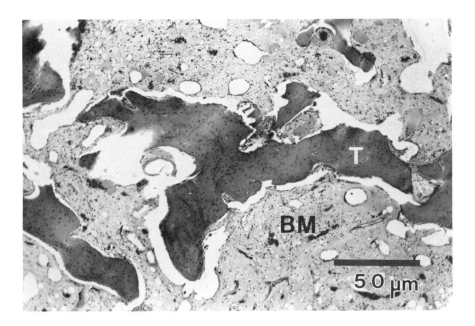

FIGURE 10.   Light photomicrograph of cancellous bone within the diaphysis of a rat femur. Seen here are parts of trabeculae (T) surrounded by a bone marrow (BM).

from the surrounding tissues of the host by encapsulation. If they are preserved, they serve as an implant, gradually being resorbed and replaced by new host bone. Bone structure must be understood before these concepts can be applied to clinical problem solving using bone and its analogs. In the following section, the basic development and structure of bones is reviewed.

By 8 weeks, bone formation has begun in the developing embryo.[52] There are essentially two types of bones in the body. The first type is *flat bones* which include the clavicle, and bones of the face and skull vault.[4,85,86] Flat bones develop by a process called *intramembranous ossification*. These bones are frequently referred to as membranous bones. This process begins with the establishment of primitive center of connective tissue. Here mesenchymal cells form strands of collagenous fibers.[52] The mesenchymal cells differentiate into *osteoblasts* which establish a center of ossification.[4,51,52,86,87] Osteoblasts synthesize a collagenous unmineralized matrix called *osteoid*. This gradually mineralizes by impregnation with calcium-phosphate salts. Once mineralized, osteoid is called *bone matrix*. When the original collagenous matrix is enveloped peripherally by mineral, a *trabecula* is formed (Figure 10). The primary center of ossification is vascularized. As the mineralization process continues, the trabeculae fuse to form primary cancellous bone that is infiltrated with marrow containing hemopoietic tissue. A network of trabeculum is called a *primary spongiosa*. Trabecular bone is also called *cancellous bone* (Figure 10).

Developing bones of the skull are composed of cancellous bone. By appositional growth, cancellous bone is converted to dense bone called *compact or cortical bone*. When bones increase in size by appositional growth, osteogenic cells cover the trabeculae and subsequently differentiate into osteoblasts, which deposit bone mineral over the trabeculae. When these osteoblasts are embedded in bone mineral, they transform into osteocytes. Long cytoplasmic process extend out from the osteocytes. A new layer of osteoblasts form on top of the most recently synthesized bone. These cells also extend cytoplasmic processes which form gap junctions with osteocytes beneath them. This continues until the spaces between the trabeculae are filled in with compact bone. Because compact or cortical bone is vascularized and the cells communicate with each other, this bone forms a living system and is not a dormant or dead scaffold of mineral.

At birth, parietal bones of the cranial vault enlarge by appositional growth on their convex surfaces. In order to maintain their curvature, bone is simultaneously removed from the concave side. The removal of bone is accomplished by chondroclasts. These cells unlike osteoblasts are derived from monocytes. These are large multinucleated cells which have an extensive ruffled border. Their secretion dissolves mineral. This process is called bone remodeling.[51]

Skull bones do not fuse together until adulthood. Chondroid tissue (containing types I and II collagen),[88,89] and secondary cartilage can be found in the sutures between the cranial vaults,[90-92] and along the edges of the metopic sutures between the frontal bones.[93] Mechanical forces applied to the cranial vault as a result of developing brain tissue may be responsible for the formation of chondroid tissue and cartilage at the sutures.[91,92] Gradually endochondral ossification of the cranial bones proceeds while chondroid tissue of the (metopic) sutures form lamellar bone.[93] Resorption at the suture sites may proceed for several years after birth, maintaining a constant fissure. This anatomical arrangement may be necessary for rapid cranial enlargement during the early years of development.

The second type of bone in the body is the *long bone* (Figure 11). Long bones make up the limbs and axial skeleton. These bones mineralize by a process called *endochondral ossification* and are frequently referred to as cartilagenous bones. Bones in the base of the skull are included here.[85] Embryologically, evaginations or outpouchings of the epithelial walls occur at predetermined sites where the limbs will develop. These sites are called limb buds. Mesenchymal cells form centers of chondrification within the limb buds. These cells differentiate into chondrocytes and begin to produce a collagen matrix. As described previously, a perichondrium forms around these centers and the tissues grow by interstitial and appositional growth. A cartilage model of bone develops where the future bone will form.[4,51,86] Blood vessels begin to invade a centrally located area of the chondrogenic layer inducing a differentiation of the chondrocytes into osteoblasts. The perichondrium now surrounds osteoblasts instead of chondrocytes and is appropriately called the periosteum. Gradually the chondrocytes start to hypertrophy and die. The result is a collagenous matrix riddled with cavities created by the empty chondrocyte lacunae. Osteoblasts line the cartilage and start to synthesize osteoid. Eventually, the cartilage matrix which originated in the cartilage model begins to calcify, and the osteoid created by the osteoblasts also begins to calcify.

A periosteal band, or ring of initial calcification forms and is known as the *primary center of ossification*. This mineralization of the matrix causes a decrease in the effective diffusion of nutrients through the matrix and to the remaining chondrocytes of the developing cartilage model. The hypertrophic process is thus exacerbated by the onset of mineralization. The developing ring of bone is very dense *compact* or *cortical bone* (Figure 12).[87] Inside the ring of bone is the marrow chamber containing cancellous bone and hemapoietic tissue. The ring of cortical bone is called the diaphysis and is composed of an outer layer of bone near the periosteum called the outer circumferential lamella. There is also an inner layer of bone near the cancellous core of the diaphysis called the inner circumferential lamella. The inside surface of the ring of compact bone which interfaces with the marrow cavity is called the *endosteal surface*. The outer surface of the ring of compact bone is called the *periosteal surface*.

Between the inner and outer circumferential lamella is located the main structure of bone, the *osteon* or *Haversian system* (Figure 13). Flat bones also contain osteons, but not to the same extent as long bones. An osteon develops when trabeculae mineralize around a blood vessel. The blood vessel becomes circumferentially enveloped by successive layers of mineralizing osteoid. Osteons are usually arranged parallel to the longitudinal axis of the diaphysis. The canal that houses the blood vessel is called the Haversian canal. This type of bone is mature and called lamellar bone.[51,86] Each lamella has an associated ring of

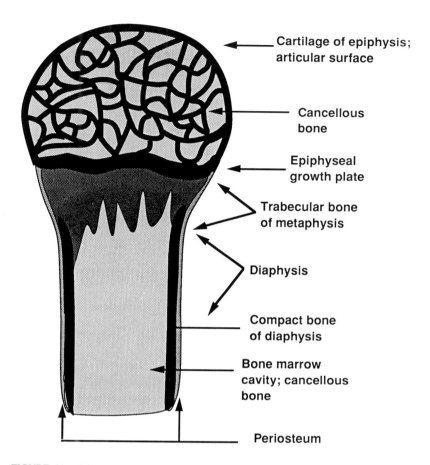

Cartilage of epiphysis; articular surface

Cancellous bone

Epiphyseal growth plate

Trabecular bone of metaphysis

Diaphysis

Compact bone of diaphysis

Bone marrow cavity; cancellous bone

Periosteum

FIGURE 11.   Diagram of long bone. Only one half of the bone is seen here. Shown are the components which make up a typical long bone. The epiphyseal ends of the bone are capped by an articular cartilage surface. Under this is cancellous bone. The epiphysis is separated from the metaphysis by the epiphyseal growth plate. This cartilagenous plate is responsible for bone elongation. Below the plate, calcifying cartilage (from the epiphyseal plate) is present as the metaphysis. Below this region is the diaphysis. Circumferentially, the diaphysis is composed of compact bone while its core contains cancellous bone. Between the walls of the cancellous bone is hemopoietic tissue of the bone marrow.

osteoblasts. Each osteoblast is contained in a lacuna. Osteoblasts become trapped by the mineralized matrix they secrete and eventually transform, and are called osteocytes. Gap junction between cytoplasmic processes provides a means of communication between osteocytes.[4] The limiting edge of the osteon is a dense line of mineral which is low in collagen.[86]

At either end of the long bone are located the epiphyses (Figure 11). During development, the epiphysis is cartilagenous but after birth, a secondary center of ossification develops resulting in cancellous bone formation at either end of the long bone. A surface of cartilage remains at either end of the bones to allow for frictionless movement between the joints, and is called the articular cartilages. Within each epiphysis, a cartilagenous plate develops and is called the epiphyseal growth plate. This plate is responsible for further bone elongation and remains active until the bone is fully mature. The epiphyseal plate is composed of zones or layers of chondrocytes (Figure 14). The uppermost layer is called the resting zone. It contains several layers of thin flat chondrocytes which are inactive. A gradual transition of the cells occurs to a zone of proliferation. In this layer cells undergo mitosis. Near the bottom of the zone, cells enlarge as they transform into cells of the mature zone. These cells are physiologically very active but they do not undergo further mitosis as do their

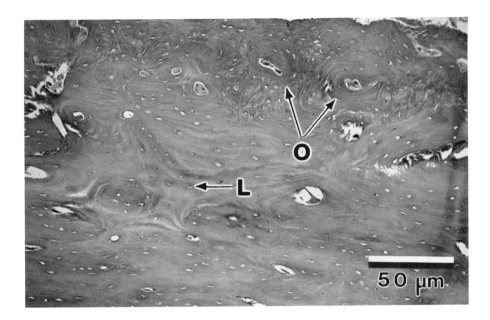

FIGURE 12.   Light photomicrograph. Seen here is cortical bone from a rat femur. Numerous lacunae (L) can be seen, each containing an osteocyte. In the upper half of the micrograph Haversian systems (osteons) can be seen (O). The central canal of the osteon contains a blood vessel surrounded by concentric lamellae of bone.

relatives in the proliferating zone. Instead, mature cells enlarge the epiphysis longitudinally, while the proliferating cells continue to move away in a vertical direction. In the collagenous matrix surrounding these cells, numerous matrix vessels bud off from the long cytoplasmic fingers of the cells. Gradually these mature cells undergo hypertrophy. The bottom zone is called the zone of calcification or maturation. Mineralization of the matrix occurs here.

The epiphyseal plate is undergoing interstitial growth in its proliferating and maturing zones, and therefore moves away from the diaphyseal shaft while simultaneously adding to the length of the diaphysis. However, the growth plate never enlarges because it is undergoing hypertrophy, necrosis, and mineralization in its lower layers. Mineralized matrix beneath the calcified zone is in the form of trabeculae as a result of the necrotic chondrocytes, and is called the metaphyseal region of the diaphysis or the metaphysis. It is invaded by capillaries and osteogenic cells from the diaphysis. These cells line the trabeculae and differentiate into osteoblasts which now synthesize new bone. In this way, the partially mineralized trabeculae of the metaphysis are transformed into solid compact bone of the diaphyseal shaft. However, the metaphysis is similar in size to the epiphysis and will be reduced in size by osteoclast resorption. As a result of this remodeling, the metaphysis will transform into the diaphysis. Bone elongation by this sequence of events, growth plate cartilage to mineralized metaphyseal trabeculae, to diaphyseal bone, perpetuates itself as a result of the epiphyseal appositional growth. It persists until adolescence when bone elongation ceases. In *short bones,* no epiphyseal plate develops since bone elongation is limited. Elongation by interstitial cartilage growth at the ends of the short bones is the mechanism by which these structures increase in size.[51]

Mineralization is an ongoing process that occurs in both the epiphyseal growth plate, the metaphysis, and the maturing matrix of the bony diaphysis. There are a number of theories about the mechanism of mineralization in these areas. In growth plate, it has been suggested that calcium ions may travel by ion exchange along sulfated proteoglycans, and that phosphate ions diffuse between the proteoglycan aggregates until they reach matrix

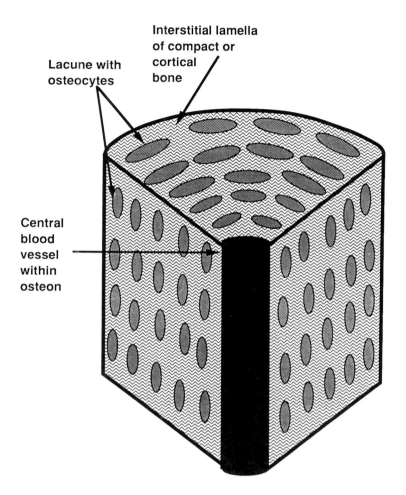

FIGURE 13. Diagram of osteon or Haversian system. Seen here is a central blood
vessel which runs through the middle (Haversian canal) of the osteon. Circumferentially located are lacunae. Inside the lacunae are osteoblasts which have deposited
interstitial lamella of bone.

vesicles.[80] Acidic phospholipids located in the vesicle membrane may then act as a binding
site for calcium ions.[94] Initially, mineral nodules may form upon or with matrix vesicles.[64,95-98] Subsequently, mineralization spreads to collagen fibrils and ultimately throughout
the matrix.[86,94] Another possibility is that mineral seeding occurs in the gap zone of collagen
fibrils,[99] and then spreads along collagen fibrils, and eventually into the matrix.

V. SUMMARY

There are several characteristics a biomaterial should have in order to serve as a skin,
cartilage, or bone substitute. Ideally, it should resemble that tissue structurally. By understanding the gross and fine structure of a tissue it becomes possible to model a facsimile.
To this end, the structure of skin, cartilage, and bone have been reviewed in the preceding
portion of this chapter.

A tissue that is injured and requires augmentation or replacement with a biomaterial or
biomedical device will function optimally if the characteristics of that material are closely
matched to the original host tissue. For this reason, it is of paramount importance to understand the mechanical properties of the original tissue as well as the replacement bio-

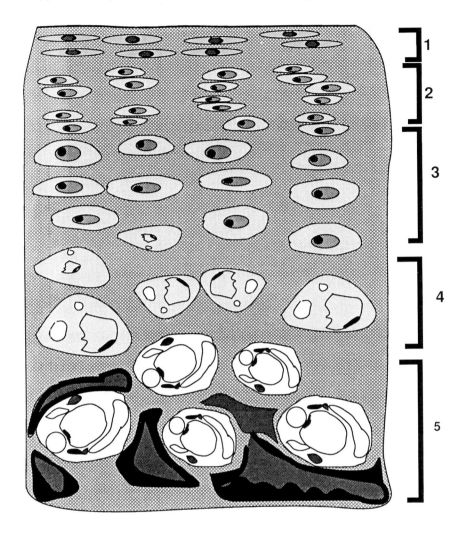

FIGURE 14.   Diagram of epiphyseal growth plate. The zones or layers of the growth plate are represented by numbers 1 to 5. They will be described in the following section. (1) The uppermost layer, or resting zone, contains inactive chondrocytes; (2) dividing chondrocytes constitute the proliferating zone; (3) maturing cells make up the maturing zone; (4) aged vacuolated cells constitute the hypertrophic zone; (5) necrotic cells embedded in a matrix undergoing calcification make up the calcifying cartilage zone.

material. With this in mind, the succeeding portion of this chapter, will review the biomechanical properties of skin, cartilage, and bone.

VI. DEFINITIONS OF MECHANICAL TERMS

It will be useful to define several mechanical parameters, and their units, which will be used frequently throughout this chapter. Figure 15 shows a typical stress-strain curve obtained by testing a strip of tissue in uniaxial tension (or compression) at a constant strain rate. Strain rate is the speed at which the strain is applied to the sample during the test.

Stress (MPa = 10^6 Pascals), on the y-axis, is the force (N = Newtons = kg m/s^2) divided by the area (m^2) of tissue; strength or ultimate stress is the peak stress value.

Strain (dimensionless, or %), on the x-axis, is the change in tissue length (deformation) divided by the initial length of the tissue; ultimate strain is encountered at failure of the tissue.

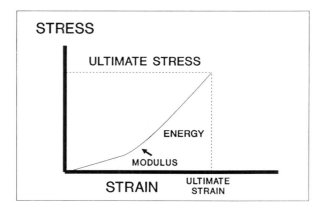

FIGURE 15. Stress-strain curve for tissue showing definitions of the ultimate material properties—stress, strain, modulus, and energy absorbed. Modulus is the slope of the linear portion of the stress-strain curve; energy absorbed is the area beneath the stress-strain curve (see text for units).

Modulus (MPa, or GPa = 10^9 Pa) is the incremental change in stress divided by the change in strain; it is the slope of the stress-strain curve. For tissues with a nonlinear stress-strain curve, the peak modulus is often reported. Note that modulus and stiffness cannot be used interchangeably: the stiffness of a material depends on its modulus, plus geometric factors. The modulus of a material can be thought of as a "normalized" stiffness.

The energy absorbed by the specimen during the test is the area beneath the stress-strain curve.

Authors reporting mechanical data for tissues have used a variety of units in the past. In this chapter, all the numerical values have been converted to the proper units described above.

VII. MECHANICAL PROPERTIES OF SKIN

Excellent reviews of the mechanical properties of skin have been given by Wilkes et al.,[100] and Silver and Doillon.[101] The mechanical properties of the skin are due primarily to the amounts and interactions of the extracellular components of the dermis: collagen fibers, elastic fibers, and interfibrillar matrix. The epidermis does not make a significant contribution to the mechanical properties of skin[102] except perhaps where the epidermis is extremely thick, such as on the palms, and the soles of the feet.

A. STRUCTURE/MECHANICAL PROPERTY RELATIONSHIPS

Collagen, the chief structural protein of the animal kingdom, can withstand high stress while undergoing small strain. In skin and other connective tissues, collagen is responsible for limiting tissue deformation. Collagen is a fibrous protein (300-kDa mol wt) which has several levels of organization in the skin from triple-helical molecule, to fibril, to fiber, to three-dimensional collagen fiber network. Collagen fibril diameters in adult human skin[103] range from 600 to 1000 A; collagen fiber diameters[104] range from 10 to 40 μm. The collagen in skin is predominantly type I, with smaller amounts of type III which become elevated during development and wound healing.[105] Collagen accounts for about 77% of the fat-free dry weight of the skin.[106] Fibrous type I collagen can withstand stress in the order of 100 MPa, strains up to 50%, with a modulus of 3 GPa.[107]

Elastin, a hydrophobic, rubbery protein[108] accounts for only 4% of the fat-free dry weight of the skin.[106] Elastin is approximately one hundredth as strong as collagen, but can reversibly

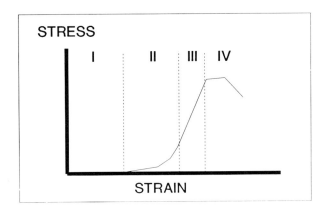

FIGURE 16. Stress-strain curve for adult human skin consists of four phases. Phase I, collagen fiber network "slack"; II, recruitment and alignment of collagen fibers; III, linear region with peak modulus; IV, failure region. (Adapted from Wilkes, G. L., Brown, I. A., and Wildnauer, R. H., *CRC Crit. Rev. Bioeng.*, 1, 453, 1973.)

withstand high mechanical strains, and is probably responsible for the "elastic recoil" of skin and other connective tissues after removal of the load.[109]

The interfibrillar matrix of skin is composed primarily of water and glycosaminoglycans (GAGs) including dermatan sulfate (54% of total GAG), hyaluronic acid (41.5% of total GAG), and chondroitin 4-sulfate (4.5% of total GAG).[110] The interfibrillar matrix is a viscous gel which does not contribute significantly to the ultimate material properties of skin. Oxlund and Andreassen[111] treated skin strips with hyaluronidase which resulted in no significant changes in the tensile strength of the skin. The interfibrillar matrix does, however, contribute to the time-dependent (viscoelastic) properties of skin.[112]

The stress-strain curve for adult human skin, shown on Figure 16, can be divided into 4 phases.[100,113] In phase I, or the "toe-region" of the curve, very small changes in stress result in large strains, as the collagen fibers are in a relatively random orientation with respect to the axis of the applied stress. The collagen fibers gradually rearrange by aligning along the axis of stretch. Skin tends to retract when excised,[114] so that Phase I of the *in vitro* stress-strain curve probably represents the normal "resting tension" of skin.

In phase II, more fibers become aligned in the direction of the applied stress ("recruitment" of fibers), and the modulus of the skin increases to a value of 16 MPa at a strain of about 60%.[115]

From this point on (phase III), the stress-strain relationship is approximately linear, with aligned collagen fibers resisting the stress. Skin is believed to operate in phases II and III *in vivo* in response to normal physiologic loads.[116]

Failure of the skin collagen network occurs (phase IV) at a stress in the range of 7 MPa (human abdominal skin)[117] to 12 MPa (guinea pig back skin),[118] at a strain of about 100%.

It is important to consider that the failure load depends equally on the material properties, and geometric characteristics of the skin. The failure load is the product of the ultimate stress and the cross-sectional area (width × thickness) of the skin tested. The thickness of the skin varies over the body, and tends to decrease with increasing age.[119] Material properties of the skin change with aging as well.[120]

B. ANISOTROPY OF SKIN

The mechanical behavior of skin is anisotropic, meaning the properties are not the same in all test directions. This phenomenon was first reported by Dupuytren[121] and carefully studied by Langer,[32] who observed that circular holes pierced in cadaver skin became elliptical. "Langer's lines" connect the major axes of the ellipses, which represent the lines of principal tension in the skin,[122] or the direction of preferred orientation of the dermal collagen fiber network.[123] The retraction of 1 in. squares removed from cadavers was 9% in the direction of Langer's lines, and 5% perpendicular to Langer's lines.[122] Gibson et al.,[123] using *in situ* measurements on live subjects, found that the skin was least extensible along Langer's lines.

The anisotropic mechanical behavior of skin should be an important factor in deciding the location and orientation of surgical incisions and skin defect excisions.

C. VISCOELASTIC PROPERTIES OF SKIN

The viscoelastic behavior of human skin was studied by Dunn and Silver[117] by subjecting strips of human abdominal skin to incremental strains, followed by periods of stress relaxation. In a perfectly elastic material, no relaxation occurs; all the strain energy is stored reversibly. In a viscoelastic material such as skin, a portion of the stress relaxes (viscous fraction), as energy is lost, and a time-independent, steady-state "elastic fraction" of the stress remains. At low strains, as collagen fiber realignment occurs, the elastic fraction is low (0.5) and increases approximately linearly with strain to a value of 0.75 at a strain of 100%. This elastic fraction of 0.75 is similar to that found for tendon,[117] suggesting that regardless of tissue type, aligned collagen fiber networks behave similarly. These data demonstrate that the viscoelasticity of skin is a function of the strain level of the skin. The elastic fraction is also a function of the test direction. Schneider et al.,[124] testing human abdominal skin in biaxial stress relaxation, reported an average elastic fraction value of 0.74 along the lateral axis and 0.78 along the superoinferior axis.

The viscosity of the skin decreases with increasing shear rate—a phenomenon termed thixotropy.[112] Based on the shear-thinning behavior of hyaluronic acid in synovial fluid,[125] thixotropy in skin is probably due to the glycosaminoglycans in the dermis.[112]

VIII. MECHANICAL PROPERTIES OF CARTILAGE

Mechanical studies on cartilage have been performed primarily on articular cartilage. Cartilage mechanical properties depend primarily on the interactions between proteoglycans, water, and collagen. The highly charged, polyanionic proteoglycan network exists in a swollen state, and is limited to a certain volume by the collagen network which encases the viscous gel (see Myers and Mow).[126] The mechanical properties of articular cartilage will be discussed in detail, followed by a summary of the properties of nasal septal cartilage.

A. STRUCTURE/MECHANICAL PROPERTY RELATIONSHIPS

The extracellular matrix of cartilagenous tissue is generally composed of water (60 to 80%), collagen fibers (60% of the dry weight), and proteoglycans (40% of the dry weight). Proteoglycans contribute to the mechanical properties in three ways: Donnan osmotic effects, excluded volume effects, and viscoelastic effects.[127,128]

Donnan osmotic effects are due to the high fixed negative charge on the glycosaminoglycan side chains of the proteoglycans, and the semipermeable collagenous network. The negatively charged proteoglycans become surrounded by counterions, cations, to preserve bulk electroneutrality. The imbalance between ionic concentrations of cartilage and the fluid outside of its semipermeable collagenous membrane cause a Donnan osmotic pressure which contributes significantly to the compressive properties of cartilage.

In the unloaded state, the Donnan osmotic pressure, which tends to expand the tissue, is limited or balanced by the intrinsic tensile stress in the collagen fiber network. When a compressive load is placed on the cartilage, fluid is squeezed out of the matrix, increasing the effective swelling pressure until equilibrium is reached with the applied load. After the

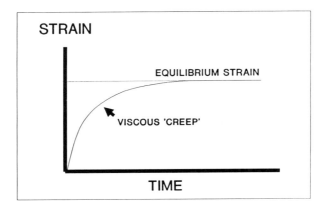

FIGURE 17.   Creep experiment for articular cartilage. A constant load is applied, and the deformation is monitored vs. time. Equilibrium is reached when the internal osmotic swelling pressure equals the applied stress. (Adapted from Myers, E. R. and Mow, V. C., *Cartilage: Structure, Function, and Biochemistry,* Academic Press, New York, 1983.)

load is removed, the tissue imbibes water until the preloaded state is reestablished (see Myers et al.;[127] Carney and Muir;[128] Comper and Laurent[129] for reviews).

"Excluded volume" effects of proteoglycans are due to their large size in the physiologic milieu. The negative fixed charge repulsions cause the proteoglycan side chains on the hyaluronic acid core to extend into the "bottlebrush" configuration. These enormous (200-MDa mol wt), extended molecules exclude other molecules from occupying that space. The collagen network may be further stabilized by these excluded volume effects.

Discussion of the complex electromechanical properties of cartilage is beyond the scope of this chapter (see Grodzinsky[130] for review). Briefly, mechanical stress on cartilage results in the development of electric potentials across the cartilage, and vice versa. This effect is due to electrokinetic[129] and other electromechanical phenomena.[131] The electric fields which develop as a result of mechanical stress may be important in maintaining normal tissue architecture and directing repair of injured tissues (see, e.g., Brighton et al.).[132]

B. VISCOELASTIC PROPERTIES OF CARTILAGE

Cartilage, like skin and other connective tissues, is a viscoelastic material. The ability of cartilage to dissipate the energy of mechanical impacts is enhanced by viscoelasticity. In a slow-loading situation, water is squeezed out of the tissue, which recovers reversibly upon load removal, if the amount of surrounding fluid is sufficient. The results of a constant-load (creep) experiment are shown on Figure 17. The tissue strain increases gradually as fluid flows from the tissue, until a plateau value (equilibrium strain) is reached when the osmotic swelling pressure of the tissue exactly matches the applied stress. During rapid loading and unloading, however, the material behaves more elastically, because there is not enough time for fluid flow to occur.[133] A perfectly elastic material would respond to a constant stress by instantaneously deforming to an equilibrium strain.

C. NASAL SEPTAL CARTILAGE

For craniofacial cartilages, i.e., nasal and auricular cartilages which do not support appreciable loads, mechanical failure is not usually a concern so that the modulus is probably the most important material property. The ultimate stress, modulus, and strain for human nasal septal and auricular cartilage are shown in Table 3. Glasgold et al.[134] reported compressive moduli for human nasal septal cartilage as a function of age, sex, and sterilization/stor-

TABLE 3
Ultimate Material Properties of Human Cartilage

Cartilage type	Test type	Strength (MPa)	Modulus (MPa)	Ultimate strain (%)
Nasal[134]	Compression	3	19	70
Auricular[135]	Tension	3	20[a]	30

[a] Estimated from published stress-strain curve.

age methods. The stress-strain curve for human nasal septal cartilage was found to be nonlinear, and a "lower stiffness" and "upper stiffness" (peak modulus) were calculated. The peak modulus for control specimens was 19.3 MPa, similar to the tensile modulus of skin. Freeze-drying or irradiation-sterilizing the samples, followed by a month storage, significantly increased (almost doubled) their peak modulus. Other sterilization/storage techniques, including merthiolate and Alcide EXPOR® chemosterilant, did not significantly alter the compressive modulus of the samples.

Human auricular cartilage, an elastic cartilage, was tested in tension by Yamaguchi and Katake.[135] The strength (3 MPa) and modulus (20 MPa) were very similar to those values for nasal septal cartilage tested in compression by Glasgold et al.[134]

Mechanical data are important when considering tissue banking for cartilage autografts and allografts. It is clearly desirable to match the biomechanical properties of graft tissues to those of the recipient site whenever possible. In addition, the shape of nasal cartilage seems to be influenced by internal "interlocked" stresses (see Fry;[136] Murakami et al.[137]). The shape of deformed cartilage can be corrected by morselization,[138] or full-thickness incisions on the concave surface, or "wedge" shaped incisions on the convex surface of the deformed cartilage.[137]

IX. MECHANICAL PROPERTIES OF BONE

Bone is a hard connective tissue designed to provide mechanical support for locomotion, and protection for the soft structures of the body. The mechanical properties of bone vary according to the function and anatomic site of the bone.[139] Bone is a mechanically complex material, due to its unique structure (composite material), and protein-mineral interactions (biphasic material). In addition, bone continuously remodels in response to the stress it encounters in daily activities (Wolff's Law),[140] making its mechanical properties a function of its mechanical environment.[141,142] Most studies of mechanical properties of bone have been performed on the long weight-bearing bones of the limbs. Bone mechanical properties have been determined in tension, compression, bending, shear, and torsion (see discussion by Nordin and Frankel).[143] A general overview of the mechanical properties of bone will be given, followed by a summary of the mechanical properties of craniofacial bone. See the book by Evans[144] for a comprehensive review of the mechanical properties of bone.

A. STRUCTURE/MECHANICAL PROPERTY RELATIONSHIPS

Mature bone is composed primarily of the mineral hydroxylapatite (67% of the fat-free dry weight) and collagen (30% of the fat-free dry weight). Collagen, a rope-like protein, is the prime tension carrier but cannot withstand appreciable compressive forces. McCutchen[145] suggests that hydroxylapatite "struts" within collagen fibers might increase the tensile modulus of bone collagen. Hydroxyapatite ($Ca_{10}(PO_4)_6OH_2$) also acts as a "filler" to enable the protein/mineral composite to withstand great compressive forces. Hydroxyapatite has a density of 3.15 and a hardness[146] of 5 Mohs, a compressive strength of 100 MPa, and a stiffness of 130 GPa.[147] Collagen has a tensile strength of about 100 MPa and a stiffness of 3 GPa.

Depending on the anatomic site, bone is basically composed of different proportions of two distinct types of tissue: cortical and cancellous bone. Cortical bone is sometimes referred to as compact bone; cancellous bone has been called spongy or trabecular bone. These two types of bone tissue differ in mechanical properties, mainly because of the difference between their relative porosities. The porosity of cortical bone is 5 to 30%; the porosity of cancellous bone is 30 to 90%.[148]

1. Cortical Bone

According to Katz,[149] four levels of structure are important in cortical bone mechanical properties:

1. The molecular level (i.e., properties of collagen, hydroxyapatite)
2. The ultrastructural level (collagen/hydroxylapatite interactions)
3. The microstructural level (woven vs. plexiform vs. Haversian bone)
4. The macrostructural level (size and shape of the whole bone)

Using ultrasonic techniques, Katz et al.[149] reported that the modulus of cortical bone is greatest in the longitudinal direction (30 GPa), and least in the radial direction (17 GPa), with the tangential modulus in between (21 GPa). The modulus of plexiform bone was reported to be greater than that of Haversian bone.[149] Haversian or osteonal bone, however, is a "tough" material (resists fatigue failure), partially due to crack-propagation resistance of the cement line.[150] The ultimate strength of cortical bone is greatest in compression (200 MPa), weaker in tension (125 MPa), and lowest in shear loading (60 MPa).[151]

A number of studies have attempted to clarify the relative roles of porosity, density, mineralization, or collagen fiber architecture on the mechanical properties of cortical bone. Modulus decreases with increasing porosity according to a power law[152] with a coefficient of 0.55. Modulus has been found to increase in a roughly cubic relationship with calcium content and volume fraction.[153] With respect to tensile strength, however, collagen fiber orientation is an important factor, while mineralization seems to be a poor predictor of tensile strength.[154]

2. Cancellous Bone

Cancellous (trabecular) bone mechanical properties were recently reviewed by Goldstein.[155] The material properties of trabecular bone vary with the anatomic location of the bone tested.[156] The modulus of trabecular bone is 20 to 50% of that for cortical bone.[155] Cancellous bone material properties are strain-rate sensitive, according to a power law with the strain rate raised to the 0.06 power.[148] The ultimate compressive strength of cancellous bone is about 10 MPa.[148]

Bone, like other connective tissues, is viscoelastic—its mechanical properties depend on the loading rate or the time following load application.[144,157] In addition, the mechanical properties of bone depend on the age of the animal.[158]

Bone tissue is an electromechanical transducer—stress application results in an induced voltage across the bone.[159] See Pollack[160] for a review of piezoelectricity and other electromechanical phenomena in bone tissue.

B. CRANIOFACIAL BONE

Currey[161] proposed that long bones are "designed" for high stiffness, impact resistance, and fatigue failure resistance. The mechanical role of the skull vault, however, is impact resistance; the role of the mandible is to support static loads.[161] The structure and mechanical properties of the craniofacial bones, therefore, are somewhat different than those of the

TABLE 4
Mechanical Properties of Bone

Site	Test direction	Modulus of elasticity (GPa)	Tensile strength (MPa)	Compressive strength (MPa)
Long bones[a]	Longitudinal	18	136	150
Skull[163]	Tangential radial	5.6	48[b]	96
		2.4	37[b]	74

[a] Average of tibia, fibula, and femur; data from Yamada.[162]
[b] Calculated as one half of compressive strength; based on Evans and Lissner.[164]

tubular long bones of the appendicular skeleton (see Table 4). The flat bones of the skull are composed of inner and outer cortical layers, separated by a weak, porous cancellous layer (diploe).

Compared to the amount of biomechanical data available for the appendicular and axial skeleton, there is a paucity of data on the mechanical properties of human craniofacial bone.[144] Some of the earlier studies were performed on embalmed cadaveric skull bone, presumably because fresh bone was not available.[164]

The mechanical properties of "fresh" craniofacial bone (see Table 4) have been addressed by several groups.[163,165,166] The compressive strength and modulus of the skull bones are greater in the tangential than in the radial direction,[163] because in the radial direction the weak diploe layer partially supports the load.[144] The energy-absorbing capacity (area beneath the stress-strain curve), however, is greater in the radial than the tangential direction.[163]

The stress-strain curves for human cortical skull bone are strain-rate dependent.[165,166] The ultimate strength and modulus increase, and the ultimate strain decreases, with increasing strain-rate. Wood[166] and Evans[144] suggest that cortical skull bone (not the diploe) behaves isotropically in the tangential direction. This is probably due to the relatively "random" orientation of the calvarial osteons.[166] Cortical bone from long bones, on the other hand, is highly anisotropic due to the preferred orientation of the osteons.[166]

Material properties of fetal cranial bone were reported by Kriewall.[167] Moduli tested in bending were on the order of 1 to 2 GPa, and 3 to 4 GPa, when the gross collagen fiber direction was perpendicular and parallel to the test direction, respectively.

Other biomechanical studies on the human face and skull have addressed impact tolerance[168] or computer-modeling of stress distribution in response to various loads.[169,170]

It is important to note that the mechanical response of tissues *in vivo* are influenced by the surrounding tissues. For example, bones have been shown to absorb 40% more energy to fracture when covered by a layer of skin.[171]

X. SUMMARY

The structure and mechanical properties of skin, cartilage, and bone are quite different (see Figure 18), reflecting the diverse structures and mechanical environments of these tissues. For the interested reader, phenomenological modeling of the mechanical behavior of different connective tissues has been discussed by Viidik[172] and Silver.[173]

Skin is a connective tissue which contains strong collagen fibers, and resilient elastin fibers, in a viscous matrix. Collagen fibers tend to lie in preferential directions (Langer's lines), and can align in the direction of an applied load. Skin behaves viscoelastically (time-dependent) and anisotropically (test direction dependent). These factors should be considered during surgical reapproximation of dermal tissues. Cartilage is a "spongelike" material whose mechanical behavior is largely dependent on fluid flow through a viscous, charged

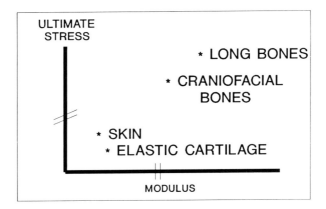

FIGURE 18.   Schematic comparing ultimate stress and modulus for skin, cartilage, and bone. Note the axes are broken to indicate that bone values are orders of magnitude greater than those for skin and cartilage.

matrix. Collagen fibers encase the swollen matrix, limiting its shape in the unloaded state. Bone is a most complex composite material whose mechanical properties vary from site to site, according to the functional demands and local architecture. Cortical and cancellous bone combine to form structures optimized for various mechanical roles, from high bending strength and modulus of the femur, to impact resistance in the skull.

In this chapter, we have reviewed the structure and mechanical properties of skin, cartilage, and bone. The bioengineer and surgeon must be familiar with structure/mechanical property relationships of tissues, in order to effectively design and implant biomaterials for repair of injured tissues.

REFERENCES

1. **Briggaman, R. A.**, Control of differentiation of epidermal structures, in *Morphogenesis and Malformation of the Skin. Birth Defects*, Original Article Series, Blandau, R. J., Ed., Alan R. Liss, New York, 1981, 17(2), 39.
2. **Holbrook, K. A. and Smith, L. T.**, Ultrastructural aspects of human skin during the embryonic, fetal, premature, neonatal and adult periods of life, in *Morphogenesis and Malformation of the Skin. Birth Defects*, Original Article Series, Blandau, R. J., Ed., Alan R. Liss, New York, 1981, 17(2), 9.
3. **Smith, L. T. and Holbrook, K. A.**, Development of dermal connective tissue in human embryonic and fetal skin, in *Scanning Electron Microscopy*, Johari, O., Ed., AMF O'Hare, Chicago, 4, 1745, 1982.
4. **Bloom, W. and Fawcett, D. W.**, *A Textbook of Histology*, 11th ed., Dreibelbis, D., Ed., W. B. Saunders, Philadelphia, 1986.
5. **Elias, P. M., Goerge, J., and Friend, D. S.**, Mammalian epidermal barrier layer lipids: composition and influence on structure, *J. Invest. Dermatol.*, 69, 535, 1977.
6. **Jarrett, A.**, The epidermis and its relations with the dermis, in *The Physiology and Pathophysiology of the Skin*, Jarrett, A., Ed., Academic Press, London, 1973, 3.
7. **Maltoltsy, A. G.**, Desmosomes, filaments and keratohyalin granules: their role in the stabilization and keratinization of the epidermis, *J. Invest. Dermatol.*, 65, 127, 1975.
8. **Jarrett, A.**, Normal epidermal keratinization, in *The Physiology and Pathophysiology of the Skin*, Jarrett, A., Ed., Academic Press, London, 1973, 161.
9. **Jarrett, A.**, Disorders of keratinization: psoriasis and ichthyosos, in *The Physiology annd Pathophysiology of the Skin*, Jarrett, A., Ed., Academic Press, London, 1973, 215.
10. **Winkelmann, R. K.**, The Merkel cell system and a comparison between it and the neurosecretory or APUD cell system, *J. Invest. Dermatol.*, 69, 41, 1977.

11. **Hashimoto, K.,** Fine structure of the Merkel cell in human oral mucosa, *J. Invest. Dermatol.,* 58, 381, 1972.

12. **Holbrook, K. A., Byers, P. H., and Pinnell, S. R.,** The structure and function of dermal connective tissue in normal individuals and patients with inherited connective tissue disorders, in *Scanning Electron Microscopy,* Johari, O., Ed., AMF O'Hare, Chicago, 4, 1731, 1982.

13. **Riley, P. A.,** Melanin and melanocytes, in *The Physiology and Pathophysiology of the Skin,* Vol. 1, Jarrett, A., Ed., Academic Press, London, 1974, 1104.

14. **Szabo, G.,** The regional anatomy of the human integument with special reference to the distribution of hair follicles, sweat glands and melanocytes, *Philos. Trans. R. Soc. London Ser. B,* 252, 447, 1967.

15. **Katz, S., Tamaki, K., and Sacks, D. H.,** Epidermal Langerhans cells are derived from cells originating in the bone marrow, *Nature (London),* 282, 324, 1979.

16. **Shelley, W. B. and Lennart, J.,** The Langerhans cell: its origin, nature and function, *Acta Dermatol. (Stockholm),* Suppl. 79, 7, 1978.

17. **Stingl, G., Katz, I. S., Clement, L., Green, I., and Shevack, E. M.,** Immunologic functions of Ia-bearing epidermal Langerhans cells, *J. Immunol.,* 121, 2005, 1978.

18. **Silberg, I., Baer, R. L., and Rosenthal, S. A.,** The role of Langerhans cells in contact hypersensitivity. A review of findings in man and guinea pigs, *J. Invest. Dermatol.,* 66, 210, 1976.

19. **Epstein, E. H. and Munderloh, N. H.,** Human skin collagen. Presence of type I and type III at all levels of the dermis, *J. Biol. Chem.,* 253, 1336, 1978.

20. **Fleischmajer, R., Gay, S., Meigel, W. N., and Perlish, J. S.,** Collagen in the cellular and fibrotic stages and scleroderma, *Arthritis Rheum.,* 21, 418, 1980.

21. **Cotta-Pereira, G., Rodrigo, F. G., and Bittencourt-Sampaio, S.,** Oxytalan, elaunin, and elastic fibers in the human skin, *J. Invest. Dermatol.,* 66, 143, 1976.

22. **Junqueira, L. C. U., Montes, J. S., Martins, J. E. C., and Joazeiro, P. P.,** Dermal collagen distribution. A histochemical and ultrastructural study, *Histochemistry,* 79, 397, 1983.

23. **Craig, A. S., Eikenberry, E. F., and Parry, D. A. D.,** Ultrastructural organization of skin: classification on the basis of mechanical role, *Connect. Tissue Res.,* 16, 213, 1987.

24. **Smith, L. T., Holbrook, K. A., and Bryers, P. H.,** Structure of the dermal matrix during development and in the adult, *J. Invest. Dermatol.,* 79, 93, 1982.

25. **Hoffman, P., Linker, A., and Meyer, K.,** *Arch. Biochem. Biophys.,* 69, 453, 1957.

26. **Loewi, G. and Meyer, K.,** *Biochim. Biophys. Acta,* 37, 453, 1958.

27. **Flint, M. H., Craig, A. S., Reilly, H. C., Gillard, G. C., and Parry, D. A. D.,** Collagen fibril diameters and glycosaminoglycan content of skins-indices of tissue maturity and function, *Connect. Tissue Res.,* 13, 69, 1984.

28. **Scott, J. E., Orford, C. R., and Hughes, E. W.,** Proteoglycancollagen arrangements in developing rat tail tendon, *Biochem. J.,* 195, 573, 1981.

29. **Parry, D. A. D., Barnes, G. R. G., and Craig, A. S.,** A comparison of the size distribution of collagen fibrils in connective tissues as a function of age and a possible relation between fibril size distribution and mechanical properties, *Proc. R. Soc. London Ser. B.,* 203, 305, 1978.

30. **Merrilees, M. J. and Flint, M. H.,** Ultrastructural study of tension and pressure zones in a rabbit flexor tendon, *Am. J. Anat.,* 157, 87, 1980.

31. **Parry, D. A. D. and Craig, A. S.,** Growth and development of collagen fibrils in connective tissues, in *Ultrastructure of the Connective Tissue Matrix,* Ruggeri, A. and Motta, P. M., Eds., Martinus Nijhoff, Boston, 1984, 34.

32. **Langer, K.,** Zur Anatomie und Physiologie der Haut. I. Uber die spaltbarkeit der cutis, *S. B. Akad. Wiss. Wien,* 44, 19, 1861.

33. **Gibson, T.,** The physical properties of skin, in *Reconstructive Plastic Surgery,* Vol. 1, 2nd ed., Converse, J. M. and McCarthy, J. G., Eds., W. B. Saunders, Philadelphia, 1977, 301.

34. **Converse, J. M.,** Introduction to plastic surgery, in *Reconstructive Plastic Surgery,* Vol. 1, 2nd ed., Converse, J. M. and McCarthy, J. G., Eds., W. B. Saunders, Philadelphia, 1977, 301.

35. **Serri, F. and Huber, W. M.,** The development of the sebacious glands in man, in *Advances in Biology of the Skin,* Vol. 4, Montagna, W., Ellis, R., and Silver, A., Eds., Pergamon Press, Elmsford, NY, 1963, 1.

36. **Montagna, W.,** The sebacious glands in man, in *Advances in Biology of the Skin,* Vol. 4, Montagna, W., Ellis, R., and Silver, A., Eds., Pergamon Press, Elmsford, NY, 1963, 19.

37. **Horner, W. E.,** On the odoriferous glands of the negro, *Am. J. Med. Sci.,* 21, 13, 1846.

38. **Nicolaides, N.,** Human skin surface lipids—Origin, composition and possible function, in *Advances in Biology of the Skin,* Vol. 4, Montagna, W., Ellis, R., and Silver, A., Eds., Pergamon Press, New York, 1963, 167.

39. **Szabo, G.,** The number of eccrine sweat glands in human skin, in *Advances in Biology of the Skin,* Vol. 3, Montagna, W., Ellis, R., and Silver, A., Eds., Pergamon Press, Elmsford, NY, 1962, 1.

40. **Robinson, S.,** The regulation of sweating in exercise, in *Advances in Biology of the Skin,* Vol. 3, Montagna, W., Ellis, R., and Silver, A., Eds., Pergamon Press, Elmsford, NY, 1962, 152.

41. **Winklemann, R. K.,** Cutaneous vascular patterns, in *Advances in Biology of the Skin,* Montagna, W., Ellis, R., and Silver, A., Eds., Pergamon Press, Elmsford, NY, 1961, 1.

42. **Winklemann, R. K.,** Dermal nerve networks, in *Nerve Endings in Normal and Pathological Skin,* Arhur, C., Ed., Charles C. Thomas, 1960, 18.

43. **Thorogood, P. D. and Hinchcliffe, J. R.,** An analysis of the condensation process during chondrogenesis in the embryonic chick hind limb, *J. Embryol. Exp. Morphol.,* 33, 581, 1975.

44. **Ede, D. A.,** Cellular condensations and chondrogenesis, in *Cartilage: Development, Differentiation and Growth,* Vol. 2, Hall, B. K., Ed., Academic Press, New York, 1983, 143.

45. **Fell, H. B.,** The histogenesis of cartilage and bone in the long bone of the embryonic fowl, *J. Morphol.,* 40, 417, 1925.

46. **Fell, H. B. and Canti, R. B.,** Experiments on the developments *in vitro* of the avian knee joint, *Proc. R. Soc. London, Ser. B.,* 316, 1935.

47. **Ede, D. A., Flint, O. P., Wilby, O. K., and Colquhoun, P.,** The development of precartilage condensations in limb-bud mesenchyme of normal and mutant embryos *in vivo* and *in vitro,* in *Vertebrate Limb and Somite Morphogenesis,* Ede, D. A., Hinchcliffe, J. R., and Balls, M., Eds., Cambridge University Press, New York, 1977, 161.

48. **Solursh, M.,** Cell-cell interactions and chondrogenesis, in *Cartilage: Development, Differentiation and Growth,* Vol. 2, Hall, B. K., Ed., Academic Press, New York, 1983, 121.

49. **Urist, M. R.,** The origin of cartilage: investigations in quest of chondrogenic DNA, in *Cartilage: Development, Differentiation and Growth,* Hall, B. K., Ed., Academic Press, New York, 1983, 2.

50. **Kosher, R. A.,** The chondroblast and the chondrocyte, collagens of cartilage, in *Cartilage: Structure, Function and Biochemistry,* Vol. 1, Hall, B. K., Ed., Academic Press, New York, 1983, 59.

51. **Ham, A. W. and Cormack, D. H.,** *Histophysiology of Cartilage, Bone and Joints,* Lippincott, New York, 1979, chap. 14-16.

52. **Patten, B. M. and Carlson, B. M.,** Connective tissues and the skeletal and muscular systems, in *Foundations of Embryology,* 3rd ed., Wiley, W. J. and Hepburn, C. A., Eds., McGraw-Hill, New York, 1974, chap. 16.

53. **Serafini-Fracassini, A. and Smith, J. W.,** Cartilagenous epiphyseal plates, in *The Structure and Biochemistry of Cartilage,* Churchill Livingstone, New York, 1974, 138.

54. **Silver, F.,** Microscopic and macroscopic structure of tissues, in *Biological Materials: Structure, Mechanical Properties, and Modeling of Soft Tissues,* W. Welkowitz, Ed., New York University Press, New York, 1987, chap. 3.

55. **Gibson, T.,** Transplantation of cartilage, in *Reconstructive Plastic Surgery,* Vol. 1, 2nd ed., Converse, J. M. and McCarthy, J. G., Eds., W. B. Saunders, Philadelphia, 1977, 301.

56. **Stockwell, R. A.,** *Biology of Cartilage Cells,* Harrison, R. J. and McMinn, R. M. H., Eds., Cambridge University Press, Cambidge, 1979, 1.

57. **Sheldon, H.,** Transmission electron microscopy of cartilage, in *Cartilage, Structure, Function and Biochemistry,* Vol. 1, Hall, B. K., Ed., Academic Press, New York, 1983, 87.

58. **Schenk, R. K., Eggli, P. S., and Hunziker, E. B.,** Articular cartilage morphology, in *Articular Cartilage Biochemistry,* Kuettner, K. E., Schleyer, R., Hascall, V., Eds., Raven Press, New York, 1986, 3.

59. **Engfeldt, B. and Hjertquist, S. O.,** Studies on the epihyseal growth zone, *Virchows Arch. B (Cell Pathology),* 1, 222, 1968.

60. **Clark, I. C.,** Articular cartilage: a review and electron microscopy study. II. The territorial fibrillar architecture, *J. Anat.,* 118, 261, 1974.

61. **Boyde, A. and Jones, S. J.,** Scanning electron microscopy of cartilage, in *Cartilage: Structure, Function and Biochemistry,* Vol. 1, Hall, K., Ed., Academic Press, New York, 1983, 105.

62. **Zimny, M. L. and Redler, I.,** Chondrocytes in health and disease, in *Scanning Electron Microscopy/ IITRI,* Johari, O. and Corvin, I., Eds., Inst. Technol. Res. Inst., Chicago, 1974, 805.

63. **Laczko, J., Levai, G., Verga, S., and Gyarmati, J.,** Preparation of the tibial growth organ of young rats for scanning electron microscopy, *Mikroskopie,* 31, 57, 1975.

64. **Arsenault, A. L., Ottensmeyer, F. P., and Heath, I. B.,** An electron microscopic and spectroscopic study of murine epiphyseal cartilage: analysis of fine structure and matrix vesicles preserved by freezing and freeze substitution, *J. Ultrastruct. Mol. Struct. Res.,* 98, 32, 1988.

65. **Engfeldt, B., Hultenby, J., and Muller, M.,** Ultrastructure of hyaline cartilage, *Acta Pathol. Microbiol. Immunol. Scand.,* Sect. A, 94, 313, 1986.

66. **Hunziker, E. B., Herman, W., Schenk, R. K., Muller, M., and Moor, H.,** Cartilage ultrastructure after high pressure freezing, freeze substitution and low temperature embedding, I. Chondrocyte ultrastructure, implications for the theories of mineralization and vascular invasion, *J. Cell Biol.,* 98, 267, 1984.

67. **Lash, J. W. and Vasan, S. N.,** Glycosaminoglycans of cartilage, in *Cartilage: Structure, Function and Biochemistry,* Vol. 1, Hall, B. K., Ed., Academic Press, New York, 1983, 215.

68. **Mayne, R., and von der Mark, K.,** Collagens of cartilage, in *Cartilage: Structure, Function and Biochemistry,* Vol. 1, Hall, B. K., Ed., Academic Press, New York, 1983, 181.

69. **Iozzo, R. V.,** Biology of disease. Proteoglycans: structure, function, and role in neoplasia, *Lab. Invest.,* 53(4), 373, 1985.

70. **Mayne, R. and Irwin, M. H.,** Collagen types in cartilage, in *Articular Cartilage Biochemistry,* Kuettner, K. E., Schleyer, R., Hascall, V., Eds., Raven Press, New York, 1986, 23.

71. **Silver, F.,** Connective tissue structure, *Biological Material Structure, Mechanical Properties, and Modeling of Soft Tissues,* W. Welkowitz, Ed., New York University Press, New York, 1987, chap. 2.

72. **Stockwell, R. A.,** *Biology of Cartilage Cells,* Harrison, R. J. and McMinn, R. M. H., Eds., Cambridge University Press, London, 1979, 32.

73. **Poole, A. R., Pidoux, I., Reiner, A., and Rosenberg, L.,** An immunoelectron microscope study of the organization of proteoglycan monomer, link protein, and collagen in the matrix of articular cartilage, *J. Cell Biol.,* 93, 921, 1982.

74. **Heinegard, D. and Paulsson, M.,** Structure and metabolism of proteoglycans, in *Connective Tissue Biochemistry,* Piez, K. and Reddi, H., Eds., Elsevier, New York, 1984, 277.

75. **Rosenberg, L. C. and Buckwalter, J. A.,** Cartilage proteoglycans, in *Articular Cartilage Biochemistry,* Kuettner, K. E., Ed., Raven Press, New York, 1986, 59.

76. **Rosenberg, L.,** Structure of cartilage proteoglycans, in *Dynamics of Connective Tissue Macromolecules,* Burleigh, P. M. C. and Poole, A. R., Eds., North-Holland, Amsterdam, 1975, chap. 5.

77. **Kempson, G. L., Muir, S., Swanson, A. V., and Freedman, M. A. R.,** Correlations between stiffness and chemical constituents of cartilage of the human femeral head, *Biochem. Biophys. Acta,* 215, 70, 1970.

78. **Wasserman, A. J., Doillon, C. J., Glasgold, A. I., Kato, Y. P., Christiansen, D., Rizvi, A., Wong, E., Goldstein, J., and Silver, F. H.,** Clinical applications of electron microscopy to the study of collagenous biomaterials, in *Scanning Microscopy,* Johari, O., Ed., Vol. 2, AMF O'Hare, Chicago, 1988, 1635.

79. **Wasserman, A. J., Doillon, C. J., Glasgold, A. I., Kato, Y. P., Christiansen, D., and Silver, F. H.,** An electron histochemical and ultrastructural evaluation of human nasal septal cartilage grafts stored in merthiolate and alcide, in *Proc. 46th Annual Meeting Electron Microscopy Society of America,* Bailey, G. W., San Francisco Press, 244, 1988.

80. **Hargest, T. E., Gay, C. V., Scharer, H., and Wasserman, A. J.,** Vertical distribution of cells and matrix of epiphyseal growth plate cartilage determined by quantitative electron probe analysis, *J. Histochem. Cytochem.,* 4(33), 275, 1985.

81. **Clark, I. C.,** Articular cartilage a review and electron microscopy study. I. The interterritorial fibrillar architecture, *J. Bone Jt. Surg.,* 53B, 732, 1971.

82. **Morris, I. R.,** Functional anatomy of the upper airway, *Airway Management Anesth.,* 6(4), 639, 1988.

83. **Hall, B. K.,** Tissue interactions and chondrogenesis, in *Cartilage: Development, Differentiation and Growth,* Vol. 2, Brian, K. Hall, Ed., Academic Press, New York, 1983, 187.

84. **Benjamin, M., Evans, E. J., and Copp, L.,** The histology of tendon attachments of bone to man, *J. Anat.,* 149, 89, 1986.

85. **Pritchard, J. J.,** General histology of bone, in *The Biochemistry and Physiology of Bone,* Bourne, G. H., Ed., Academic Press, New York, 1972, chap. 1.

86. **Bouvier, M.,** The biology and composition of bone, in *Bone Mechanics,* Cowin, S. C., Ed., CRC Press, Boca Raton, FL, 1989, chap. 1.

87. **Cowin, S. C., Van Burskirk, W. C., and Ashman, R. B.,** Properties of Bone, in *Handbook of Bioengineering,* Skalak, R. and Chien, S., Eds., McGraw-Hill, New York, 1987, chap. 2.

88. **Goret-Nicaise, M.,** Identification of collagen type I and type II in chondroid tissue, *Calcif. Tissue Int.,* 36, 682, 1982.

89. **Goret-Nicaise, M. and Dhem, A.,** Presence of chondroid tissue in the symphyseal region of the growing human mandible, *Acta Anat.,* 113, 189, 1982.

90. **Pritchard, J. J., Scott, J. H., and Girgis, F. G.,** The structure and development of cranial and facial sutures, *J. Anat.,* 90, 73, 1956.

91. **Persson, M.,** Structure and growth of facial sutures, *Odontol. Revy.* 24(Suppl. 26), 1, 1973.

92. **Persson, M., Magnusson, B. C., and Thilander, B.,** Sutural closure in rabbit and man: a morphological and histochemical study, *J. Anat.,* 123, 313, 1978.

93. **Manzannares, M. C., Goret-Nicase, M., and Dhem, A.,** Metopic sutural closure in the human skull, *J. Anat.,* 161, 203, 1988.

94. **Vogel, J. J. and Boyan-Salyers, B. D.,** Acidic lipids associated with the local mechanism of calcification, *Clin. Orthop. Relat. Res.,* 118, 230, 1976.

95. **Arsenault, A. L. and Hunziker, E. B.,** Electron microscopic analysis of mineral deposits in the calcifying epiphyseal growth plate, *Calcif. Tissue Int.,* 42, 119, 1988.

96. **Landis, W. J.,** A study of calcification in the leg tendons from the domestic turkey, *J. Ultrastruct. Mol. Struct. Res.,* 94, 217, 1986.

97. **Bonucci, E.,** The locus of initial calcification in cartilage and bone, *Clin. Orthop.,* 78, 108, 1971.

98. **Katchburian, E.,** Membrane-bound bodies as initiators of mineralization of dentine, *J. Anat.,* 116, 285, 1973.

99. **Glimcher, M. J.,** Composition, structure and organization of bone and other mineralized tissues and the mechanism of calcification, in *Handbook of Physiology,* Vol. 7, American Physiology Society, Washington, D.C., 7, Endocrinology, 1976, 25.

100. **Wilkes, G. L., Brown, I. A., and Wildnauer, R. H.,** The biomechanical properties of skin, *CRC Crit. Rev. Bioeng.,* 1, 453, 1973.

101. **Silver, F. H. and Doillon, C. J.,** Skin: structure-mechanical property relationships, Biomechanics Symposium, New York, American Society of Mechanical Engineers, 1987, 249.

102. **Wildnauer, R. H., Bothwell, J. W., and Douglas, A.,** Influence of water content on the biomechanical properties of stratum corneum, *J. Invest. Dermatol.,* 35, 436, 1970.

103. **Fleischmajer, R. S., Gay, S., Perlish, J. S., and Cesarini, J. P.,** Immunoelectron microscopy of type III collagen in normal and sclerodermal skin, *J. Invest. Dermatol.,* 75, 189, 1980.

104. **Brown, I. B.,** Scanning electron microscopy of human dermal fibrous tissue, *J. Anat.,* 113, 159, 1972.

105. **Bailey, A. J., Bazin, S., Sims, T. J., LeLous, M., Nicoletis, C., and Delaney, A.,** Characterization of the collagen of human hypertrophic and normal scars, *Biochim. Biophys. Acta,* 405, 412, 1975.

106. **Weinstein, G. D. and Boucek, R. J.,** Collagen and elastin of the human dermis, *J. Invest. Dermatol.,* 35, 227, 1960.

107. **Park, J. B.,** *Biomaterials,* Plenum Press, New York, 1979.

108. **Franzblau, C. and Farris, B.,** in *Cell Biology of Extracellular Matrix,* E. D. Hay, Ed., Plenum Press, New York, 1981, 65.

109. **Oxlund, H., Manschot, J., and Viidik, A.,** The role of elastin in the mechanical properties of skin, *J. Biomech.,* 21, 213, 1988.

110. **Shetlar, M. R., Shetlar, C. L., Chien, S. F., Linares, H. A., Dobrkofsky, M., and Larson, D. L.,** The hypertrophic scar. Hexosamine containing components of burn scars, *Proc. Soc. Exp. Biol. Med.,* 139, 544, 1972.

111. **Oxlund, H. and Andreassen, T. T.,** The roles of hyaluronic acid, collagen and elastin in the mechanical properties of connective tissues, *J. Anat.,* 131, 611, 1980.

112. **Finlay, J. B.,** Thixotropy in human skin, *J. Biomech.,* 11, 333, 1978.

113. **Ridge, M. D. and Wright, V.,** The rheology of skin. A bioengineering study of the mechanical properties of human skin in relation to its structure, *Br. J. Dermat.,* 77, 639, 1965.

114. **Harkness, R. D.,** Mechanical properties of skin in relation to its biological function and its chemical components, in *Biophysical Properties of Skin. A Treatise on Skin,* Vol. 1, Elden, H. R., Ed., Wiley Intersciences, New York, 1971, 393.

115. **Dunn, M. G., Silver, F. H., and Swann, D. A.,** Mechanical analysis of hypertrophic scar tissue: structural basis for apparent increased rigidity, *J. Invest. Dermatol.,* 84, 9, 1985.

116. **Gibson, T., Kenedi, R. M., and Craik, J. E.,** The mobile micro-architecture of skin. A bio-engineering study, *Brit. J. Surg.,* 52, 764, 1965.

117. **Dunn, M. G. and Silver, F. H.,** Viscoelastic behavior of human connective tissues: relative contribution of viscous and elastic components, *Connect. Tissue Res.,* 12, 59, 1983.

118. **Doillon, C. J., Dunn, M. G., and Silver, F. H.,** Relationship between mechanical properties and collagen structure of closed and open wounds, *J. Biomech. Eng.,* 110, 352, 1988.

119. **Hall, D. A., Blackett, A. D., Zajac, A. R., Switala, S., and Airey, C. M.,** Changes in skinfold thickness with increasing age, *Age Ageing,* 10, 19, 1981.

120. **Leveque, J. L., de Rigal, J., Agache, P. G., and Monneur, C.,** Influence of ageing on the *in vivo* extensibility of human skin at low stress, *Arch. Derm. Res.,* 269, 127, 1980.

121. **Dupuytren, G.,** Traité théorique et Pratique des Blessures par Armes de Guerre, Vol. 1, Maison, Paris, 1834, 66.

122. **Ridge, M. D. and Wright, V.,** The directional effects of skin. A bioengineering study with particular reference to Langer's lines, *J. Invest. Dermatol.,* 46, 341, 1966.

123. **Gibson, T., Stark, H., and Evans, J. H.,** Directional variation in extensibility of human skin *in vivo, J. Biomech.,* 2, 201, 1969.

124. **Schneider, D. C., Davidson, T. M., and Nahum, A. M.,** *In vitro* biaxial stress-strain response of human skin, *Arch. Otolaryngol.,* 110, 329, 1984.

125. **Dintenfass, L.,** Rheology of complex fluids and some observations on joint lubrication, *Fed. Proc.,* 25, 1054, 1966.

126. **Myers, E. R. and Mow, V. C.,** Biomechanics of cartilage and its response to biomechanical stimuli, in *Cartilage: Structure, Function, and Biochemistry,* Hall, B. K., Ed., Academic Press, New York, 1983.

127. **Myers, E. R., Armstrong, C. G., and Mow, V. C.,** Swelling pressure and collagen tension, in *Connective Tissue Matrix,* Hulkins, D. W. L., Ed., Macmillan, London, 1984, 161.

128. **Carney, S. L. and Muir, H.,** The structure and function of cartilage proteoglycans, *Physiol. Rev.,* 68, 858, 1988.

129. **Comper, W. D. and Laurent, T. C.,** Physiological function of connective tissue polysaccharides, *Physiol. Rev.,* 58, 255, 1978.

130. **Grodzinsky, A. J.,** Electromechanical and physicochemical properties of connective tissues, *CRC Crit. Rev. Biomed. Eng.,* 9, 133, 1983.

131. **Frank, E. H. and Grodzinsky, A. J.,** Cartilage electromechanics. I. Electrokinetic transduction and the effects of electrolyte pH and ionic strength, *J. Biomech.,* 20, 615, 1987.

132. **Brighton, C. T., Black, J., and Pollack, S. R.,** *Electrical Properties of Bone and Cartilage,* Grune & Stratton, New York, 1979.

133. **Mow, V. C., Roth, V., and Armstrong, C. G.,** Biomechanics of joint cartilage, in *Basic Biomechanics of the Skeletal System,* Frankel, V. H. and Nordin, M., Eds., Lea & Febiger, Philadelphia, 1980, chap. 2.

134. **Glasgold, M. J., Kato, Y. P., Christiansen, D., Hauge, J. A., Glasgold, A. I., and Silver, F. H.,** Mechanical properties of septal cartilage homografts, *Otolaryngol. Head Neck Surg.,* 99, 374, 1988.

135. **Yamaguchi, T. and Katake, K.,** Study on strength of auricular cartilages of men and animals, *J. Kyoto Pref. Med. Univ.,* 67, 420, 1960.

136. **Fry, H. J. H.,** Cartilage and cartilage grafts: the basic properties of the tissue and the components responsible for them, *Plast. Reconstr. Surg.,* 40, 426, 1967.

137. **Murakami, W. T., Wong, L. W., and Davidson, T. M.,** Applications of the biomechanical behavior of cartilage to nasal septoplastic surgery, *Laryngoscope,* 92, 300, 1982.

138. **Rubin, F. F.,** Permanent change in shape of cartilage by morselization, *Arch. Otolaryngol.,* 89, 601, 1969.

139. **Currey, J. D.,** Mechanical properties of bone tissues with greatly differing functions, *J. Biomech.,* 12, 313, 1979.

140. **Wolff, J. L.,** Das Gesetz der Transformation der Knochen, A. Hirschwald, Berlin, 1892.

141. **Carter, D. R.,** Mechanical loading histories and cortical bone remodeling, *Calcif. Tissue Int.,* 36, S19, 1984.

142. **Frost, H. M.,** Vital biomechanics: proposed general concepts for skeletal adaptations to mechanical useage, *Calcif. Tissue Int.,* 42, 145, 1988.

143. **Nordin, M. and Frankel, V. H.,** Biomechanics of whole bones and bone tissue, in *Basic Biomechanics of the Skeletal System,* Frankel, V. H. and Nordin, M., Eds., Lea & Febiger, Philadelphia, 1980, chap. 2.

144. **Evans, F. G.,** *Mechanical Properties of Bone,* Charles C. Thomas, Springfield, IL, 1973.

145. **McCutchen, C. W.,** Do mineral crystals stiffen bone by straight-jacketing its collagen?, *J. Theor. Biol.,* 51, 51, 1975.

146. **Mason, B. and Barry, L. G.,** *Elements of Mineralogy,* W. H. Freeman, San Francisco, 1968.

147. **Vincent, J. F. V.,** *Structural Biomaterials,* John Wiley & Sons, New York, 1982.

148. **Carter, D. R. and Hayes, W. C.,** The compressive behavior of bone as a two-phase porous structure, *J. Bone Jt. Surg.,* 59A, 954, 1977.

149. **Katz, J. L., Yoon, H. B., Lipson, S., Maharidge, R., Meunier, A., and Christel, P.,** The effects of remodeling on the elastic properties of bone, *Calcif. Tissue Int.,* 36, S31, 1984.

150. **Burr, D. B., Schaffler, M. B., and Frederickson, R. G.,** Composition of the cement line and its possible mechanical role as a local interface in human compact bone, *J. Biomech.,* 21, 939, 1988.

151. **Reilly, D. and Burstein, A.,** The elastic and ultimate properties of compact bone tissue, *J. Biomech.,* 8, 393, 1975.

152. **Schaffler, M. B. and Burr, D. B.,** Stiffness of compact bone: effects of porosity and density, *J. Biomech.,* 21, 13, 1988.

153. **Currey, J. D.,** The effect of porosity and mineral content on the Young's modulus of elasticity of compact bone, *J. Biomech.,* 21, 131, 1988.

154. **Martin, R. B. and Ishida, J.,** The relative effects of collagen fiber orientation, porosity, density, and mineralization of bone strength, *J. Biomech.,* 22, 419, 1989.

155. **Goldstein, S. A.,** The mechanical properties of trabecular bone: dependence on anatomic location and function, *J. Biomech.,* 20, 1055, 1987.

156. **Evans, F. G. and King, A. L.,** Regional differences in some physical properties of human spongy bone, in *Biomechanical Studies of the Musculoskeletal System,* Evans, F. G., Ed., Charles C. Thomas, Springfield, IL, 1961, 49.

157. **Currey, J. D.,** Mechanical properties of bone, *Clin. Orth. Rel. Res.,* 73, 210, 1970.

158. **Kiebzak, G. M., Smith R., Gundberg, C. C., Howe, J. C., and Sacktor, B.,** Bone status of senescent male rats: chemical, morphometric, and mechanical analysis, *J. Bone Miner. Res.,* 3, 37, 1988.

159. **Fukada, E. and Yasuda, I.,** On the piezoelectric effect of bone, *J. Phys. Soc. Jpn.,* 10, 1158, 1957.

160. **Pollack, S. R.,** Bioelectrical properties of bone. Endogenous electrical signals, *Orthop. Clin. N. Am.,* 15, 3, 1984.

161. **Currey, J. D.,** What should bones be designed to do?, *Calcif. Tissue Int.,* 36, 57, 1984.

162. **Yamada, H.,** *Strength of Biological Materials,* Evans, F. G., Ed., Williams & Wilkins, Baltimore, 1970.

163. **McElhaney, J. H., Fogle, J. L., Melvin, J. W., Haynes, R. R., Roberts, V. L., and Alem, N. M.,** Mechanical properties of cranial bone, *J. Biomech.,* 3, 495, 1970.

164. **Evans, F. G. and Lissner, H. R.,** Tensile and compressive strength of human parietal bone, *J. Appl. Physiol.,* 10, 493, 1957.

165. **Roberts, V. L. and Melvin, J. W.,** The measurement of the dynamic mechanical properties of human skull bone, *Appl. Polym. Symp.,* 12, 235, 1969.

166. **Wood, J. L.,** Dynamic response of human cranial bone, *J. Biomech.,* 4, 1, 1971.

167. **Kriewall, T. J.,** Structural, mechanical, and material properties of fetal cranial bone, *Am. J. Obstet. Gynecol.,* 143, 707, 1982.

168. **Hodgson, V. R.,** Tolerance of the facial bones to impact, *Am. J. Anat.,* 120, 113, 1967.

169. **Endo, B. and Adachi, K.,** Biomechanical simulation study on the forms of the frontal bone and facial bones of the recent human facial skeleton by using a two-dimensional frame model with stepwise variable cross-section members, *Okajimas Folia Anat. Jpn.,* 64, 335, 1988.

170. **Tanne, K., Miyasaka, J., Yamagata, Y., Sachdeva, R., Tsutsumi, S., and Sakuda, M.,** Three-dimensional model of the human craniofacial skeleton: method and preliminary results using finite element analysis, *J. Biomed. Eng.,* 10, 246, 1988.

171. **Currey, J. D.,** The effect of protection on the impact strength of rabbits' bones, *Acta Anat.,* 71, 87, 1968.

172. **Viidik, A., Danielsen, C. C., and Oxlund, H.,** On fundamental and phenomenological models, structure and mechanical properties of collagen, elastin, and glycosaminoglycan complexes, *Biorheology,* 19, 437, 1982.

173. **Silver, F. H.,** *Biological Materials: Structure, Mechanical Properties, and Modeling of Soft Tissues,* New York University Press, New York, 1987, chap. 7.

Chapter 4

REPAIR OF SKIN, CARTILAGE, AND BONE

Frederick H. Silver and J. Russell Parsons

TABLE OF CONTENTS

I. INTRODUCTION

Biomaterials are used to repair wounds created by mechanical trauma and to augment tissues. In both of these cases surgical intervention is necessary to properly install medical devices. Creation of a wound in any fashion sets into motion a series of events leading to healing or to chronic inflammation. Chronic inflammation associated with the presence of an implant can lead to implant destruction and/or a foreign body response that may impair the function of a medical device. Therefore it is essential to understand normal repair of skin, cartilage, and bone and the events that are necessary to ensure proper function of facial implants.

II. SOFT-TISSUE REPAIR

A. REPAIR OF SKIN

Repair of defects that involve the dermis occurs exclusively by the deposition of scar tissue through the wound healing process. Healing of skin occurs via a complex series of events including inflammatory, proliferative, and remodeling phases as described in Figure 1. Immediate events that are associated with the formation of a wound include leakage of blood components from severed vessels, activation of blood clotting and platelet aggregation, protein denaturation at the site of the injury, bacterial and viral contamination of the wound, and implant introduction into the wound. Responses to these stimuli include local accumulation of inflammatory cells (neutrophils, monocytes, and lymphocytes), activation of several biological systems (blood clotting, fibrinolytic, immune, and kinin), release of cellular (lymphokines, monokines), and other regulatory factors.[1] These processes are described in more detail below.

B. CARTILAGE REPAIR

Much of our knowledge concerning cartilage repair relates to articular cartilage that lines joint surfaces. Articular cartilage as well as cartilages in the nose fall into the classification of hyaline cartilages. Repair of hyaline cartilage found in joints has been studied extensively in order to optimize surgical reconstruction of these structures after injury associated with trauma, contact sports, and osteoarthritis.

The degree to which articular cartilage can repair itself is a function of the wound depth and location, proximity to blood vessels, age, and protection against abrasion. There is considerable disagreement concerning the extent of restoration of the joint surface; however, is clear that it is incomplete.[2,3]

Superficial laceration to articular cartilage results in little or no local bleeding and therefore formation of a fibrin clot or formation of granulation tissue[3] does not occur. Healing under these conditions occurs only by division of chondrocytes adjacent to the defect. Little or no closure of superficial wounds is observed despite transient proliferation of chondrocytes.[2-4] By electron microscopy the base of the defect can show an ultrathin cover of what has been described as fine collagen fibers.[5]

Deep lacerations that penetrate subchondral bone result in damage to blood vessels, bleeding, and initiation of wound healing.[3] Repair tissue in these defects consists of fibrocartilage containing type I collagen and not type II collagen, which is found in normal cartilage.[6] The mechanism of repair of deep cartilage wounds is similar to the manner by which the dermal component of skin is repaired as described below.

C. GENERAL MECHANISM FOR REPAIR OF SKIN DERMIS AND FIBROCARTILAGE

Repair of the dermis and deep cartilage wounds occurs as a result of disruption of blood vessels and leakage of plasma components into tissue. Activation of blood clotting leads to

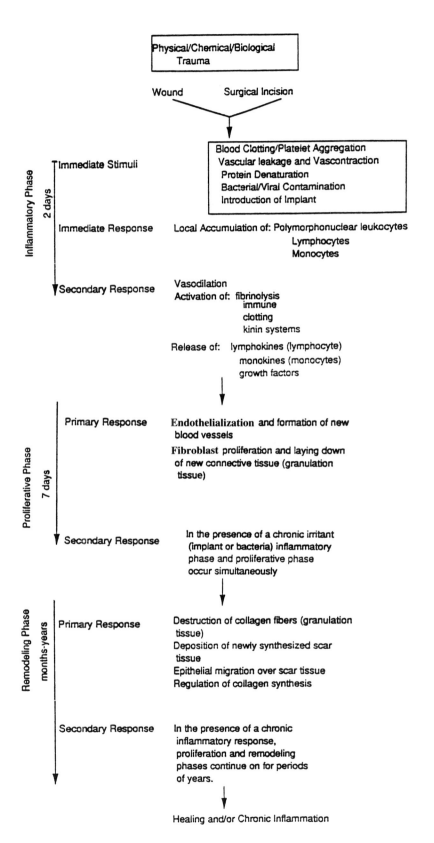

FIGURE 1.   Events that characterize wound healing.

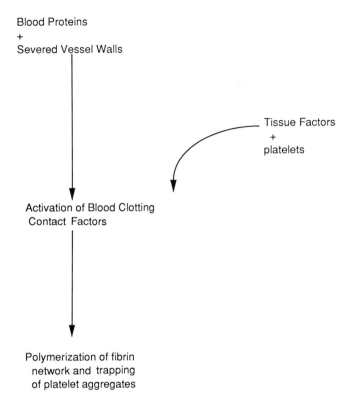

FIGURE 2.   Formation of fibrin network from soluble proteins involved in blood coagulation.

the formation of an insoluble fibrin network (Figure 2) and the activation of the complement, kinin, and fibrinolysis systems (Figure 3). Denatured proteins, bacteria, and blood cells become entrapped in a network of fibrin. These components are removed via activation of fibrinolysis (fibrin) and complement (bacteria) systems. Tissue repair occurs as the fibrin network is digested during the proliferative phase.

Shortly after wounding occurs, there is an increase in hyaluronic acid in the wound;[7] a model recently has been developed suggesting that specific binding of hyaluronic acid (a glycosaminoglycan found in skin and other tissues) to fibrin results in the formation of a matrix that plays a role in tissue repair processes during the granulating and remodeling stages.[8] Fibronectin, a glycoprotein found in plasma, is cross-linked to fibrin, the fibrous component of a clot, via the plasma enzyme transglutaminase.[9,10] This promotes neutrophil chemotaxis[11] and adhesion[12] in the wound. In time, local accumulation of inflammatory cells including neutrophils, lymphocytes, and macrophages occurs. Elaboration of factors from macrophages,[13,14] such as Interleukin 1, which has been shown to induce cartilage degradation,[15] is believed to trigger release of collagenase from fibroblasts and cause tissue lysis. Fibroblasts have been reported to respond to culture medium conditioned by stimulated mononuclear cells by a five- to tenfold increase in collagenolytic activity.[16] Inflammation is prolonged in the presence of macrophages, monocytes, and infectious organisms, and may be a direct result of fibroblast-inflammatory cell interactions and release of active collagenases.

The proliferative phase of soft tissue wound healing involves formation of new blood vessels and laying down of new connective tissue, termed granulation tissue, and occurs after invasion of fibroblasts. Fibronectin present in the wound is chemotactic for fibroblasts,[17,18] and thereby the presence of fibronectin from blood or tissue attracts cells into

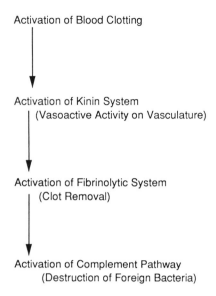

Activation of Blood Clotting

Activation of Kinin System
(Vasoactive Activity on Vasculature)

Activation of Fibrinolytic System
(Clot Removal)

Activation of Complement Pathway
(Destruction of Foreign Bacteria)

FIGURE 3. Activation of kinin, fibrinolysis, and complement
pathways as a result of blood clotting activity.

the wound area. Fibroblasts present in the wound synthesize types I, III, and V collagens[19,20] and proteoglycans.[21] Inhibition of angiogenesis by administration of protamine sulfate delays the deposition of granulation tissue.[22]

In the presence of an implant that biodegrades during the proliferative phase or causes a moderate amount of chronic inflammation, proliferation of new connective tissue cells and deposition of granulation occur simultaneously with a prolonged inflammatory phase.[1] If inflammation predominates over proliferation then little or no new connective tissue is deposited. When the inflammatory response is prolonged, host tissue is damaged and the wound becomes larger. If inflammation is only a minor component of the response, then the remodeling phase is initiated.

Cellular response can be significantly affected by the presence of an implant. In the proliferative and inflammatory stages of healing, an implant of any material must be considered a "stimulus" for the various cells involved in the inflammatory process. The stimulus is thought to be largely one of chemotaxis, although foreign body mediated chemotaxis is poorly understood.[23] At the site of an implant, during healing, contact between phagocytes and the implant surface (either bulk or particulate) is inevitable. This contact will be followed by degeneration of at least some of the contacting cells irregardless of the "inertness" of the foreign body. This cell degeneration, or perhaps simply contact with certain materials, is thought to result in emission of chemotactic agents. Black[24] has suggested that serum protein interactions with the implant surface may activate complement and produce hapten complexes, in turn activating an immune response. In any event, the migration of phagocytes is enhanced and is no longer a random occurrence. Upon arriving at the implant site, the macrophage elaborates chemical mediators that activate the proliferation of fibroblasts, and promotes fibroblastic synthesis of collagen and liberation of lytic enzymes, primarily collagenase. This collagenase degrades the collagen in the wound area to lower peptide fragments, which may also act as chemotactic agents for more macrophages and fibroblasts.[25] The attraction or chemotaxis may become chronic, and phagocytes, particularly macrophages, can become a chronic cell type in tissues at or near the interface of the implant. Thus, if the macrophage involvement is maintained, fibrosis may proceed to a point of significant pathology.[26] Ultimately, some of these mononuclear cells evolve into histocytes which, in combination with mesenchymal cell derived fibroblasts, generate a collagenous tissue "wall" about the implant.[26] Another chronic response to some materials involves coalescence of macrophages to form foreign body giant cells.

It is presently unknown how or which chemotactic agents are elaborated in response to foreign materials, or if the process is multifactorial, depending on the particular class of material, nature of the wound, and surrounding tissue.[23] It is generally agreed that the response to a material is in proportion to the degree to which the material is a chemical or physical irritant. For instance, some pure metals and alloys which tend to produce corrosion products *in vivo* have long been known to evoke more severe reactions than "inert" metals or alloys.[24] Williams et al.[27] have studied the chemotactic effects of various metal ions, such as titanium, aluminum, cobalt, and nickel; they speculated that the strength of chemotaxis correlated with the degree of cellularity and the extent of the encapsulating layer about the bulk metals upon implantation. If this line of reasoning is correct, then chemotaxis in concert with proliferation and migration of monocytes and macrophages may be a fundamental mechanism that determines the extent of the acute and chronic inflammatory/foreign body response to various implant materials. In addition, as discussed above, these macrophages may produce factors which activate fibroblasts to produce lytic enzymes, further degrading the tissue about the implant.

Remodeling of granulation tissue occurs during the final phase of wound healing by fibroblast phagocytosis of preformed collagen fibrils[28-30] leading to collagen fiber reorientation.[31] Once the underlying soft tissue is repaired, in skin, epithelial migration over the wound begins.

D. EPITHELIALIZATION OF SKIN WOUNDS

Reepithelialization via migratory activity at the wound margins begins within 6 hours for gingival epithelium,[32] and 24 hours in human epidermis,[33] and is believed to involve fibronectin[34] and factors such as epidermal growth factor.[35] Epithelial cells migrate beneath the dessicated portion of a blood clot and the upper layer of granulation tissue.[36,37]

Factors that attract epidermal cells include interleukin 1 secreted by macrophages and epidermal cells[38] as well as a factor secreted by smooth muscle cells.[39] Epidermal cells appear to produce a plasminogen activator that activates the fibrinolysis system and enables them to move through a fibrin network.[40,41] Basal epidermal cells use fibronectin-rich tissue as substratum for attachment and migration during reepithelialization,[36,42] and express fibronectin receptors on their cell membranes during wound healing.[43,44]

Factors that stimulate epidermal cell mitosis include epidermal growth factor,[45] eye-derived growth factor,[46] epidermal cell-derived factor,[47] and partially purified platelet-derived growth factor.[48]

III. HARD-TISSUE HEALING

The healing of bone is a regenerative process rather than a connective tissue (scar) repair that was discussed above for skin and cartilage. Bone regeneration occurs through two distinct mechanisms; namely, endochondral and membranous formation. Endochondral bone formation is what occurs in the epiphyseal plate of a long bone and is responsible for long bone growth. This type of bone originates with a cartilage analog that is gradually transformed through a complex series of events into calcified tissue.[49] A similar sequence of events has been described in the healing of bone wounds (fractures, etc.). An organized cartilagenous structure as in the epiphyseal plate is not formed. However, cartilage which ultimately calcifies does indeed form, and studies have examined the physiologic similarities in growth plate calcification and bone healing.[50]

Membranous bone growth does not require a cartilage analog structure. This type of bone is formed by mesenchymal cells which have differentiated into osteoblasts.[50] These cells lay down osteoid which ultimately calcifies. Membranous bones include the calvarium, facial bones, clavicle, mandible, and bone immediately subperiosteal (appositional bone). Membranous or appositional bone formation occurs in bone healing along the undersurface of the periosteum in the vicinity of bone disruption.[51]

Given the above information, bone healing must be considered a mixture of endochondral and membranous or appositional formation. The stages of repair include induction, inflammation, soft callus, callus calcification, and remodeling.[51] The inductive phase begins shortly following bone disruption and may last until the stage of inflammation is complete. During induction, viable cells in the region of disruption are induced to form new bone. These cells may arise from the periosteum or endosteum, or maybe activated osteocytes. These indigenous bone associated cells are modulated to become new osteoblasts. A second source of cells includes fibroblasts, endothelial cells, muscle cells, and various primative mesenchymal cells which may differentiate into cartilage and bone forming cells under the appropriate stimulus. The exact nature of the differentiative stimulus is not clearly understood, but may be associated with the depression of pH and formation of a region of relative hypoxia about the bone "wound".[51]

Osteoinductive proteins capable of promoting differentiation of cells preferentially into bone forming cells are also associated with bone tissue. Appropriate acid demineralization of bone yields a collagenous matrix (Demineralized Bone Matrix, DBM) in which embedded noncollagenous inductive proteins remain active. When implanted these proteins are readily accessible to surrounding inducible cells.[51,52] Various active fractions of the osteoinductive proteins have been isolated from demineralized bone and purified to various degrees.[53-55] These fractions have been termed Bone Morphogenetic Protein (BMP) by Urist et al.[53] Currently, much applied research is directed toward development of clinically applicable methods of utilizing DBM and osteoinductive factors to stimulate bone healing.[56,57]

Under normal circumstances of bone healing, the inflammatory phase also begins almost immediately after bone disruption and persists until significant cartilage and/or bone formation has been initiated. The exact interval is poorly defined but may last up to a week (see Figure 4). It is during this stage that a hematoma is formed attendant to local disruption of vascular supply. As in soft tissue healing, macrophages appear at this time to remove nonviable tissue. The appearance of macrophages is associated with the activation of osteoclasts and osteolytic activity. The activation of osteoclasts may be the result of elaboration of factors from macrophages, as in the case of activation of fibroblasts in soft tissue wound healing.

As with soft tissue, the presence of an implant can result in the persistence of inflammation. Depending on the relative compatibility of the implant material, this inflammation may become a chronic inflammatory foreign body response with the appearance of significant numbers of giant cells. If this material is suitably inert, the local response becomes that of quiescent inflammation with formation of a layer of organized fibrous tissue "walling off" the implant from adjacent bone.[24] If this is the case, the predominate cell type within the layer is fibroblastic with an occasional macrophage or giant cell. Analogous to soft tissue, the fibrous layer thickness, cellularity, and cell differential are all indicative of the "compatibility" of the implant material.[24] It should be noted, however, that externally applied stress and/or relative motion of an implant may also affect the local tissue response.

The phase of soft callus formation is important in the healing of bone, particularly long bone fractures (see Figure 4). It is during this phase that the fracture is actually spanned and stabilized by callus. Callus formation is achieved by a combination of appositional osteoid formation beneath the periosteum and formation of significant cartilage at the fracture site. Osteoid and cartilage proliferate and gradually begin to ossify. After 3 to 4 weeks the soft callus has sufficient rigidity to prevent gross motion of a fracture.

During the hard callus phase, the soft callus analog is gradually converted to fiber bone, and osteoclasts remain active in removing dead bone and beginning the remodeling process

Cell and Tissue Types in Fracture Healing

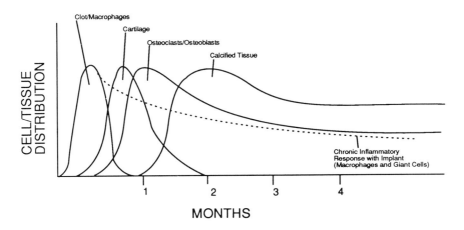

Phases of Fracture Healing

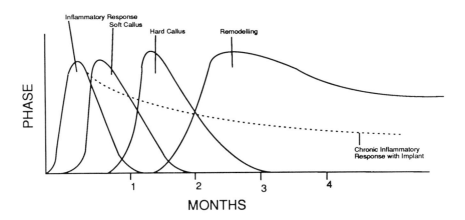

FIGURE 4. The phases of fracture healing as a function of time and the distribution of cell and tissue types as a function of time are illustrated. The inflammatory phase occurs during the first week of healing and is characterized by the presence of clot, various inflammatory cell types (neutrophils, monocytes, lymphocytes), and macrophages. The introduction of an implant can result in the persistence of inflammation in the vicinity of the implant. This inflammatory response may become chronic. The soft callus phase is characterized by the appearance of appositional osteoid and the formation of significant cartilage. After 3 to 4 weeks the soft callus begins to ossify and the stage of hard callus formation begins. The callus analog is gradually converted to fiber bone with a significant increase in osteoblastic and osteoclastic activity. Once the conversion to fiber bone is completed, the bone wound/fracture is clinically healed. For a major long bone fracture in the adult human, the time to achieve this stage may be 3 to 4 months. In the final stage of healing, fiber bone is gradually remodeled through coordinated osteoclastic and osteoblastic activity. This phase may require years.

(see Figure 4). Once the callus is converted to fiber/woven bone, the defect or fracture is clinically healed. In the adult human, the average time to achieve this stage is 3 to 4 months for a major long bone fracture.[51]

The final stage in bone healing is that of remodeling (see Figure 4). In this stage, fiber bone is gradually remodeled through coordinated osteoclastic and osteoblastic activity to lamellar bone. It is through the remodeling process that the original bony geometry is approximately restored. The guiding stimulus for remodeling is thought to be externally applied stress as originally described in "Wolff's Law".[59] The presence of an implant, in addition to potentially producing a chronic foreign body response, may induce an inappropriate remodeling response. Most structural implants are fabricated from rigid metals, with moduli at least an order of magnitude stiffer than bone. Consequently, stress states in the local vicinity of an implant may be significantly altered (reduced). This can result in loss of bone, termed "stress protection atrophy".[60] For instance, "stress protection atrophy" is thought to play a major role in loss of bone in the vicinity of bone plates and in the proximal femur with subsequent loosening of the femoral component in total hip arthroplasty. Of course, other factors affect the stability and service life of implants, notably including the chronic and acute tissue response to the implant materials.

In summary, implant survival and proper functioning in both soft and hard tissue applications requires formation of a stable implant-tissue interface by rapid migration of cells, followed by cell attachment, replication, and synthesis of appropriate connective tissue/bone components. Excessive inflammation involving polymorphonuclear and mononuclear cells ultimately leads to destruction of the interface and failure of the implant. An understanding of the role of inflammatory cells interacting with implant materials, and possibly modulating the behavior of other cell types, may be key in understanding the inherent biocompatibility of these materials.

REFERENCES

1. **Silver, F. H. and Doillon, C. J.,** *Biocompatibility: Interactions of Biological and Implantable Materials, Vol. 1, Polymers,* VCH Publishers, New York, 1989, 97.
2. **Sokoloff, L.,** *The Biology of Degenerative Joint Disease,* University of Chicago Press, Chicago, 1969, 61.
3. **Rosenberg, L.,** Biological basis for the imperfect repair of articular cartilage following injury, in *Soft and Hard Tissue Repair,* Hunt, T. K., Heppenstall, R. B., Pines, E., and Rovee, D., Praeger Press, New York, 1984.
4. **DePalma, A. F., McKeever, C. D., and Subin, D. K.,** Process of repair of articular cartilage demonstrated by histology and autoradiography with titrated thymidine, *Clin. Orthop.,* 86, 45, 1969.
5. **Fuller, J. A. and Ghadially, F. N.,** Ultrastructural observations on surgically produced partial thickness defects in articular cartilage, *Clin. Orthop.,* 86, 193, 1972.
6. **Campbell, C. J.,** The healing of cartilage defects, *Clin. Orthop. Rel. Res.,* 64, 45, 1969.
7. **Bentley, J. P.,** Rate of chondroitin sulfate formation in wound healing, *Ann. Surg.,* 165, 186, 1967.
8. **Weigel, P. H., Fuller, G. M., and LeBoeuf, R. D.,** A model for the role of hyaluronic acid and fibrin in the early events during the inflammatory response and wound healing, *J. Theoret. Biol.,* 119, 219, 1986.
9. **Mosher, D. F.,** Fibronectin, *Prog. Hemostasis Thromb.,* 5, 111, 1980.
10. **Grinnell, M. H., Billingham, R. E., and Burgess, L.,** Distribution of fibronectin during wound healing *in vivo, J. Invest. Dermatol.,* 76, 181, 1981.
11. **Jarstrand, C., Ahlgren, T., and Berghen, L.,** Fibronectin increases the motility, phagocytosis and NBT (nitroblue tetrazolium)-reduction of granulocytes, *J. Clin. Lab. Immunol.,* 8, 59, 1982.
12. **Vercellotti, G. M., McCarthy, J., Furcht, L. T., Jacob, H. S., Moldown, C. F.,** Inflamed fibronectin: an altered fibronectin enhances neutrophil adhesion, *Blood,* 62, 1063, 1983.
13. **Jankanen, M. and Penttinen, R.,** Enhanced fibroblast collagen production by a macrophage-derived factor (CEMF), *Biochem. Biophys. Res. Commun.,* 108, 447, 1982.
14. **Huybrechts-Godin, G., Peeters-Joris, C., and Vaes, G.,** Partial characterization of the macrophage factor that stimulates fibroblasts to produce collagenase and to degrade collagen, *Biochim. Biophys. Acta,* 51, 846, 1985.
15. **Pettipher, E. R., Higgs, G. A., and Henderson, B.,** Interleukin I induces leukocyte infiltration and cartilage proteoglycan degradation in the synovial joint, *Proc. Natl. Acad. Sci. U.S.A.,* 83, 8749, 1986.
16. **Richards, D. and Rutherford, R. B.,** The effects of interleukin I on collagenolytic activity and prostaglandin-E secretion by human periodontal-ligament and gingival fibroblast, *Arch. Oral Biol.,* 33, 237, 1988.

17. **Gauss-Muller, V., Kleinman, H. K., Martin, G. R., and Schiffman, E.,** Role of attachment factors and attractants in fibroblast chemotraxis, *J. Lab. Clin. Med.,* 96, 1071, 1980.
18. **Postlethwaite, A. E., Keski-oja, J., Balian, G., and Kang, A. H.,** Induction of fibroblast chemotaxis by fibronectin. Localization of the chemotactic region to a 140,000 molecular weight non-gelatin-binding fragment, *J. Exp. Med.,* 153, 494, 1981.
19. **Shuttleworth, C. A. and Forrest, L.,** Pepsin-solubilized collagen of guinea pig dermis and dermal scar, *Biochim. Biophys. Acta,* 365, 454, 1974.
20. **Stenn, K. S., Madri, J. A., and Roll, F. J.,** Migrating epidermis produces AB2 collagen and requires continued collagen synthesis for movement, *Nature,* 277, 229, 1979.
21. **Swann, D. A., Garg, H. G., Hondry, C. J., Hermann, H., Siebert, E., Sotmman, S., and Stafford, W.,** Isolation and partial characterization of dermatan sulfate proteoglycans from post-burn scar tissues, *Collagen Rel. Res.,* 8, 295, 1988.
22. **McGrath, M. H. and Emery, J. M.,** The effect of inhibition of angiogenesis in granulation tissue on wound healing and the fibroblast, *Ann. Plastic Surg.,* 15, 105, 1985.
23. **Pizzoferrato, A., Vespucci, A., Ciapetti, G., and Stea, S.,** Chemotactic behavior of macrophages under biomaterials influence, in *Techniques of Biocompatibility Testing,* Vol. 2, Williams, D. F., Ed., CRC Press, Boca Raton, FL, 1984.
24. **Black, J.,** *Orthopaedic Biomaterials in Research and Practice,* Churchill Livingstone, New York, 1988.
25. **Korn, J. H., Halushka, P. V., and LeRoy, E. C.,** Mononuclear cell modulation of connective tissue function, *J. Clin. Invest.,* 65, 543, 1980.
26. **Lord, G. H.,** Regulation and reasons for biocompatibility testing, in *Techniques of Biocompatibility Testing,* Vol. 1, Williams, D. F., Ed., CRC Press, Boca Raton, FL, 1986.
27. **Williams, D. F.,** Analysis of soft tissue response to biomaterials, in *Techniques of Biocompatibility Testing,* Vol. 1, Williams, D. F., Ed., CRC Press, Boca Raton, FL, 1984.
28. **Ten Cate, A. R. and Deporter, D. A.,** The degradative role of the fibroblast in the remodeling and turnover of collagen in soft connective tissue, *Anat. Rec.,* 182, 1, 1975.
29. **Baur, P. S., Barrat, G. F., Brown, G. M., and Parks, D. H.,** Ultrastructural evidence for the presence of "fibroblasts and myofibroclasts" in wound healing tissues, *J. Trauma,* 19, 744, 1979.
30. **Melcher, A. H. and Chan, J.,** Phagocytosis and digestion of collagen by gingival fibroblasts *in vivo:* a study of serial sections, *J. Ultrastruct. Res.,* 77, 1, 1981.
31. **McGaw, Wm. and Ten Cate, R.,** A role for collagen phagocytosis by fibroblasts in scar remodeling: an ultrastructural stereologic study, *J. Invest. Dermatol.,* 81, 375, 1983.
32. **Martinez, I. R.,** In *Epidermal Wound Healing,* Maibach, H. I. and Rovee, D. T., Eds., Year Book Publishers, Chicago, 1972, 323.
33. **Viziam, C. B., Matoltsy, A. G., and Mescon, H.,** Epithelization of small wounds, *J. Invest. Dermatol.,* 43, 499, 1964.
34. **Nishida, K. T., Nakagawa, K. S., Awata, T., Ohashi, Y., Watanste, K., and Manabe, R.,** Fibronectin promotes epithelial migration of culture rabbit cornea *in situ, J. Cell Biol.,* 97, 168, 1983.
35. **Sporn, M. B. and Robertson, A. B.,** Peptide growth factors and inflammation, tissue repair and cancer, *J. Clin. Invest.,* 78, 329, 1986.
36. **Donaldson, D. J. and Mahan, J. T.,** Keratinocyte migration and the extracellular matrix, *J. Invest. Dermatol.,* 90, 623, 1988.
37. **Ross, R. and Odland, G.,** Human wound repair. II. Inflammatory cells, epithelial mesenchymal interrelations and fibrogenesis, *J. Cell Biol.,* 39, 152, 1968.
38. **Luger, T. A. and Oppenheim, J.,** Characteristics of IL 1 and epidermal cell derived thymocytes activating factor, *Adv. Inflam. Res.,* 5, 1, 1983.
39. **Martinet, N., Harne, L. A., and Grotendorst, G. R.,** Identification and characterization of chemoattractants for epidermal cells, *J. Invest. Dermatol.,* 90, 122, 1988.
40. **Grondahl-Hansen, J., Lund, L. R., Ralfkiaer, E., Ottevanger, V., and Dano, K.,** Urokinase- and tissue-type plasminogen activators in keratinocytes during wound reepithelialization *in vivo, J. Invest. Dermatol.,* 90, 790, 1988.
41. **Morioka, S., Lazarus, G. S., Baird, J. L., and Jesse, P. J.,** Migrating keratinocytes express urokinase-type plasminogen activator, *J. Invest. Dermatol.,* 88, 418, 1987.
42. **Takashima, A. and Grinnell, F.,** Human keratinocyte adhesion and phagocytosis promoted by fibronectin, *J. Invest. Dermatol.,* 83, 352, 1984.
43. **Grinnel, F., Toda, K.-I., and Takashima, A.,** Activation of keratinocyte fibronectin receptor function during cutaneous wound healing, *J. Cell Sci.,* Suppl. 8, 199, 1987.
44. **Takashima, A., Billingham, R. E., and Grinnell, F.,** Activation of rabbit keratinocyte fibronectin receptor function *in vivo* during wound healing, *J. Invest. Dermatol.,* 86, 585, 1986.
45. **Green, H., Kehinde, O., and Thomas, J.,** Growth of cultured human epidermal cells into multiple epithelia suitable for grafting, *Proc. Natl. Acad. Sci. U.S.A.,* 76, 5665, 1979.

46. **Fourtanier, A. Y., Courty, J., Muller, E., Courbis, Y., Prurieras, M., Barritault, D.,** Eye-derived growth factor isolated from bovine retina and used for epidermal wound healing *in vivo, J. Invest. Dermatol.,* 87, 76, 1986.

47. **Eisinger, M., Sadan, S., Silver, I. A., and Flick, R. B.,** Growth regulation of skin cells by epidermal cell-derived factors: implications for wound healing, *Proc. Natl. Acad. Sci. U.S.A.,* 85, 1937, 1988.

48. **Lynch, S. E., Nixon, J. C., Colvin, R. B., and Antoniades, H. N.,** Role of platelet-derived growth factor in wound healing: synergistic effects with other growth factors, *Proc Natl. Acad. Sci. U.S.A.,* 84, 7696, 1987.

49. **McClean, F. C. and Urist, M. R.,** *Bone,* University of Chicago Press, Chicago, 1968.

50. **Ketenjian, A. Y. and Arsenis, C.,** *Clin. Orthop.,* 107, 266, 1975.

51. **Heppenstall, R. B.,** Fracture healing, in *Soft and Hard Tissue Repair,* Hunt, T. K., Heppenstall, R. B., Pines, E., and Rovee, D., Eds., Praeger Press, New York, 1984.

52. **Urist, M. R. and Strates, B. S. W.,** Bone formation in implants of partially and wholly demineralized bone matrix: including observations on acetone-fixed intra and extracellular proteins, *Clin. Orthop.,* 71, 271, 1970.

53. **Urist, M. R., Jurist, J. M., Dubuc, F., Strates, B. S.,** Quantitation of new bone formation in intramuscular implants of bone matrix in rabbits, *Clin. Orthop.,* 68, 279, 1970.

54. **Urist, M. R., Huo, Y. K., Brownell, A. G., Hohl, W. M., Buyske, J., Lietze, A., Tempst, P., Hunkapiller, M., DeLange, R. J.,** Purification of bovine bone morphogenetic protein by hydroxyapatite chromatography, *Proc. Natl. Acad. Sci. U.S.A.,* 81, 371, 1984.

55. **Sampath, T. K. and Reddi, A. H.,** Distribution of bone inductive proteins in mineralized and demineralized extracellular matrix, Biochem. Biophys. Res. *Commun.,* 119, 949, 1984.

56. **Urist, M. R. and Strates, B. S.,** Bone morphogenetic protein, *J. Dent. Res.,* 50, 1392, 1971.

57. **Glowacki, J., Kaban, L. B., Sonis, S. T., Rosenthal, R. K., and Mulliken, J. B.,** Physiological aspects of bone repair using demineralized bone, in *Soft and Hard Tissue Repair,* Hunt, T. K., Heppenstall, R. B., Pines, E., Rovee, D., Eds., Praeger Press, New York, 1984, 265.

58. **Damien, C. J., Wesiman, D. S., Benedict, J. J., Winfield, A. M., and Parsons, J. R.,** Demineralized bone matrix with and without the addition of an osteogenic factor: a comparative analysis in bone and muscle, 15th Ann. Meet. of the Society for Biomaterials, Orlando, FL, April-May, 1989.

59. **Treharne, R. W.,** Review of Wolff's Law and its proposed means of operation, *Orthop. Rev.,* 10, 35, 1981.

60. **Woo, S. L.-Y., Akeson, W. H., Coutts, R. D.,** A comparison of cortical bone atrophy secondary to fixation with plates with large differences in bending stiffness, *J. Bone Jt. Surg.,* 62A, 68, 1980.

Chapter 5

ETIOLOGY OF SCARRING AND WRINKLE FORMATION

Dale P. Devore

TABLE OF CONTENTS

I. INTRODUCTION

Skin is perhaps the most complex organ of the body and more than any other reveals changes and defects that are hidden by other organs and tissues. One of the most obvious changes during aging is the accentuation of skin wrinkling. The wrinkle is still not adequately explained and its anatomy does not appear to be different than surrounding tissues.[1] Dermal scars are visible defects that occur due to an imperfect healing process.[2] While few scars create functional disability, they are of major concern, particularly if located on the facial area. This chapter will discuss the dynamics of scar formation and attempt to provide insight on changes associated with wrinkling, especially during the aging process.

II. DYNAMICS OF SCAR FORMATION

Cutaneous wounds heal by two primary mechanisms: (1) superficial wounds affecting only the epidermis heal by simple reepithelialization; (2) wounds which penetrate the dermal layers and the subcutaneous tissue are repaired by formation of scar tissue. Scar tissue results from a series of phenomena that occur during normal wound repair. The scar itself is a normal consequence of somewhat imperfect repair mechanisms. The stages of wound repair have been described in several different ways but always include the following: a vascular phase, an inflammatory phase, formation of granulation tissue, matrix remodeling, and reepithelialization (see Chapter 4).[3] Chvapil and Koopmann[2] differentiated the stages of wound repair into: the cellular-humoral phase, the phase of glycosaminoglycan accumulation, the phase of collagen deposition and polymerization, and the phase of scar remodeling. An understanding of the processes involved in wound repair can have important implications in the treatment and eventual appearance of the scar. The development of scar tissue is outlined in Figure 1.

A. WOUND HEALING PROCESS

Injury to the skin initiates an immediate vascular response characterized by a transient period of vasoconstriction, followed by a more prolonged period of vasodilation. Blood components infiltrate the wound site, endothelial cells release, exposing fibrillar collagen, and platelets attach to these exposed sites. As platelets become activated, components are released which initiate events of the intrinsic coagulation pathway. At the same time, a complex series of events trigger the inflammatory pathways generating soluble mediators to direct subsequent stages of the healing process.

The first cells that respond are the polymorphonuclear leukocytes and macrophages. Both cell types infiltrate the wound simultaneously. The polymorphonuclear leukocyte remains for several days and is then largely replaced by the macrophage. The macrophage is key to healing dynamics, not only assisting in bacterial phagocytosis and tissue debridement, but perhaps more importantly, functioning to direct subsequent stages of the healing process. As the macrophage becomes activated, it releases proteases, growth factors, and chemotactic factors. Factors released by activated macrophages stimulate proliferation of fibroblasts and endothelial cells, and promote the formation of granulation tissue. An excellent review of growth factors in wound healing has been prepared by P. ten Dijke and K. K. Iwata.[4]

Granulation tissue is composed of inflammatory cells, fibroblasts, and new blood vessels in the matrix of collagen, glycosaminoglycans, and glycoproteins. The fibroblast is critical to the formation of granulation tissue. It produces fibrillar collagen, other matrix components, and enzymes required for remodeling of the wound. Remodeling occurs immediately and continues for months after reepithelialization. Remodeling increases tensile strength and decreases scar tissue bulk and greatly influences the final appearance of the healed scar.

The scar itself is primarily composed of collagen. Bailey et al.[5] suggest that the formation

```
INJURY TO SKIN, FULL THICKNESS
     o Release of blood components
     o Activation of coagulation cascade
     o Release of platelet factors; TGF-B, PDGF, FGF

HEMOSTASIS ACHIEVED
     o Clot becomes infiltrated with inflammatory cells
          PMN's
          Macrophages
               release TGF-B, PDGF-like mediators
               of collagen production
          Lymphocytes
               lymphokines secreted including,
               EGF, TGF-A

PREGRANULATION TISSUE
Clot containing, PMN's, macrophages, lymphocytes, some
type IV collagen
     o Fibroblasts attracted to site, possibly several
       subpopulations; synthesis of type I and type III
       collagen, fibronectin
     o Endothelial cells attracted to site, initiation
       of neovascularization
     o Epithelial cell migration, reepithelialization
       stimulated by serum and platelet factors

GRANULATION TISSUE
Containing fibroblasts, macrophages, and neovascular
in a loose network of collagen, fibronectin, and
hyaluronic acid
     o Formation of matrix
          dissolution of granulation tissue, formation
          of connective tissue
               collagen production stimulated by TGF-B,
               PDGF, FGF, EGF, and other factors

MATRIX
Disorderly collagen array, minimal tensile strength

     Remodeling of Matrix
          Loss of type III collagen, loss of fibronectin
          Old collagen replaced with new collagen

TISSUE SCAR
     o Continues to mature and reestablish equilibrium
       between synthesis and degradation of matrix
```

FIGURE 1. Development of tissue scar.

of collagen during wound repair follows the same course as in the development of embryonic skin and subsequent postnatal development. While the parallel is clear in the case of hydroxylation and cross-linking, it seems to differ in the case of collagen types. In both human infant dermis and in guinea pig dermis, type III collagen synthesis is greater than type I collagen synthesis during early phases of development. In healing wounds, type I collagen predominates throughout the healing process. Once collagen is secreted, it undergoes intramolecular and intermolecular cross-linking to form collagen fibers that polymerize and provide increase in scar tensile strength. Collagen bundles grow in bulk and organize from a random pattern to lie parallel to the skin surface.

Like normal skin, the collagen and other matrix components in the wound are constantly being remodeled. Mature scar tissue in humans shows low metabolic activity even after 20 years,[6] although the activity is generally at a lower rate than in normal skin.[7]

As mentioned previously, a scar is an imperfect substitute for the original tissue. Scars

TABLE 1
Classification of Tissue Scars

Depressed Scars
  Acne-related
    Depressed
    Ice pick
  Nonacne-related
    Dermal atrophy
    Dermal and subdermal
    Dermal with subcutaneous defect
Hypertrophic
Keloid

are imperfect in mechanical properties and in nutritional and functional characteristics. The tensile strength of scar tissue reaches only 75 to 80% of the tensile strength of normal skin[8] and scars form a barrier to normal diffusion of oxygen and nutrients.

There are various classifications of tissue scars as shown in Table 1. Acne scars are moderate, well-marginated craters or depressions. The ice pick scar is a less common acne scar variant. These scars are irregular and deep. Acne scars may develop into more serious hypertrophic or keloid scars. Nonacne-related depressed scars include scars from simple lacerations, surgical incisions, and dermal atrophy. Hypertrophic and keloids are more pronounced scars that are raised above the skin surface. These pathologic scars will be discussed in more detail.

B. PATHOLOGICAL SCARS

In the early stages of wound repair, scars have an excessive amount of matrix tissue. As remodeling occurs, the collagen fibers and matrix organize to increase tensile strength and the scar bulk diminishes. Maturation of the scar brings a balance between synthesis and degradation of collagen and matrix components. If this balance is interrupted by a slight deficiency in degradation or an increase in the rate of synthesis, the collagen content of the healing wound would be abnormally increased. This loss of control in normal wound repair could lead to the development of keloid or hypertrophic scars.

Hypertrophic scars contain excess collagenous matrix but conform to the shape of the original wound. Keloids, on the other hand, contain excessive quantities of matrix, and extend beyond the boundaries of the wound, no longer conforming to the shape of the original wound.[9]

Hypertrophic scars seem to be self-limiting and can be revised with excellent results. Keloids, however, are unsightly, and at times, painful, abnormal overreactions in wound repair. These scars provide a significant challenge to treatment and management. It is difficult to differentiate keloids from hypertrophic scars in early phases of development. With time, the keloid becomes increasingly pronounced as collagen accumulation continues. There are distinct histological differences between the keloid and hypertrophic scars. Most evident is the appearance of brightly eosinophilic collagen bundles in the keloid occurring in haphazard bundles. Morphological evaluation by Knapp et al.[10] showed that in keloids, discrete collagen fiber bundles were absent, and fibers were in poorly connected sheets in a random arrangement. Brown and Gibson[11] observed a similar arrangement in hypertrophic scars. Larson et al.[12] observed that the diameter of collagen fibers in hypertrophic scars was smaller than found in normal dermis.

1. Possible Causes of Abnormal Scar Formation

The most striking feature of both keloids and hypertrophic scars is the constant increase in collagen accumulation over long periods of time. Normal scars accumulate collagen for

TABLE 2
Possible Causes of Abnormal Scar Tissue

Subpopulations of high collagen producing fibroblasts
Excess quantities of fibroblast mitogens
Reduced collagenase activity, high levels of inhibitors or low levels of activators
Absence or reduced levels of fibroblast deactivation factors, e.g., interferons[41]

about 21 d after which collagen levels remain constant.[13] Continuing accumulation of collagen in keloids and in hypertrophic scars must result from either increased synthesis, reduced degradation, or a combination of both processes.

Several studies have demonstrated an elevated rate of collagen synthesis in hypertrophic and keloid scar tissue. Craig et al.[14] showed in organ culture, that the rate of collagen synthesis was three to four times higher than in normal scar at 6 months after injury. The rate of synthesis falls over a period of years reaching the level of a mature normal scar after 2 to 3 years in keloids and after 4 to 5 years in hypertrophic scars. Other evidence of increased collagen synthesis has been provided by Knapp et al.[10] who showed that the activity of lysyl oxidase was three times higher in keloids and hypertrophic scars than in normal tissue of the same patient. Cohen and co-workers[15] indicated that prolyl hydroxylase activity was significantly higher in keloids than in hypertrophic scars, and that activity was higher in hypertrophic scars than in skin adjacent to hypertrophic scar. Collagen synthesis in keloids was twenty times higher than in normal skin, and three times higher than in hypertrophic scars.

Studies of collagenase activity have been conducted by Cohen and co-workers[15] and by Milsom and Craig.[16] The former demonstrated that collagenase activity in keloids and hypertrophic scars was increased over that of normal skin. Keloids showed twice the activity of hypertrophic scars. The latter investigators showed that collagenase activity in keloids and hypertrophic scars, in general, was no different than in normal scars, although several specimen of keloids and hypertrophic scars showed increased collagenase activity. Based on the evidence presented above, it seems that both keloids and hypertrophic scars develop due to excessive collagen synthesis. The reason for this abnormal accumulation of fibrous tissue is still not understood. However, possible causes of such abnormal scar tissue are provided in Table 2.

Shakespeare and van Rentergham[17] suggest that the failure of epidermal cells to anchor the fibrous tissue of a healing wound may contribute to the lack of control of collagen synthesis and degradation in hypertrophic scars. Kischer[18] indicated that epidermis seems to exhibit activity in cell regulation, and Odland and Ross[19] showed that the basal cells of epidermis exhibit fibrinolytic activity.

The failure to adequately control collagen synthesis likely results from aberrant cellular regulation. Keloid fibroblasts grown in cell culture produce more collagen than normal skin fibroblasts. Uitto et al.[20] have reported an over production of type I procollagen from keloid fibroblasts. Diegelmann, et al.[21] suggest that a subpopulation of high collagen-producing fibroblasts is present in keloids. This subpopulation may become dominant due to selectivity prompted by appropriate changes in a healing wound, such as pH, oxygen tensions, or lactate levels. Selectivity for these fibroblasts may also be due to activity of specific mitogenic factors, such as FGF, EGF, etc.

Regulation of collagen biosynthesis is complex and beyond the scope of this discussion. In general, understanding of such regulation during wound repair is still primitive. Continued research on the biosynthesis of collagen will lead to a better understanding of control mechanisms in normal tissue. This knowledge will eventually lead to methods to facilitate wound repair and hopefully to retard the development of keloid and hypertrophic scars.

III. WRINKLE FORMATION

Investigations into wrinkle formation and treatment of wrinkles has generally been of great interest to the medical community. The increasing elderly population and the concern for self-image and youthfulness, as evidenced by the more than 10 billion dollars spent annually on cosmetics, has resulted in increased interest in better understanding wrinkle formation, particularly during the aging process.

A. ANATOMY OF WRINKLES

Kligman and co-workers[22] examined histological preparations of skin specimen from autopsy material and from living subjects. Specimen from living subjects included excised skin from areas of temporal frown lines, "crow's" feet, fine criss-crossed wrinkles, and crinkled skin. There were no histological differences between the wrinkles and surrounding tissues in any of the specimen. When examined by scanning electron microscopy, the three-dimensional network of the fibrous structure was identical in the wrinkle and in the surrounding tissue. These results confirmed earlier conclusions of Wright and Shellow,[23] and Montagna and Carlisle[24] who also found no histological differences between wrinkles and surrounding skin. Kligman et al.[22] concluded that wrinkles are configurational changes without specific histological alterations. Lavker et al.[25] compared the skin surface patterns of young and old subjects. In young skin, the skin surface patterns consisted of intersecting creases creating interwoven, regular geometric patterns. Protected areas of skin in older subjects were well preserved although somewhat more shallow and less angular. The formation of these patterns is not known. However, it is likely that they are magnified during aging.

B. FORMATION OF WRINKLES

Early investigators indicated that wrinkles formed as a result of atrophy of the papillary dermis and flattening of the epidermis.[26] Lorincz[27] expanded this pathology by stating that wrinkles were worsened during aging as the horny layer became more brittle, a result of reduced water binding capacity. Kligman et al.,[22] finding no chemical or architectural changes in wrinkles, attributed wrinkling to progressive failure of the elastic system to smooth out creases formed by mechanical stress on the skin. The elastic system keeps the skin tight and allows it to conform to physical deformations. Montagna and Carlisle[24] observed profound changes in the elastic network in individuals 50 years and older. The terminal elastic fiber arcades became progressively thicker and more irregular. Eventually, the entire elastic fiber system in the papillary dermis began to shrink with distal branches failing to reach the epidermis. These changes were similar, but less severe than changes noted in sun-exposed areas of skin. In these areas, large-scale changes in the elastic fibers in the papillary dermis were noted even in individuals in their late 20s and 30s. In some cases the integrity of elastic fibers was lost, the fibers forming a thick amorphous layer with no visible fine fibers.

A similar relationship between wrinkles and loss of elastic tissue was observed by Shelly and Wood.[28] They evaluated large areas of fine wrinkled skin in a woman of age 40. The most unique finding was a complete absence of elastic fibers from the mid-dermal zone of the skin. Absence of elastic tissue has been observed in postacne scars[29] in varieties of elastoses,[30] and in wrinkling.[31-32]

1. Pathology of Elastic Fibers in Aging

Recent studies have examined elastin gene expression as a function of age. Analyses indicated that levels of elastin messenger RNA remained constant to about age 45.[33] However, elastin messenger RNA levels were greatly reduced in cultures from an individual 61 years old. This result supports information showing that elastin production dramatically declines

TABLE 3
Causes of Wrinkle Formation

Degradation of elastic fiber network
Loss of functional elastic fibers due to reduced elastin production
Loss of water-binding capacity

in human skin fibroblasts from persons 70 years and older.[34] Uitto[35] suggests a decline in elastin gene expression could contribute to the loss of functional elastic fibers during aging. One result of this loss would be the accentuation of wrinkles and the development of new wrinkles.

2. Changes in Other Extracellular Matrix Components

Elastic fibers are not the only extracellular matrix component altered during aging. Smith et al.[36] reported an increase in insoluble collagen and in the total collagen and a decrease in soluble collagen. Aged collagen appears to exhibit increased cross-linking, a finding consistent with increased mechanical stability and with increased shrinkage temperature.[37]

Changes in glycosaminoglycans during cutaneous aging have also been reported. There appears to be a decrease in glycosaminoglycan content with aging,[38] particularly for hyaluronic acid.[39] Proteoglycans and hyaluronic acid are responsible for hydration of dermis via their water-binding capacity. Reduced levels of these matrix components could result in reduced dermal hydration and contribute to an increasingly rigid, less elastic skin which is more prone to exhibit wrinkling.

3. Effects of Solar Radiation on Wrinkling

Many of the manifestations of aging processes on skin wrinkling are accentuated by exposure to solar radiation. As discussed above, the elastic fiber system undergoes extensive degradation when skin is exposed to solar radiation. The integrity of the elastic fiber is lost and increasing masses of very thick and irregular fiber structures are noted. Lavker et al.[25] found that skin surface patterns were markedly altered when skin of older individuals was exposed to solar radiation. There was only minimal alteration of skin surface patterns in unexposed areas of the same individuals. The manifestations of exposure to solar radiation was recently reviewed by Gilchrest.[40] Clinical, and recent histological findings, show that photoaging is responsible for most unwanted age-associated changes in the skin, such as coarseness and wrinkling. As was discussed previously, the most detrimental effect of photoaging was the damage to elastic fibers as evidenced by thickened, irregular, amorphous elastic fibers.

Likely causes of wrinkle formation are shown in Table 3. Wrinkling of skin is an inevitable manifestation of aging which can be significantly accelerated by continuous exposure to solar radiation. Anatomical examination has failed to clearly distinguish wrinkled skin from surrounding nonwrinkled tissue. However, recent histological and biochemical analysis have shown significant deterioration of the elastic fiber network and a progressive decrease in collagen solubility in aging skin. Aging skin is characterized by wrinkling and increased coarseness. It appears that wrinkle development occurs as skin loses its ability to recover from mechanical stress.

REFERENCES

1. **Kligman, A. M. and Balin, A. K.,** Aging of human skin, in *Aging and The Skin,* Balin, A. K. and Kligman, A. M., Eds., Raven Press, New York, 1989, 1.
2. **Chvapil, M. and Koopmann, C. F., Jr.,** Scar formation: Physiology and pathological states, *Otolaryngol. Clin. North Am.,* 17, 265, 1984.
3. **Goslen, J. B.,** Physiology of wound healing and scar formation, in *Facial Scars-Incision, Revision, and Camouflage,* Thomas, J. R. and Holt, G. R., Eds., C. V. Mosby, St. Louis, 1989, 10.
4. **ten Dijke, P. and Iwata, K. K.,** Growth factors for wound healing, *Biotechnology,* 7, 793, 1989.
5. **Bailey, A. J., Brazin, S., Sims, T. J., Lelous, M., Nicoletis, C., and Delauny, A.,** Characterization of the collagen of human hypertrophic and normal scars, *Biochim. Biophys. Acta,* 405, 412, 1975.
6. **Jackson, D. S.,** Dermal scar, in *Collagen in Health and Disease,* Weiss, J. B. and Jayson, M. I. V., Eds., Churchill Livingstone, Edinburgh, 1982, 446.
7. **Craig, R. D. P., Shofield, J. D., and Jackson, D. S.,** Collagen biosynthesis in normal and hypertrophic scars and keloid as a function of the duration of the scar, *Br. J. Surg.,* 62, 741, 1975.
8. **Levenson, S. M., Geever, E. G., and Crawley, L. V.,** The healing of rat skin wounds, *Ann. Surg.,* 161, 293, 1965.
9. **Peacock, E. E., Madden, J. W., Jr., and Trier, W. C.,** Biologic basis for the treatment of keloids and hypertrophic scars, *South. Med. J.,* 63, 755, 1970.
10. **Knapp, T. R., Daniels, J. R., and Kaplan, E. N.,** Pathological scar formation. Morphologic and biochemical correlates, *Am. J. Pathol.,* 86, 47, 1977.
11. **Brown, I. A. and Gibson, T.,** Pathological aspects of wound healing, in *Wound Healing,* Gibson, T. and van der Muelen, J. C., Eds., Foundation International Cooperation in Medical Sciences, Rotterdam, The Netherlands, 1975, 134.
12. **Larson, D. L., Linares, H. A., Baur, P., Willis, B., Abston, S., and Lewis, S. R.,** Pathological aspects of skin healing in burns, in *Wound Healing,* Gibson, T. and van der Meulen, J. C., Eds., Foundation International Cooperation in Medical Sciences, Rotterdam, The Netherlands, 1975, 122.
13. **Madden, J. W. and Peacock, E. S.,** Studies on the biology of collagen during wound healing. III. Dynamic metabolism of scar collagen and remodeling of dermal wounds, *Ann. Surg.,* 174, 511, 1971.
14. **Craig, R. D. P., Schofield, J. D., and Jackson, D. S.,** Collagen biosynthesis in normal skin, normal hypertrophic scar and keloid, *Eur. J. Clin. Invest.,* 5, 69, 1975.
15. **Cohen, I. K., Keiser, H. R., and Sjoerdsman, A.,** Collagen synthesis in human keloid and hypertrophic scar, *Surg. Forum,* 22, 488, 1971.
16. **Milson, J. P. and Craig, R. D. P.,** Collagen degradation in cultured keloid and hypertrophic scar tissue, *Br. J. Dermatol.,* 89, 635, 1973.
17. **Shakespeare, P. G. and van Renterghem, L.,** Some observations on the surface structure of collagen in hypertrophic scars, *Burns,* 11, 175, 1985.
18. **Kischer, C. W.,** Fine structure of granulation tissue from deep injury, *J. Invest. Dermatol.,* 72, 147, 1979.
19. **Odland, G. and Ross, R.,** Human wound repair. I. Epidermal regeneration, *J. Cell Biol.,* 39, 135, 1968.
20. **Uitto, J., Perejda, A. J., Abergel, R. P., Chu, M. L., and Ramirez, R.,** Altered steady-state ratio of Type I/III procollagen mRNA's correlates with selectively increased Type I procollagen biosynthesis in cultured keloid fibroblasts, *Proc. Natl. Acad. Sci. U.S.A.,* 82, 5935, 1985.
21. **Diegelmann, R. F., Linbald, W. J., and Cohen, I. K.,** Fibrogenic process during tissue repair, in *Collagen, Vol. II, Biochemistry and Biomechanics,* Nimni, M. E., Ed., CRC Press, Boca Raton, FL, 1988, 113.
22. **Kligman, A. M., Zheng, P., and Lavker, R. M.,** The anatomy and pathogenesis of wrinkles, *Br. J. Dermatol.,* 113, 37, 1985.
23. **Wright, E. T. and Shelow, L. R.,** The histopathology of wrinkles, *J. Soc. Cosmet. Chem.,* 24, 81, 1965.
24. **Montagna, W. and Carlisle, K.,** Structural changes in aging human skin, *J. Invest. Dermatol.,* 73, 47, 1979.
25. **Lavker, R. M., Kwong, F., and Kligman, A. M.,** Changes in skin surface patterns with age, *J. Gerontol.,* 35, 348, 1989.
26. **Wells, G. C.,** Senile changes of the skin, *J. Am. Gerontol. Soc.,* 2, 535, 1954.
27. **Lorincz, A. L.,** The physiology of aging skin, *Ill. Med. J.,* 117, 59, 1960.
28. **Shelley, W. B. and Wood, M. G.,** Wrinkles due to idiopathic loss of mid-dermal elastic tissue, *Br. J. Dermatol.,* 97, 441, 1977.
29. **Dick, G. F., Ashe, B. M., Rodgers, E. G., Diercks, R. C., and Goltz, R. W.,** Study of elastolytic activity of *Propionibacterium acnes* and *Staphilococcus epidermidis* in acne vulgaris and in normal skin, *Acta Derm. Venereol.,* 56, 279, 1976.
30. **Jarrett, A.,** The elastic tissue of the dermis, in *The Physiology and Pathophysiology of the Skin,* Jarrett, A., Ed., Academic Press, New York, 1974, 973.
31. **Ross, R. and Bornstein, P.,** Elastic fibers in the body, *Sci. Am.,* 224, 44, 1971.

32. **Montagna, W. and Parakkal, P. F.,** *The Structure and Function of Skin,* Academic Press, New York, 1974, 108.
33. **Fazio, M. J., Olsen, D. R., and Kuivaniemi, H.,,** Isolation and characterization of human elastin cDNAs, and age-associated variation in elastin gene expression in cultured skin fibroblasts, *Lab. Invest.,* 58, 270, 1988.
34. **Sephel, G., Buckley, A., and Davidson, J. M.,** Development initiation of elastin gene expression by human fetal skin fibroblasts, *J. Invest. Dermatol.,* 88, 732, 1987.
35. **Uitto, J., Fazio, M. J., and Olsen, D. R.,** Molecular mechanisms of cutaneous aging, *J. Am. Acad. Dermatol.,* 21, 614, 1989.
36. **Smith, J. G., Jr., Davidson, E. A., Sams, W. M., Jr., and Clark, R. D.,** Alteration in human dermal connective tissue with age and chronic sun damage, *J. Invest. Dermatol.,* 39, 347, 1962.
37. **Bentley, J. D.,** Aging of collagen, *J. Invest. Dermatol.,* 73, 80, 1979.
38. **Clausen, B.,** Influence of age on chondroitin sulfates and collagen of human aorta, myocardiun, and skin, *Lab. Invest.,* 12, 538, 1963.
39. **Fleischmajer, R., Perlish, J. S., and Bashey, R. I.,** Human dermal glycosaminoglycans and aging, *Biochim. Biophys. Acta,* 279, 265, 1972.
40. **Gilchrest, B. A.,** Skin aging and photoaging: an overview, *J. Am. Acad. Dermatol.,* 21, 610, 1989.
41. **Berman, B. and Duncan, M. R.,** Short-term keloid treatment *in vivo* with human interferon alpha-2b results in a selective and persistent normalization of keloid fibroblast collagen, glycosaminoglycan, and collagenase production *in vitro, J. Am. Acad. Dermatol.,* 21, 694, 1989.

Chapter 6

PHYSICAL CHARACTERISTICS AND BIOCOMPATIBILITY OF IMPLANT MATERIALS

G. Richard Holt

TABLE OF CONTENTS

I. INTRODUCTION

Before an implant can be applied to clinical utilization, there must be a great deal of preliminary work involved to properly characterize the properties of the material and to test its biological performance under *in vitro* and *in vivo* conditions. The field of implant technology has rapidly enlarged, both in the sophistication of the techniques of material assays and in the knowledge of the host tissue response to a given material to be used as a human implant. The result of this expanded interest is a wider and more complex armamentarium of soft tissue and bone for utilization in facial plastic and reconstructive surgery.

The contributors to this field include a wide variety of scientists, engineers, and clinicians, including specialists in clinical medicine and dentistry, chemistry and chemical engineering, biomaterials science and processing, biomedical engineering, and pathology. Indeed, a multidisciplinary approach is often necessary to research, test, and apply current technology to a given clinical need. It is this camaraderie that makes biomaterials applied research so interesting and rewarding.

II. CHARACTERIZATION OF BIOMATERIALS

The characteristics of the bulk material are very important when properly applied to the need of the implant. It must be remembered that the bulk characteristics of a material may differ from the actual surface characteristics that are present at the tissue-implant interface. This difference is due to the alteration of the surface by design or by natural reaction to cause the formation of a slightly different exterior material. However, the primary or first characterization of importance is to describe the material in terms of composition, strength, biodegradability, mechanical analyses, and fatigue.

A. METALLIC IMPLANTS

Metallic devices may be composed of ''pure'' metal or, more commonly, may be an alloy of several metals (Table 1). An alloy is developed to improve the bulk qualities of the pure base metal by adding certain other metals whose properties help achieve a more successful biocompatibility or better mechanical properties. The most commonly used metals in facial implants include titanium, stainless steel, and tantalum with other metals such as chromium, aluminum, cobalt, copper, nickel, and tungsten included in alloys to improve their properties and/or behavior.

Metals are crystalline materials with a well-defined and orderly three-dimensional arrangement of their atoms and molecules. Most metals have a basic cubic or hexagonal shape seen at the electron microscopic level to form a lattice structure which is characteristic of the metal. The lattice structure can be changed to some degree by heating, cooling, hardening, or deformation—all planned to achieve a better change in the physical properties of the metal to achieve a certain result. Natural defects in the lattice structure exist and may lead to changes in the properties of the metal by substitution of other atoms to form alloys. Large structural defects can lead to permanent deformation of a metal and its failure to hold up under external stresses.

Metallurgic evaluations are carried out on materials in a very uniform and consistent fashion in order to generate comparative information on various metals. Common tests utilized to characterize a metallic biomaterial include: elastic modulus, tensile strength, percent of elongation, compressive strength, shear strength and modulus, and strain. Engineering stress represents the material's ability to handle a given load per cross-sectioned area and is particularly important to match with the loading characteristics of dental and other maxillofacial implant needs. Stress vs. strain curves are generated experimentally for these implant materials and yield the properties of the bulk material itself regardless of its

TABLE 1
Biomaterials as Facial Implants

Category	Biomaterial	Clinical application
Metals and metallic alloys	Stainless steel	Mandibular joint prostheses
	Cobalt alloys	Fracture fixation plates and screws
	Pure titanium and titanium alloys	Mandibular bone trays
	Platinum-iridium	Cranioplasty
	Gold	Implantable electrodes
		Eyelid implants
		Osseointegrated implants
Polymers	Polymethylmethacrylate (PMMA)	Cranioplasty
	Silicone elastomers	Bone cements and tissue adhesives
	Polytetrafluoroethylene (Teflon)	Intraocular lenses
	GORE-TEX®	Blood vessel prostheses
	Polyurethanes	Artificial skin
	Polycarbonates	Soft-tissue augmentation
	Dacron	Joint prosthesis coatings
Ceramics	Bioglass	Middle ear ossicular replacements
	Hydroxyapatite	Joint prosthesis coatings
	Aluminum oxide	Cranioplasty
		Mandibular bone replacement
		Artificial ocular prostheses
Biological materials	Polyglycolic acid	Sutures
	Polylactic acid	Timed-release drug delivery systems
	Collagen	Dermal augmentation
	Freeze-dried bone and cartilage	Artificial skin
		Bone and cartilage augmentation

shape or thickness. It is important to use these data to predict, prior to *in vivo* testing, what the response of the material will be to the many mechanical forces which will be placed on the implant by its use and positioning in the host tissues. Thus, the forces of shear, compression, tension, torsion, and bending, all must be known before selecting the appropriate material to function as an implant under those conditions. It is also important to perform long-term *in vitro* loading studies to determine the response of a material to chronic wear, over a long time period of potential implantation. Most metals will undergo "relaxation" with time which may also lead to "fatigue" and failure of the implant with chronic loading. A more brittle metal such as stainless steel may wear well initially but can undergo fatigue failure with long-term implantation. Additionally, all metals undergo some form of corrosion when exposed to the physiologic fluid environment of the recipient tissues, and this action will lead to chronic failure in many metals. Stainless steel is quite resistant to corrosion due to the presence of many other elements in its alloy composition, such as chromium, nickel, molybdenum, and manganese, in addition to its iron base. However, this also leads to a material that can undergo plastic deformation with time.

Titanium and its alloys are generally held to be among the most biocompatible metallic implants utilized today. Titanium is lightweight, very resistant to corrosion, and has demonstrated a high degree of tissue acceptance in long-term implantations (Figures 1 and 2). Commercially pure titanium appears to have a better biocompatibility than the most commonly used alloy Ti-6A1-4V (89% titanium, 6% aluminum, 4% vanadium). Titanium is a rather soft metal, and if not anchored in bone, can be deformed by external loading forces. When used in mandibular reconstruction and as anchoring screws for bony facial applications, its long term response to implantation is excellent.

Tantalum and vanadium have both been used in the past for mandibular reconstruction as bone trays, but both have inferior mechanical properties when compared to titanium. Their strength is low and they may fatigue rapidly, thus necessitating their removal after

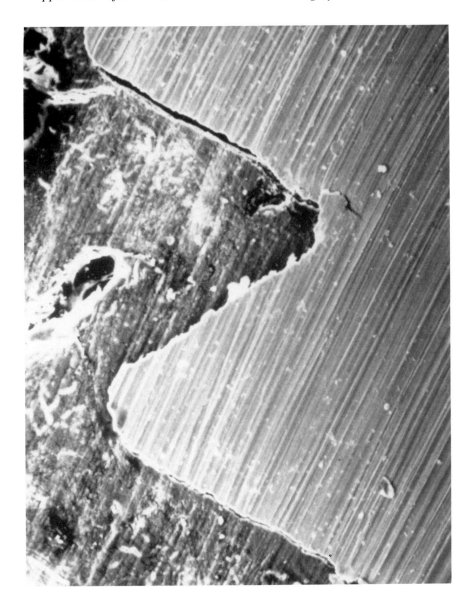

FIGURE 1.   High power SEM (magnification × 160,000) demonstrating a close approximation of trabecular bone to the titanium implant surface. There is some ordered collagen fibers and a ground substance matrix between the implant and bone over a small surface contact area.

mandibular healing has occurred. Because of their mechanical properties, some metallic implants, such as stainless steel, may have a better stress response than the surrounding bone; this can lead to stress-shielding of the bone, a condition not conducive to allowing the natural bone kinetics to occur during new bone formation. Thus, the metal implants may need to be removed after they have performed their stabilizing task so that the proper bone growth and development may occur.

B. CERAMICS

Like metals, ceramics have a lattice-structure microscopically. These ceramics are called oxide or special ceramics. Glasses, on the other hand, have an amorphous structure which is much less ordered on the atomic level. Most biological implants are glass ceramics which

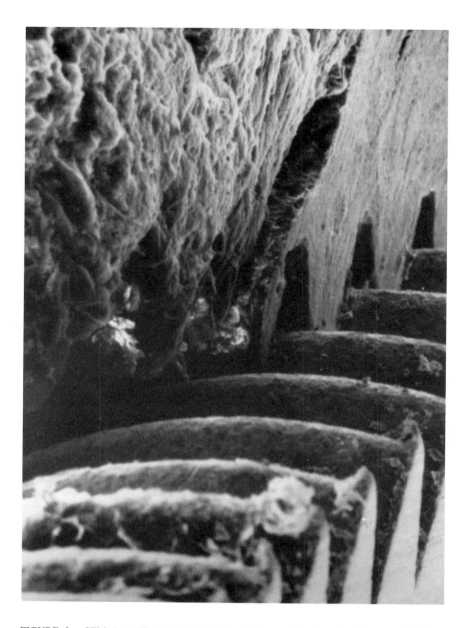

FIGURE 2. SEM (magnification × 80,000) with tangential view showing remodeled bone conforming to the configuration of the titanium implant threads. Some gap between bone and implant is due to preparation artifact as well as a small layer of adsorbed proteins.

are composed of the base element of silica, SiO_2, and other crystalline materials embedded in the noncrystalline glass. These glass ceramics are very thermal-resistant and can be utilized where thermal shock could occur. In general, the longevity of glass ceramics in the body is good—they are well tolerated and quite biocompatible. However, because of the peculiar grain size and distribution they are very susceptible to crack propagation due to stress concentration. Clinically, this is seen as a ''brittle'' material which will not bend but will fracture with stress and strain forces. This property limits their use in the head and neck region to areas where force loading is minimized, such as an ossicular implant. They are also used in dental implants as alumina compounds. Here, the implant has been designed so that the shape facilitates the application of biomechanical stresses without undue fracture.

Another form of a ceramic is the bioreactive ceramic compound, hydroxyapatite. This material, initially a powder form which is constituted into a paste for dental and intraosseous replacement, is marketed as a resorbable osteogenic bone-densifying implant material. Because it is composed of elements found in the ground substance of bone (calcium, phosphorus), it is capable of providing a substrate upon which osteoneogenesis can occur, if the tissues are capable. Its use as a load-bearing preformed device is still under clinical investigation.

C. POLYMERS

While ceramics and metals have, in general, a stronger stress-strain capability than human bone, polymers are more flexible and thus weaker. In fact, none of the man-made implant materials to date can exactly reproduce the biomechanical properties of bone. However, polymers still have a growing place in human implantation, partly due to the fact that varying their synthesis can result in widely diverse mechanical properties. This is due to the fact that the properties of polymers are related to their structural and chemical composition, which in turn is due to the length and type of the polymerization process and their cross-linking to form higher molecular weight polymers. This allows a wide range of polymer properties, from soft and weak to hard and brittle. For the implant scientist, a polymer can thus be chosen which provides the necessary characteristics for the job required. Because the polymer industry is large and diverse in the United States, much knowledge and technology is available for application to medical devices. The most commonly used medical polymers include the polyurethanes, silicones, and polymethyl methacrylate. These polymers possess properties of reasonable strength and good biocompatibility. When used as porous fibers, as in polytetrafluoroethylene (Teflon®), nylon, polylactide and polyglycolide (sutures), their properties allow for weaving and suture production. Expanded PTFE (GORE-TEX®) has excellent biocompatibility when woven into patches for soft-tissue augmentation or vascular repair.

For the most part, except for suture materials, the mechanical stresses placed on polymer implants are small and nonchronic. When used as a mandibular replacement device (Nylon), the polymer must be tested for the same mechanical tolerances as metals, including tensile strength, modulus of elasticity, stress, and strain. Impact testing can also be used if the material (such as methyl methacrylate) is to be used as a cortical bone replacement device in the skull. Internal defects during molding and processing should be investigated for quality control and to prevent the build-up of internal stresses over time and subsequent cracking with device failure. Polymers can be manufactured either by thermoplastic molding, where the material is formed in the heat-softened state in a mold; or by thermosetting, where the insoluble polymers are cured by cross-linking. Suture material is formed by extrusion of the polymer through small holes, producing a fiber that is elongated and thinned to the proper diameter before cooling.

III. SURFACE PROPERTIES OF BIOMATERIALS

As mentioned in the previous section, the surface of the prepared implant may have a very different microscopic and macroscopic appearance and reactivity than the bulk material. Titanium, for example, forms a layer of titanium oxide on its surface immediately after machining when exposed to air. This layer, approximately 100 Å thick, acts like a ceramic and helps produce its excellent tissue biocompatibility. In fact, the titanium oxide layer continues to slowly thicken over time of implantation in the tissues.

Various methods of surface texturing are being applied to implants in an attempt to improve the implant's stability. For example, creating ridges or pores on the surface by "etching" or "sputtering" the surfaces gives small areas of surface relief of about 500 μm. There appears to be a critical size to the surface relief characteristics, for if the size is too small, there is ineffective surface area for matrix adsorption; with larger pore sizes, there will be "dead space" areas not filled with matrix for cell adhesion.

Surface contamination of an implant which occurs during handling or processing can adversely affect the tissue biocompatibility. For this reason, the surface must be analyzed prior to implantation or after any failure of implantation to determine what type of contamination may have contributed to the implant failure. Proper preparation of the surface, especially with radio frequency glow-discharge cleaning cannot only clear the implant surface of unwanted particles and chemicals, it can also increase the free surface energy, thus exposing more ionic groups which facilitate initial protein adsorption upon contact with the tissues, and subsequent formation of a substrate for cellular attachment.

It is thus important to study the surface characteristics of biomaterials for a number of reasons. First and foremost, the implant in surface-tissue interface is the most important relationship in the biocompatibility of a biomaterial *in vivo*. The fate of the implant will depend upon the events and processes that take place on, or adjacent to, its surface. Additionally, it is the collective properties of the surface which determine what type of host reaction will occur. Second, it allows an investigation of the correlation between surface properties and cellular reaction to it. Third, it is often characteristic of biomaterials that the surface properties will be different from the bulk internal material properties. Knowledge of the surface also allows one to understand why a given biomaterial behaves in a certain way.

Surface analysis also provides a means of quality control over the material processing, handling, and preparation prior to implantation. A problem with any of these processes could lead to implant failure or morbidity and mortality to the host. Proper attention to Good Laboratory Practices and Standards is mandatory in both experimental and clinical investigations. Surface analysis of the biomaterials is one parameter to gauge the quality control on these practices.

Not all of the techniques of surface analysis will necessarily be applicable to every biomaterial. Judicious selection of the appropriate technique is warranted to achieve the goal of demonstrating fitness and suitability of particular biomaterials for their intended functions. Without knowledge of the actual surface properties of implanted materials as they present themselves *in vivo*, there can be no confidence in the interpretation of the results of clinical or experimental trials or of the reason for success or failure. In summary, surface analysis methods are valuable in gaining knowledge of biomaterials in:

1. Unknown identification
2. Detection of surface contamination
3. Quality assurance
4. Assurance of reproducibility, and correlation of surface property and tissue response

Several techniques are commonly used to characterize the surface of an implant.

A. ELECTRON SPECTROSCOPY FOR CHEMICAL ANALYSIS (ESCA)

ESCA has the potential to provide more useful information than other surface analysis techniques because of its high information content, its strong surface localization, and its high technology. ESCA is also known as X-ray photoelectric spectroscopy because of the emission of low energy X-rays during the experiment. The outer 10 to 20 atomic layers of the surface are characteristically the sources of the photoemission peaks being assayed, and thus the ESCA can "view" the outer 100 Å of the surface, taking into account the binding energy and peak shape, and the intensity of the signal. It is helpful in providing the following information about a surface:

- Surface elements
- Oxidation states for most atoms

- Surface charge and electrical binding
- Nondestructive depth profiling
- Identification of specific organic surface groups

B. STATIC SECONDARY ION MASS SPECTROSCOPY (SIMS)

SIMS is a surface analysis technique that is capable of providing detailed chemical information on the biomaterial's surface. Its probe size determines that area of analysis more accurately than most other methods because ion scattering effects are negligible. Since there is a high signal to background ratio with SIMS, it is excellent for faster element mapping and spatial resolution. The sampling depth for static SIMS is approximately 10 Å. Thus, from the characteristic mass pattern on the spectroscopy recording, the structural units of organic surface contamination can often be made.

C. AUGER ELECTRON SPECTROSCOPY (AES)

AES can provide information on the composition-depth profiles of surface, particularly on thin fibrous and surface coatings—a very helpful technique for industry. By scanning with AES, areas of stains and contaminations can be identified before performing a surface analysis of a biomaterial. Because of its ability to extend its depth of analysis to 2000 Å of material surface thickness, AES can provide composition information at a greater depth than SIMS. It is a highly quantifiable technique and has a narrow range of sensitivities. On the negative side, the electron beam can occasionally cause surface damage and subsequent data artifact. This technique is used primarily for elemental surface analysis.

D. SCANNING ELECTRON MICROSCOPY (SEM)

SEM is capable of providing a great deal of information about the surface of an implant as well as the implant-tissue interface for *in vivo* studies from explantation. Most SEM units are also equipped with energy dispersion X-ray analyzers that permit nondestructive elemental analysis of the material being studied. SEM can identify surface tears, defects, or inclusions, as well as confirm the presence or absence of bacteria on the sample's surface. When used in conjunction with light microscopy, SEM is useful in evaluating the surface texture of the implant. Damage to the sample is avoided with SEM so it is a nondestructive surface evaluation technique.

It is very important to utilize surface analysis techniques in the evaluation of implantable devices so as to be absolutely certain of the surface chemistry, charge, reactivity, and contamination of a biomaterial prior to implantation. All investigators and clinicians in this field have a moral obligation to the patient to utilize only those implants that have been well characterized and meet high standards of surface suitability. This cannot in itself ensure excellent biocompatibility, but it will lessen the chance for an adverse reaction which might lead to injury to the recipient host.

IV. BIOCOMPATIBILITY

In general, cells do not adhere directly to the surface of a synthetic (nonbiological) implanted material. Some substance, normally present in the extracellular matrix, serves as a substrate upon which to bind the cell and surface together. A substrate is not only important in initial cell adhesion, but also for the later proliferation and spreading of the cell population. The type of substrate required for cell adhesion varies with the type of cell; differentiated cells such as chondroblasts, osteoblasts, and epithelial cells utilize a different substrate than fibroblasts, which are less well differentiated.

Many cells form tight adhesions to the substrate surface, known as focal contacts. Focal contacts occur typically in cells of low motility, such as fibroblasts and epithelial cells. The composition of the substrate or the adsorbed layer of protein on the material's surface is crucial for the development of these tight cellular adhesions. Such proteins as fibronectin, vitronectin, and cold insoluble globulin (which may be the circulating form of fibronectin), and possibly proteoglycans, provide the necessary substratum for this attachment. Thus, focal contacts represent sites of adhesion to specific extracellular matrix (ECM) proteins that have been adsorbed onto the implant surface. The ECM contains collagen, elastin and fibronectin, interwoven into a hydrated substance formed by a network of glycoaminoglycan (GAG) chains. The GAGs are a heterogeneous group of long, negatively charged polysaccharide chains that link proteins to form giant proteoglycan molecules. An interaction with a cell membrane receptor provides the linkage for a cellular attachment to an adsorbed ECM on a biomaterial surface. Thus, the tissue cells do not adhere directly to an implant surface, but rather via a complex series of protein attachments.

Adsorption of proteins at the implant-tissue surface is inevitable. Possible explanations for this spontaneous activity include: (1) adsorption lowers the surface free energy; (2) the amphipathic character of the protein molecules with their polar/nonpolar ambivalence; and (3) the macromolecular nature of proteins and their associated limits on solubility may cause their adsorption. The protein molecules themselves have certain surface characteristics that are pertinent to causing a driving force toward protein adsorption onto an implant surface: negative and positive charges, hydrophobic domains, and charge transfer, or aromatic side chains, all of which are available for interaction with the surface. There appear to be four types of interactions which may be the driving forces for protein adsorption to biomaterial surfaces:

1. Hydrophobic interactions
2. Electrostatic bonding
3. Hydrogen bonding
4. Charge transfer

When implants are placed in the soft tissues of the facial region, the primary tissue reaction includes protein adsorption and subsequent cellular attachment. The predominant cell that attaches to the protein layer in this situation is the fibroblast. Within the first week of implantation, the fibroblast lays down immature collagen, either on the surface of the implant, or in the interstices, if the implant is porous. Thus, with few exceptions, the uniform response to a soft tissue implant is the production of a fibrous capsule or ingrowth of collagen fibers to secure the implant in position. A smooth implant such as silicone is more likely to elicit a dense ''capsule'' formation than a porous one because of the failure to develop invading fibrous bonds which secure it in place. If an implant is too highly reactive, has surface contamination, or is biodegradable, then the host-tissue response is likely to be one of high macrophage activity, increased vascularity, breakdown of the implant and overlying skin, and subsequent extrusion. Thus, the appearance of inflammatory cells (neutrophils, macrophages) appear to herald a ''poor'' biological response to the material.

When an implant is placed in bone, it is also generally held that protein adsorption is the first significant event to occur when blood comes in contact with it. Normally, the gap between implant and bone is small *in vivo,* with a tolerance of less than 100 μm. When the hole is drilled into the bone to receive the implant, care must be taken not to excessively heat the bone above 45° to 50°C as this may be the critical temperature at which osteoblasts will die.

Once in the bone, the implant is subjected to a rapid host response. The first stage of healing is characterized by the formation of a small hematoma and a circulatory change due to the liberation of a cascade of chemical breakdown products which, functioning as mediators, act on the blood vessels and attract cells from the blood and surrounding tissues. Because cortical bone is very avascular, the majority of blood products come from the endosseous or marrow-containing space of the bone. As the gap between the implant and the bone tissue should be narrow in this type of surgical implantation, this space limits the amount of hematoma formation.

The second stage of bony repair around an implant is characterized by organization tissue, regeneration, and repair. The duration and number of processes involved are related to the amount of damage and the geometry of the implantation site.

The multitude of the extracellular products and processes as well as the occurrence and function of cells in the implantation bed can be affected by soluble chemical products (ions), soluble or insoluble particles derived from the implant as well as by the biomechanical influence of the implant itself. The surface of the implant as it penetrates the bone can be in contact with both osteoid (nonmineralized) and lamellar (mineralized) bone.

The third stage of repair comprises remodeling mechanisms, involving the interface between implant and tissue, and occurs over weeks to months. It is at this time that stress shielding of the surrounding bone should not occur due to the implant, so that proper stresses can be transmitted to the bone immediately adjacent to the implant. Bone-binding intensity can be measured by the shear or torque forces required to produce failure. It is assumed that bone is the main contributor toward tensile strength of bonding and that other tissues are less important. The area of bone at the interface can be used for the calculation of bone specific tensile strength and determined in N/mm^2 or MPa.

The basal lamina in contract with a bone implant contains type IV collagen, laminin, and proteoglycans. These constituents of the ground substance are deposited in, or adjacent to, the mineralized layer. Mineralization of the ground substance seems to be important for transmission of compression as well as for sheer and tensile loads.

An implant cannot with certainty be regarded as biocompatible unless there is experimental, histologic evidence in animal studies or in removed clinical implants of an overall direct bone-implant contact. The histologic examination provides the best evidence of the type of implant attachment. Examination at the light microscopic level answers the most important questions of the interfacial arrangements; namely, whether most of the implant surface is in direct bone contact. A properly integrated implant at the cortex should have a minimal direct bone contract of 90 to 95% of the implant's surface. This high degree of bone integration should completely surround the circumference of a cylindrical implant.

Electron microscopy of the intact bone-to-metal interface is a complicated procedure. Because of the different moduli of elasticity between the bulk metal and the tissues, *in vivo* sections have resulted in accidental splitting of the interface, with the possibility that interfacial tissue is removed in the sectioning procedure. Because of this difficulty, techniques have been developed to remove the implant from the bone with a sufficient core of bone around it to leave the interface intact. Under those conditions, scanning electron microscopy and transmission electron microscopy can be performed after proper specimen preparation.

A characteristic finding in a failed implant is the interposition of fibrous tissue between the proteoglycans layer and the endosteal bone. The width of this connective tissue layer may be as great as 10^6 Å and may have a large space of disordered bone between it and the normal-appearing Haversian bone. This in-growth of connective tissue has the disadvantage of weakening the prosthetic attachment and allowing macromotion at the bone implant interface. While micromotion is helpful in bone remodeling, the larger excursions of the implant after loading will result in its loosening and extrusion. While the proteoglycans monolayer is quite important, it loses its advantage when connective tissue is interposed between it and the bone.

By far the greatest success with osseous biocompatibility to date has been achieved with the Branemark titanium osseointegration techniques. For the successful achievement of osseointegration, the pioneers have addressed six important parameters which influence the interaction between the implant and the tissue host. They are

1. Material biocompatibility
2. Implant design (macrostructure)
3. Implant surface (microstructure)
4. Status of the implant bed
5. Surgical techniques
6. Loading conditions

The proper attention to the above aspects of implant technology and technique epitomizes the high degree of success which can be achieved with implants in general and bone implants in particular.

V. SUMMARY

The biocompatibility of an implantable material is a complex and multifaceted topic. Early research and characterization of the mechanical properties of the bulk material will allow the proper selection of the material for the clinical need or application. Then, the surface properties must be analyzed to ensure that the implantable material will be as free as possible from surface contaminants which could adversely affect the host tissue response. Additionally, the surface chemistry of the implant must be identified to better understand the atomic and molecular-level physics which occur at the implant-tissue interface. It is known that cells do not adhere directly to an implant but rather through a protein matrix interface. Alterations of this chemistry can lead to failure of the implant.

Following the *in vitro* biomaterials testing and fabrication comes the period of biological testing. Here an animal model is usually chosen for the initial research, based on anatomic and physiologic rationale. Toxicology and tissue reaction studies are performed on implanted and explanted devices until the process has been well characterized, and safety and efficacy ensured. Application is then made to the U.S. Food and Drug Administration for clinical implant device trials and a human study, approved by an Institutional Review Board, is conducted. Following satisfactory completion of the study, the device is approved for human use and manufacturing.

While the above summary seems clear, it is by no means easy to develop an implant satisfactorily to the point of human use. It is a very long and tedious process, which is often quite costly, and one which may not lead to fruition. However, because of the need for extreme safety in implanting devices into human patients, it is a necessary one and will protect our patients from unnecessary harm. The successful development of a biocompatible device is a reflection of the best efforts in research, clinical medicine, and dentistry, and can lead to a satisfying improvement of the quality of life for our patients.

REFERENCES

BULK CHARACTERIZATION

1. **Hayashi, K.,** Mechanical properties of biomaterials: Relationship to clinical applications, in *Contemporary Biomaterials,* by Boretos, J. W. and Eden, M., Eds., Noyes Publishing, Park Ridge, NJ, 1984, 46.
2. **Hench, L. L. and Ethridge, E. C.,** Polymers and plastics, in *Biomaterials: An Interfacial Approach,* Academic Press, New York, 1982, 42.
3. **Leininger, R. I. and Bigg, D. M.,** Polymers, in *Handbook of Biomaterials Evaluation,* von Recum, A. F., Ed., MacMillan, New York, 1986, 24.

4. **Clarke, I. C. and McKellop, H. A.,** Wear testing, in *Handbook of Biomaterials Evaluation,* von Recum, A. F., Ed., MacMillan, New York, 1986, 121.

SURFACE CHARACTERIZATION

5. **Ratner, B. D. and McElroy, B. T.,** Electron spectroscopy for chemical analysis: Applications in the biomedical sciences, in *Spectroscopy in the Biomedical Sciences,* Gendreau, R. M., Ed., CRC Press, Boca Raton, FL, 1986, 107.
6. **Castner, D. G. and Ratner, B. D.,** Static secondary ion mass spectroscopy: a new technique for the characterization of biomedical polymer surfaces, in *Surface Characterization of Biomaterials,* Ratner, B. D., Ed., Elsevier, New York, 1988, 65.
7. **Walls, J. M.,** Methods of surface analysis, in *Methods of Surface Analysis,* Walls, J. M., Ed., Cambridge University Press, New York, 1988, 1.
8. **Grasel, T. G. and Cooper, S. L.,** Surface properties and blood compatibility of polyurethaneureas, *Biomaterials,* 7, 315, 1986.
9. **Baier, R. E. and Meyer, A. E.,** Surface analysis, in *Handbook of Biomaterials Evaluation,* von Recum, A. F., Ed., MacMillan, New York, 1986, 97.
10. **Kasemo, B. and Lausmaa, J.,** Biomaterial and implant surfaces on the role of cleanliness, contamination, and preparation procedures, *J. Biomed. Mater. Res.,* 22, 145, 1988.
11. **Gross, U., Schmitz, H.-J., and Strunz, V.,** Surface activities of bioactive glass, aluminum oxide and titanium in a living environment, *Ann. N.Y. Acad. Sci.,* 523, 211, 1988.
12. **Baier, R. E., Meyer, A. E., Natiella, J. R., et al.,** Surface properties determine bioadhesion outcomes: methods and results, *J. Biomed. Mater. Res.,* 18, 337, 1984.

BIOCOMPATIBILITY

13. **Burridge, K. and Fath, K.,** Focal contacts: transmembrane links between the ECM and the cytoskeleton, *BioEssays,* 10, 104, 1989.
14. **Ruoslahti, E. and Pierschbacher, M. D.,** New perspectives in cell adhesion: RGD and integrins, *Science,* 238, 491, 1987.
15. **Kleinman, H. K., Klebe, R. J., and Martin, G. R.,** Role of collagenous matrices in the adhesion and growth of cells, *J. Cell Biol.,* 88, 473, 1961.
16. **Ziats, N. P., Miller, K. M., and Anderson, J. M.,** *In vitro* and *in vivo* interactions of cells with biomaterials, *Biomaterials,* 9, 5, 1988.
17. **Grinnell, F.,** The role of fibronectin in the bioreactivity of material surfaces, in *Biocompatible Polymers, Metals and Composites,* Szycher, M., Ed., Technomic, Lancaster, PA, 1983, 673.
18. **Andrade, J. D. and Hlady, V.,** Protein adsorption and materials biocompatibility: A tutorial review and suggested hypotheses, in *Advances in Polymer Science,* Dusek, K., Ed., Springer-Verlag, Berlin, 1986, 3.
19. **Block, J.,** Reactions of Biological molecules with biomaterial surfaces, in *Biological Performance of Materials,* Marcel Dekker, New York, 1981, 45.
20. **Brash, J. L.,** Mechanism of adsorption of proteins to solid surfaces and its relationship to blood compatibility, in *Biocompatible Polymers, Metals, and Composites,* Szycher, M., Ed., Technomic, Lancaster, PA, 1983, 35.
21. **Ziats, N. P., Miller, K. M., and Anderson, J. M.,** *In vitro* and *in vivo* interactions of cells with biomaterials, *Biomaterials,* 9, 5, 1988.
22. **Williams, D. F. and Bagnall, R. D.,** Adsorption of proteins on polymers and its role in the response of soft tissues, in *Fundamental Aspects of Biocompatibility,* Williams, D. F., Ed., Vol. 2, CRC Press, Boca Raton, FL, 1981, 114.
23. **Black, J.,** Systemic effects of biomaterials, *Biomaterials,* 5, 11, 1984.
24. **Kazatchkilne, M. D. and Carreno, M. P.,** Activation of the complement system at the interface between blood and artificial surfaces, *Biomaterials,* 9, 30, 1988.
25. **VanSteenberghe, D. and Albrektsson, T.,** Clinical Osseointegration, in *Current Clinical Practice Series 29,* Branemark, P.-I., Henry, P., Holt, R., Liden, G., Eds., Excerpta Medica, Amsterdam, 1986.
26. **Albrektsson, T. and Jacobsson, M.,** Bone-metal interface in osseointegration, *J. Prosthet. Dent.,* 57, 597, 1987.
27. **Albrektsson, T., Arnebrant, T., Larsson, K., et al.,** Effect of a glycoprotein monolayer on the integration of titanium implants in bone, *Adv. Biomat.,* 6, 349, 1986.
28. **Holt, G. R., Parel, S. M., and Branemark, P.-I.,** Osseointegrated titanium implants, in *Facial Plastic Surgery: Facial Implants,* Studer, F. J., Ed., Thieme Medical Publishers, New York, 1986, 113.

Part II—Clinical Use of Tissue Grafts

Chapter 7

OVERVIEW

Alvin I. Glasgold and Frederick H. Silver

There is a considerable array of implantable materials available for use in facial plastic and reconstructive surgery. These include synthetics, autografts, heterografts, and homografts. In the following chapters, we will discuss these materials in depth in order to provide sufficient information to help in the selection of the most appropriate material for the varied uses. The second section will deal with the naturally occurring grafts, autografts, heterografts, and homografts.

Ideally, a biomaterial to be used as a facial implant should be readily available in adequate quantity at reasonable cost. It must be easy to work with, elicit minimal host reaction, and have some degree of permanence. If complications occur, they should be reversible without serious permanent consequences. The implant should be easy to remove if necessary.

In the search for an ideal implant, the most important factor may be survival. This is predicated on the host perception of the implant as a foreign body and its actions to reject, degrade, or resorb this foreign body. All the natural occurring implants can be considered potentially biodegradable by the host. Autografts are expected to elicit the least host reaction, since theoretically there should be no antigen-antibody or cell-mediated response. In fact, autografts do undergo some degree of resorption. Some bone, in particular iliac crest, undergoes significant resorption while cartilage autografts seem to undergo minimal, if any resorption. All body tissue can be considered potential autografts. Excluding skin, which is a surface graft, we have included those tissues which are in use today as facial implants. These include cartilage and bone which function as structural as well as recontouring materials—fascia, pericranium, and dura which are soft tissue replacement grafts. Fat, which is used as an injectable filler, is included with other injectable materials in the next section.

Homografts elicit more of an antigenic reaction than autografts which can affect their survival. This issue is dealt with by Donald in his discussion on cartilage homografts (see Chapter 9). Cartilage homografts are probably the most important homografts used in facial plastic surgery today. Homograft sclera has had some limited use as a soft tissue replacement and is not included. Homograft bone survival depends on its revascularization and it has not been a successful implant because of resorption. We have included a chapter on demineralized bone which is now being extensively investigated in the laboratory and has gained some degree of clinical popularity. However, based on the work done by Toriumi and Larrabee, demineralized bone undergoes significant resorption, and its widespread clinical utilization will require additional research (see Chapter 11). The concept of inductive bone formation still remains an exciting potential.

Heterografts have the least potential for survival as they elicit the greatest antigenic host reaction. This was demonstrated clinically, when for a period of time, bovine cartilage was a popular graft. Injectable collagen is a heterograft and like all other heterografts, does undergo complete resorption. It is dealt with in Chapter 15 along with injectable silicone and fat.

The recipient site may be as important as the graft characteristics in selecting an implant. Thickness of soft-tissue cover and exposure to trauma has been suggested as differentiating the nasal recipient site from other areas of the face. We do know that the incidence of graft rejection as well as the severity of the reaction to synthetic implants is greater in the nose than in other areas of the face, particularly the chin and cheeks. The route of introduction in the nose, chin, and cheek areas may all be through a potentially contaminated region. The nasal implant lies closest to the site of introduction. It has the thinnest skin cover and is frequently traumatized. We have come to accept the role of synthetic implants in most areas of the face. Most surgeons are opposed to the utilization of synthetic implants in the nose, preferring the possibility of some implant absorption, which may occur with natural implants rather than risk the potentially severe consequence associated with synthetic implant rejection.

With the availability of septal cartilage within the surgical field, this has become the most logical choice of grafting material for nasal reconstruction. Its only failing is nonavailability due to prior surgery or limited supply. Conchal cartilage is a very acceptable second choice of cartilage autograft. The morbidity and time associated with its acquisition is minimal and should not be a deterrent. It is curved and does lack the stiffness of septal cartilage.

In the past, septal cartilage homografts were commonly used. Donors could be patients undergoing nasal surgery the same day. In these cases, the cartilage was soaked in alcohol between cases. These grafts may have persisted as live homografts. Septal cartilage was also commonly stored in Merthiolate™ or alcohol for later use. In Europe, Cialite™ (which is similar to Merthiolate™) was more commonly used. Short-term storage in these solutions did not affect the physical characteristics of the cartilage. However, if the cartilage was stored longer than 4 weeks, some degree of softening would occur. As reported by Donald's survey and review of the literature, Merthiolate™ and alcohol storage of cartilage was employed successfully by many surgeons who claim long-term survival of these grafts (see Chapter 9). Whether these grafts persisted as incorporated building blocks eliciting minimal host reaction or were replaced by host tissue was never proven. Merthiolate™, alcohol, and Cialite™, although effective preservatives, are all low level disinfectants. With the concern regarding transmission of HIV and hepatovirus, these low level disinfectants can no longer be counted on as effective disinfectants.[1] Alcide Expor™ is a compatible effective disinfectant. It penetrates cartilage and kills bacteria and viruses rapidly. Storage in Alcide Expor™ for a period of days will produce softening of cartilage. An effective disinfection protocol would be to disinfect cartilage in Alcide Expor™ solution for a period of about 3 h and then transfer it to a Merthiolate™ solution for long-term storage. This would produce effective disinfection and not lead to rapid cartilage softening. If a surgeon considers using this approach to develop his personal bank of stored cartilage, the same precautions as those used by tissue banks should be employed. Donors should be screened by a questionnaire regarding their health history and possible exposure to HIV and hepatovirus. Donors probably also should undergo HIV antibody testing.

Donald has documented the long-term survival of cartilage homografts (see Chapter 9). It might be expected that some resorption occurs, however, host fibrous tissue replacement very likely occurs maintaining the clinical effect. The extensive experience of Sailer and others in Europe using lyophilized cartilage seems to substantiate successful long-term use of cartilage homografts.[2]

Bone taken from the rib or iliac crest has been shown to resorb when utilized purely as an onlay graft to correct contour defects in unstressed areas as in the forehead, nose or malar eminence. These enchondral bone grafts fare much better when used in areas of stress. They have been successfully used as interpositional bone grafts to fill mandibular defects, particularly after cancer resection as well as in the maxillary region in orthognathic surgery and in congenital facial deformities. In these areas of stress, the enchondral bone is less likely to undergo resorption.

The recent literature, as documented by Marentette, supports the long-term survival of membranous cranial bone even when used in nonstress areas as in dorsal nasal augmentation (see Chapter 10). In the past few years, early open surgical management of mid-facial fractures has become an established procedure. Repair and stabilization of the maxillary buttresses by miniplating and interposition of bone grafts in areas of missing bone has led to the increased utilization of these grafts. Cranial bone grafts, in particular, are most commonly used because of location and frequent exposure of the skull with severe trauma.

In purely cosmetic cases, such as correction of a saddle nose deformity, in which septal or conchal cartilage is not adequate or in other areas of the face when larger grafts are needed, there are a number of autografts from which to choose. These include rib, cartilage, and bone from the iliac crest or cranium. The factors directing the choice would include the technical difficulty as well as time in harvesting a bone autograft, the morbidity to the patient, and the potential for resorption. Clearly, cranial bone is the easiest to harvest and may undergo the least resorption of all bone grafts. This choice would also be influenced by the surgeon's experience in harvesting a cranial bone graft as opposed to the convenience of utilizing an available rib homograft. One of the authors (Glasgold, A. I.) has, for many years, utilized irradiated rib cartilage (homografts) where large sturdy grafts were needed. They have been utilized to augment the nasal dorsum, increase length of the columella-lobule complex, and assist in projection of the premaxilla. The irradiated rib homograft has been invaluable in revision and noncaucasian rhinoplasty (Figure 1A to E).

There is a definite need for a reliable soft tissue graft in functional and cosmetic reconstruction of the face. In Part III, we will discuss synthetic soft tissue implants. Their major advantage is permanence and availability without an additional surgical procedure. The significant drawback to synthetics, however, is related to host reaction. This can produce rejection or significant foreign-body reaction resulting in unpredictable areas of swelling, causing an uneven or lumpy surface. Reports of the use of human connective tissue grafts are beginning to appear more frequently in the literature, but these homografts have not yet gained widespread clinical use. The major advantage to connective tissue grafts is better host acceptance, so that infection rejection and excess host inflammatory response producing uneven contours are rare. On the other hand, the ultimate fate of connective tissue, auto- or homografts within the host has not yet been clearly established. There is a question as to their survival as a living graft or their resorption and replacement with host connective tissue. Thus, in the effacement of contour defects, overcorrection of as much as 10 to 40% has been recommended. Brody and Donald in Chapter 12 describe the properties, harvesting techniques, and clinical usages of fascia, pericranium, and dura. Of these connective tissue grafts, temporalis fascia is the most easily accessible autograft, and it is surprising that is not used with greater frequency. Its utilization for closure of nasal septal perforations is becoming more common. Powell has described his clinical use of pericranium in a variety of cosmetic procedures, including augmentation of the lips, nasolabial fold, and the temporal region.[3] Synthetic implants are presently more commonly employed in these areas because of availability without an additional surgical procedure. The recent availability of homograft dura (tutuplast™) provides us with a promising soft tissue graft. Brennan has utilized tutuplast™ in approximately 50 cases, using it predominantly for dorsal nasal augmentation. His longest follow-up is approximately 2 years. Brennan states that he has seen no resorption to this date. It is supplied in 1 mm thickness and is available through Biodynamics, Inc.[4]

In order to prevent resorption and for utilization in areas where blood supply is tenuous, vascularized pedicle grafts in the form of osteocutaneous, myoosseous, and osteomyocutaneous flaps have been employed. These have been found to be valuable in reconstruction following extensive cancer surgery as well as in certain severe congenital deformities. In this regard, the use of microvascular anastomosis in flaps to insure adequate blood supply to the bone graft and prevent resorption is an excellent new addition to the surgeon's armamentarium. Because of the length of these procedures, they have very limited application at this time.

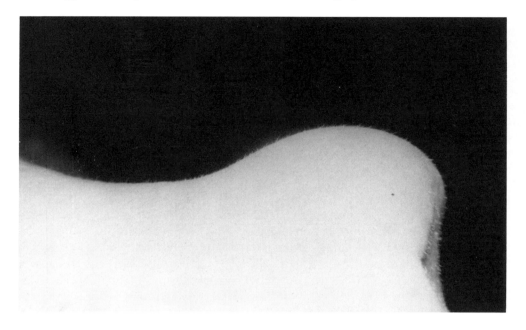

A

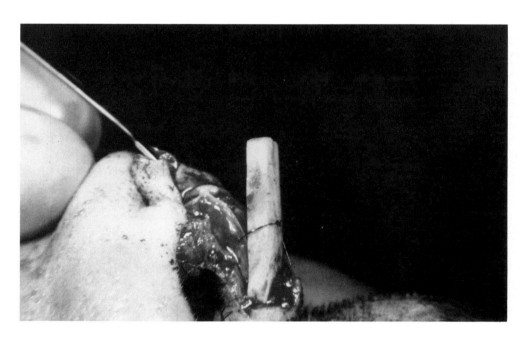

B

FIGURE 1. The use of irradiated rib cartilage homograft in revision rhinoplasty to correct a severe posttraumatic deformity. (A) Preinsertion: posttraumatic revision rhinoplasty, absent septal cartilage, retracted columella, and saddle-nose deformity. (B) Photograph of insertion through the external approach of a large columella-lobule irradiated rib homograft.

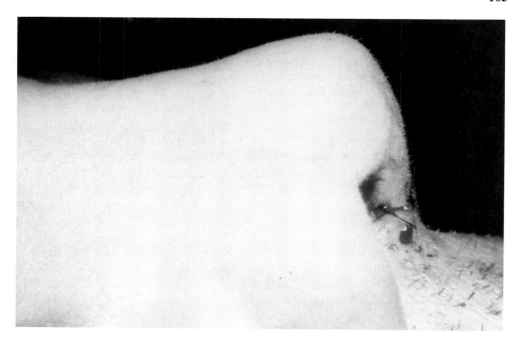

FIGURE 1C.   Postinsertion of irradiated cartilage homografts to columella-lobule complex as in (B) as well as for dorsal augmentation.

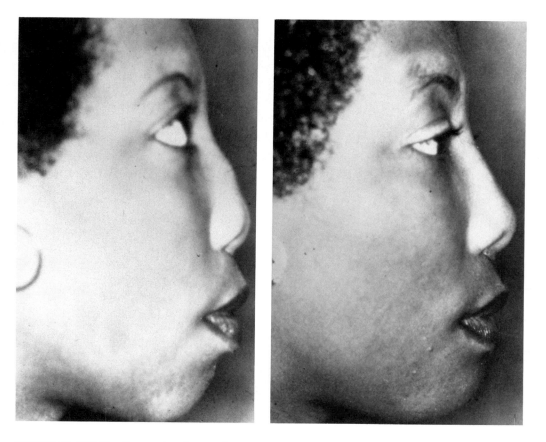

FIGURE 1D AND E.   Preoperative photograph: noncaucasian extreme anterior nasal flattening. Three years post-insertion of irradiated cartilage homograft as in (A), plus dorsal augmentation and premaxillary augmentation with irradiated cartilage.

REFERENCES

1. **Glasgold, M. J., Glasgold, A. I., and Silver, F. H., et al.,** The mechanical properties of septal cartilage homografts, Otolaryngology, Head & Neck Surg., *J. Am. Acad. Otolaryngol.,* Head and Neck Foundation, 99(4), 374, 1988.
2. **Sailer, H. F.,** *Transplantation of Lyophilized Cartilage in Maxillofacial Surgery: Experimental Foundations and Clinical Success,* S. Karger, New York, 1983, 42.
3. **Powell, B. P. and Riley, R. W.,** Pericranial free grafts in the face, *Arch. Otolaryngol. Head Neck Surg.,* 115, 187, 1989.
4. **Brennan, G. H.,** Personal communication.

Chapter 8

CARTILAGE AUTOGRAFTS

Alvin I. Glasgold and Mark J. Glasgold

TABLE OF CONTENTS

I. INTRODUCTION AND HISTORICAL BACKGROUND

Cartilage grafts have gained increasing popularity in facial plastic surgery. Although in most areas of the face alloplasts are well accepted, their history as nasal grafts has been a problem. Possibly because of thinness of the nasal covering and the susceptibility of the nose to trauma and infections, alloplasts have become inflamed and are extruded in some patients early; in others, many years after implantation. Although the incidence of rejection of alloplasts may not be high, the severity of the reaction in the nose, and the subsequent scarring and tissue distortion has made each of these events a potential clinical disaster.

Host extrusion of cartilage grafts has not been a significant problem. Cartilage homografts are mildly antigenic when implanted in humans. They are generally well accepted by the host and undergo minimal resorption in the early years postimplantation.[1-4] There is some concern regarding their 10-year survival.[5] In comparison, cartilage autografts do not undergo any significant resorption over long periods of time and thus can be considered a permanent replacement graft.

Peer and Dupertius, two of the earlier pioneers of cartilage grafts, demonstrated that cartilage autografts survive as living tissue in the host.[6,7] They also observed growth of these autografts when used in young hosts,[8,9] though these results have not been duplicated by others.[10] Peer implanted septal cartilage autografts in humans. Microscopic studies after 3 years revealed the presence of chondrocytes and no visible evidence of resorption.[6] He made similar histologic observations on autogenous ear cartilage which had been implanted for 3 years and autogenous rib which had been implanted for 12 years. These studies showed no evidence of cartilage resorption.[11] Gibson and Davis demonstrated that cartilage autografts showed some mild degree of erosion and resorption when the surface of the graft was cut. This process of erosion and resorption was of short duration and was complete within a few weeks of transplantation.[12]

There are several factors which seem important in the survival of cartilage grafts. Infection or the presence of blood in the field increases the tendency for graft resorption.[13] Elimination of a dead space in which blood or fluid accumulates is therefore important. The graft should be handled gently to avoid surface nicks which may increase resorption. Rib autografts have a tendency to warp, which is particularly evident when they are placed over the nasal dorsum.[14]

The problem of warping was examined by Peer who diced cartilage to eliminate warping,[15] however, this produced so much surface area that significant resorption occurred. Gibson and Davis advocated the technique of balanced cross-sectional carving which solved the problem of warping.[16] Although perichondrium does seem to have protective properties, it does not seem necessary for survival and could increase the tendency for the graft to warp.[16,17]

It is not necessary for cartilage grafts to be in contact with adjacent cartilage for survival.[12] It has generally been assumed that an adequate covering of soft tissue is important for survival of a cartilage graft. Cartilage autografts, however, seem to survive well under the thin covering of the nasal dorsum. Cartilage autografts are usually encapsulated with fibrous tissue which fixes them to the adjacent tissue, resulting in stabilization of the graft.[18]

II. PHYSICAL AND CHEMICAL PROPERTIES OF CARTILAGE

Cartilage is an avascular structure. It is composed of chondrocytes sitting within a chondromucoprotein matrix containing no blood vessels and surrounded by an avascular perichondrium. Chondrocytes are the living element in cartilage and are responsible for the production of the matrix. The survival of cartilage autografts has been thought by Gibson to be due to the persistence of live chondrocytes.[17] Chondrocytes are the antigenic portion of cartilage; however, because chondrocytes are so well encased within the matrix, cartilage is weakly antigenic and is considered to be an immunologically privileged graft.[19] The matrix is composed of type II collagen and proteoglycans which combine to provide tensile strength and elasticity. Collagen fibers are modified into different alignments to serve a variety of functions.

The properties that make cartilage an ideal grafting material include its strength, elasticity, and its mild antigenicity. As has been stated in this chapter, autografts do not have to be buried deeply and can be placed directly under the skin allowing for excellent contouring, particularly under the thin skin of the nose.[20]

The firmness and resiliency of cartilage obtained from portions of the nasal septum produce grafts which are excellent supporting structures. Elasticity of cartilage harvested from the concha of the ear and that obtained from the thinner portions of the nasal septum produce excellent contour grafts. Cartilage is easy to handle, and can be carved and beveled with a knife, or smoothed with a drill or an abrasive. When implanted, it does not have to be in contact with host cartilage, nor does it require a good blood supply for survival.[21] If removal is required, this can be easily accomplished since the cartilage graft is encapsulated and is not strongly attached to the surrounding host tissue.

III. SOURCE AND HARVESTING OF CARTILAGE AUTOGRAFTS

The three major sources of cartilage autografts are the nasal cartilage, the cavum and cymba concha of the ear, and the rib.

A. NASAL SEPTAL CARTILAGE GRAFT

The septal cartilage autograft meets all of the following requirements for an ideal graft to be used in nasal surgery. It is accessible within the surgical field. It provides some variation in thickness and rigidity. It is easy to contour, elicits no host reaction, and is permanent. Its only drawback is lack of availability due to prior surgery or trauma. Large segments of septal cartilage can be removed without adversely affecting the supporting nasal structure as long as an adequate intact dorsal and caudal segment is left in place (Figure 1A and B).

Septal cartilage may be accessed endonasally through a hemitransfixion or Killian incision. When an external nasal approach is used for reconstruction, separating the medial crura allows wide exposure of the entire septum. Following cartilage removal, the mucosal lining on either side can be sutured together with a continuous weaving suture or multiple interrupted sutures. This closes the potential dead space and eliminates the need for intranasal packing post-operatively. The inferior portion of septal cartilage adjacent to the nasal spine is relatively thick and strong and provides an excellent supporting graft for use as a columella strut to support or increase tip projection. Just above this inferior portion of cartilage the septum thins out somewhat. It is still firm and a bit more flexible, having the best characteristics for grafts to be utilized within the lobule as a shield or tip replacement graft. Superiorly, the thinner more elastic portions of the septum are a good source for grafts to efface small contour defects (Figure 1C). Any smooth, straight segment of the septum can be used as a single or multilayered onlay graft to elevate a depressed nasal dorsum.

B. ALAR CARTILAGE GRAFT

The cephalic portion of the lower lateral cartilage, which is commonly removed in nasal tip surgery, can be an excellent source of cartilage autograft to fill in a contour defect in another portion of the nose. In particular, in cases of alar asymmetry, a balance can be accomplished by transecting the cephalic portion of one side and using it to build up the deficient side (see Figure 5 in Section IV.B.).

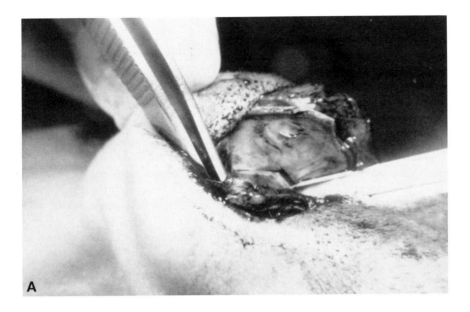

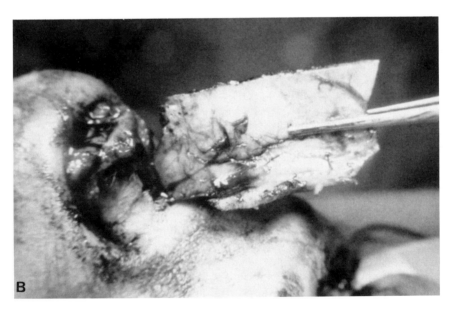

FIGURE 1.   A and B. Septal cartilage autograft accessed through the external approach. (A) Septal cartilage incision leaving adequate anterior and dorsal supporting segments; (B) removal of a large septal cartilage autograft through external approach.

C. AURICULAR CARTILAGE AUTOGRAFTS

The ear provides another excellent source of cartilage autografts. The entire cavum and cymba concha can be removed without producing a deformity of the ear. This graft can be harvested from an anterior approach, placing the incision at the depth of the antihelicle fold. The resulting scar is negligible. A bulky ear dressing can be avoided by suturing a bolus pressure dressing into the concha (Figure 2A-C). If one prefers the posterior approach, the graft can be readily obtained through an incision in the postauricular sulcus. Conchal cartilage can be harvested with or without perichondrium, being rather flexible and not as firm as the thicker portions of the septal cartilage. Conchal cartilage has been tubed and used over

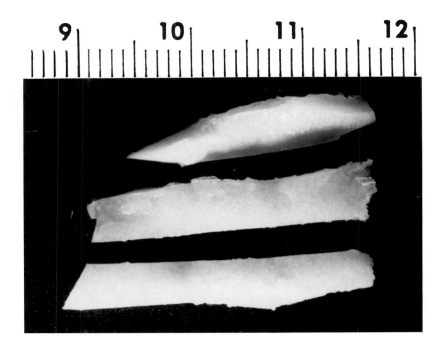

FIGURE 1C.   Graft sectioned into three segments which may be used for columella strut (bottom) and onlay grafts to nasal dorsum.

the nasal dorsum, or as a premaxillary graft to augment a retracted upper lip. When conchal cartilage is used for dorsal augmentation, it is preferable to suture together relatively similar size segments to produce the desired thickness. Conchal cartilage is ideal to recontour small defects along the nasal dorsum or to build up a deficiency of the alar of the nose. It is very useful to correct a vestibular stenosis secondary to absent alar cartilage. It may also be utilized for tip projection. It can be fashioned into a shield, or tip-projecting graft, and is also used as a tip onlay graft. Because of its curvature, it is less desirable than septal cartilage for columella struts. An additional important use of auricular cartilage is as part of a composite graft which includes cartilage perichondrium and both anterior and posterior surfaces of the skin. This is obtained from the outer curve of the ear and utilized most commonly to correct full thickness, alar, nasi, or columella defects. Auricular cartilage has also been used successfully to correct traumatic orbital floor defects.[22]

D. COSTAL CARTILAGE

Costal cartilage has been used when large segments of cartilage autografts are needed. It is harvested from the sixth or seventh rib. Although this is an excellent source of cartilage, the operating time is prolonged significantly and adds a moderate amount of morbidity. Costal cartilage, when stored at 4°C for a few days, remains viable. It must be appropriately carved to counteract its tendency to warp, which is a problem when used to correct a depressed nasal dorsum. Costal cartilage has been used to reconstruct malar and mandibular contour defects, as well as various other bony facial defects. Perhaps its most important use today is in providing the framework for total auricular reconstruction of congenital or acquired origin.[23]

IV. CLINICAL APPLICATION OF CARTILAGE GRAFTS IN FACIAL PLASTIC SURGERY

Cartilage autografts have been utilized to augment various areas of the face. By far, the most common site for cartilage grafting is in nasal reconstruction. The present trend in nasal

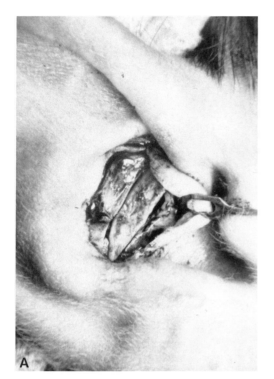
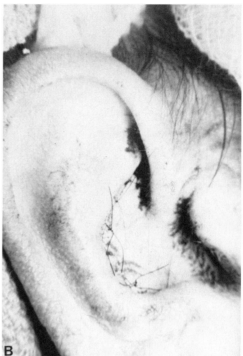

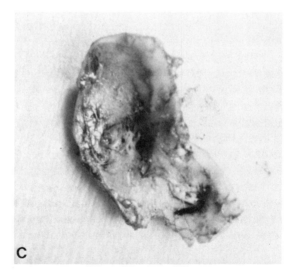

FIGURE 2.   Conchal cartilage graft removed through an anterior incision around the rim of concha. (A) Exposure and cartilage incision for removal of conchal cartilage graft; (B) closure of incision leaves minimal scar; (C) the entire concha removed for graft.

contouring is to produce a natural sculptured appearance. This has greatly increased the utilization of cartilage grafts. These grafts are used to augment, contour, and support the nasal structure. Each application produces specific effects. Familiarity with the nature of the grafts and the effect of their clinical application is necessary if the surgeon wishes to make full use of these wonderfully accessible and inexpensive materials.

A. DORSAL AUGMENTATION

Lack of projection of the nasal dorsum can occur as a congenital abnormality, a racial characteristic, and secondary to trauma or prior surgery. The use of cartilage autografts to correct this problem is a safe, reliable, and permanent method of correction.[24] Grafts augmenting the nasal dorsum may be inserted through an endonasal or external approach. The advantage of the external approach to placement of these grafts is accuracy in positioning and suture fixation of the grafts. Septal cartilage is most frequently used as a single or multiple layered graft (Figure 3A to F). When septal cartilage is not available, auricular cartilage or rib may be used. Although auricular cartilage is curved, some relatively straight segments can be obtained and sutured together with 5.0 Nylon. This layered graft can be carved to the appropriate size and shape and the edges can be beveled with a knife or an abrasive (Figure 4A and B).

B. NASAL CONTOUR DEFECTS

Small nasal contour defects can be corrected utilizing appropriate sized grafts taken from the nasal septum or the concha of the ear. These can be inserted endonasally into small exactly placed pockets or through an external approach, in which case the grafts are sutured into the proper position and retained permanently (Figure 5A to C). The curved conchal cartilage conforms to the nasal contour. When straight septal cartilage is used, light morsalization or scoring may be needed to soften and increase its flexibility. This is particularly true when dealing with alar deformities. In addition to correcting asymmetries or irregularities of the nasal base, these grafts can be inserted anywhere along the nasal dorsum to correct filling defects (Figures 6 and 7). When there is excessive narrowing of one or both sides of the nose, a cartilage strip (spreader graft) can be inserted medial to the nasal bones and/or the upper lateral cartilage. This will position the bone or upper lateral cartilage laterally. A piece of cartilage can also be contoured and layered on the outside of the bone to fill in the defect.

C. NASAL BASE GRAFTING

The nasal base is the most frequent site for cartilage grafts in the nose. The grafts inserted in the nasal base assist in tip projection, rotation, and contouring, particularly of the columella and the nasolabial angle. The various positions of nasal base grafts produce specific supporting and contouring effects which are discussed below. The columella strut, as originally advocated by Anderson, was inserted through a vertical incision at the inner margin of the columella.[24] A pocket is created intercrurally from the premaxilla to the top of the columella without entering the lobule (Figure 8A and B). The strut is rectangular and usually tapered at each end for ease of insertion into the intercrural pocket (Figure 1C). It extends down to the premaxilla, so that it is situated on a firm base, thus supporting the lobule. This same intercrural columella strut can be inserted through an external approach which is now Anderson's preferred route and achieves the same effect.[25] An intercrurally inserted columella strut supports or increases tip projection by maintaining or elongating the columella length (Figure 9). As it increases tip projection, it rotates the lobule in a cephalic direction reducing the nasal length. This effect on the lobule also produces an angulation or curvature at the columella lobule junction. It produces little effect on the nasolabial angle (Figure 10A and B). It will also correct a distorted columella (Figure 11A and B).

A columella supporting and contouring graft may also be placed in a precrural position.[26] From a similar lateral columella incision, rather than inserting the graft between the medial crura, the graft is inserted anterior to the medial crura. This places the graft directly beneath the skin of the columella. The length of the graft should extend from the premaxilla up to the columella lobule junction, without entering the lobule. This produces the same effect on tip projection and lobule rotation as when placed intercrurally. In addition, it adds a

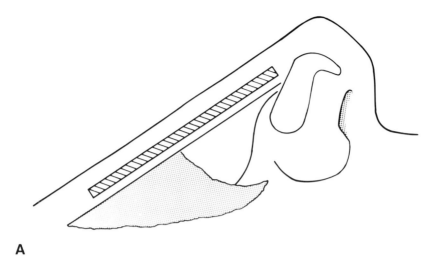

A

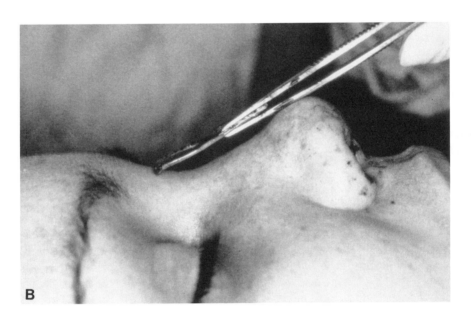

B

FIGURE 3.   Dorsal augmentation using septal cartilage autograft. (A) Illustration of position of dorsal onlay graft; (B) a photograph of dorsal onlay graft placed over defect to judge size; (C, E) front and lateral preoperative; and (D, F) front and lateral 1-year postoperative photos of correction of saddle nose defect with septal cartilage autograft. Additional small contour grafts corrected alar defects.

curvature to the columella which can, if needed, significantly alter the nasolabial angle (Figure 12A to D). The effect on the nasolabial angle and the columella curvature will depend on the thickness of the graft. It will correct a retracted columella or correct an acute nasolabial angle, and is also very useful in producing a subtle nasal change when slight rotation of the nasal base is needed without significantly changing a satisfactory tip.

The cartilage graft which was confined to the lobule was popularized by Sheehan[27] as a tip graft, and by Kamer as a shield graft.[28] This graft is placed in a tight pocket created by an endonasal incision beginning at the columella lobule junction and extending laterally along the alar margin with enough length to insert the graft. This pocket must be of exactly the right size. If extended too far superiorly, the tip will flatten and projection will be lost.

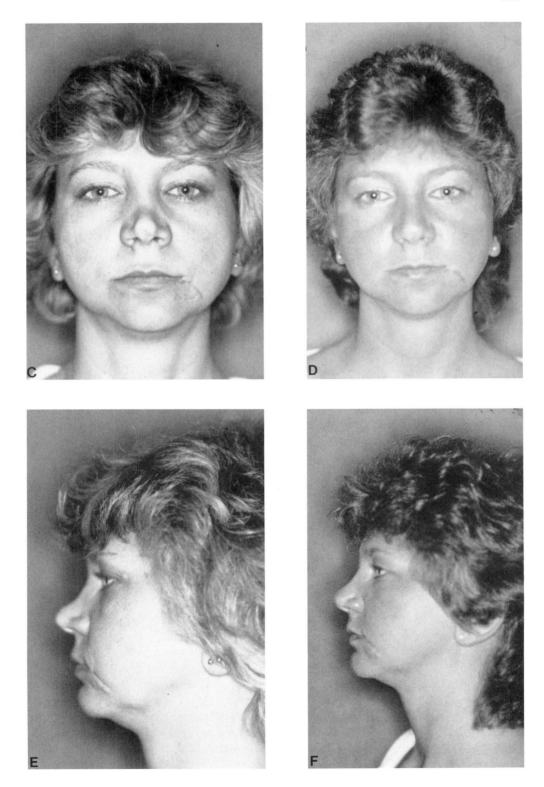

FIGURE 3C to F

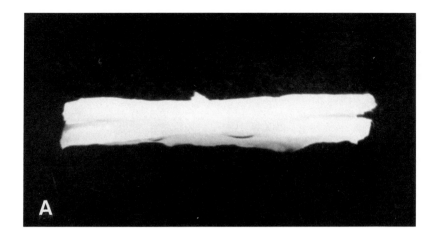

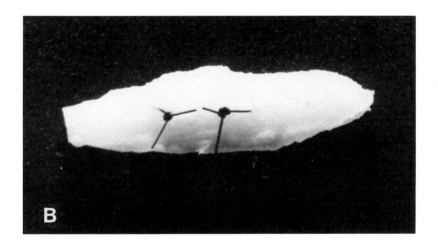

FIGURE 4.   Preparation of double-layered cartilage autograft for dorsal augmentation. (A) Side view; (B) top view illustrating position of sutures.

If extended too far inferiorly (into the columella), projection will also be lost and the inferior point of the graft will be visible on the columella. The purpose of the shield graft is to project and improve tip definition. Ideally, it elongates and narrows the lobule and defines the end point of the tip. It will appear to rotate the tip in a cephalic direction and produce an angulation at the columella-lobule junction. It does not change the columella or the nasolabial angle (Figure 13A to C). It is actually replacing and not altering the structural components of the lobule. Accurate placement of this graft through the endonasal approach is difficult. In this author's experience, graft shifting and tip asymmetries occurred in a great many cases. This problem can be eliminated by the external approach. This exposure allows proper placement and suture fixation of the graft. Suture fixation of the short tip graft confined to the area of the lobule is very time consuming.

A much simpler technique for achieving increased tip projection and narrowing, utilizes a longer graft inserted through the external approach, extending the length of the lobule and the columella. It is placed anterior to the columella. Inferiorly, a pocket created in front of the feet of the medial crura accepts the tapered bottom portion of the graft. Superiorly, the graft extends above the existing height of the alar cartilage creating a new tip defining point

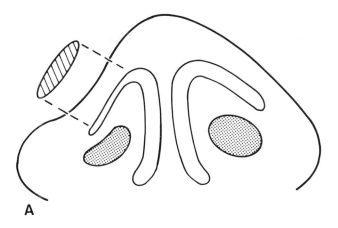

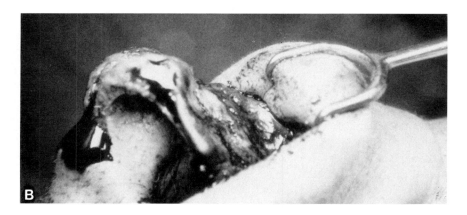

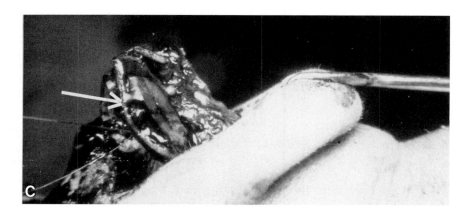

FIGURE 5. Correction of alar defects with contour grafts. (A) Illustration of placement of graft over deficient alar cartilages; (B) photograph of alar cartilage defect exposed through the external approach; (C) conchal cartilage autograft (arrow) sutured in place to recontour alar.

(Figure 14). The graft can be moved in a vertical direction to increase or decrease desired tip projection. Once placed in the inferior pocket, it is relatively easy to place a suture through the medial crura and then tie this suture in front of the graft. The graft is thus firmly fixed in position. The superior portion can then be further trimmed if desired (Figure 15A to D). The graft is ideally made from a segment of septum which has some flexibility so that

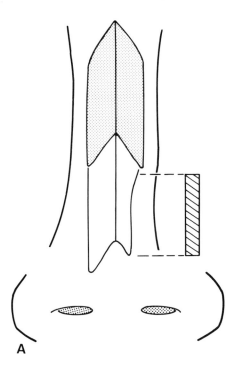

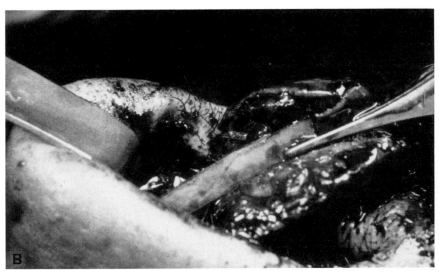

FIGURE 6.   Correction of defect of region of upper lateral cartilage. (A) Illustration of graft placement which may be lateral or medial to upper lateral cartilage; (B) photograph of graft placement.

there will be a curve to the columella lobule complex. Auricular cartilage may be used when septal cartilage is not available. As tip projection is increased with this graft, there is a tendency towards cephalic rotation. This occurs because there is a limit to the degree of stretch in the skin of the columella and the lobule. Tip blunting, which can occur with a shield graft, will not happen with this graft. Once this graft is in place and positioned, redraping of the skin will show the exact placement and position of the new tip. Because of the firm fixation, this will not tend to change postoperatively (Figure 16A to C). This graft allows the surgeon to accurately create a new tip contour without depending on the patient's

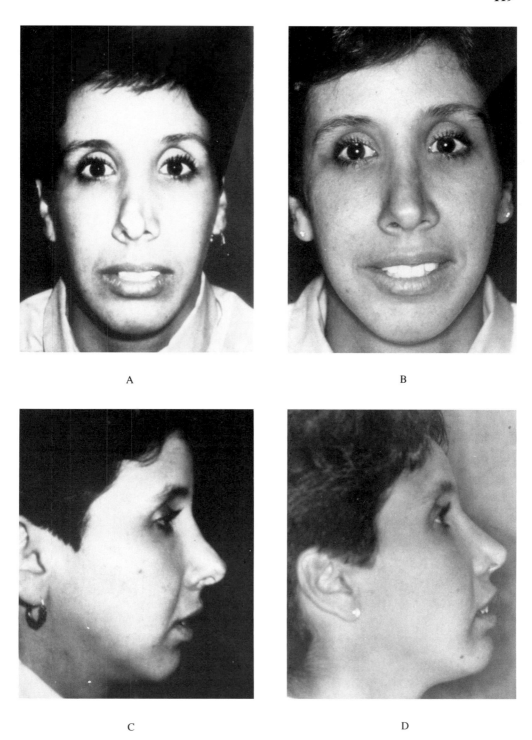

A

B

C

D

FIGURE 7. Example of use of cartilage autograft to correct contour defects of alar and lateral nasal regions. Photographs of: (A) Frontal and (C) lateral preoperative views of patient with marked deficits of alar and lateral nasal regions; (B) frontal and (D) lateral views 3 years after correction, utilizing septal cartilage autografts to recontour nose as described in text.

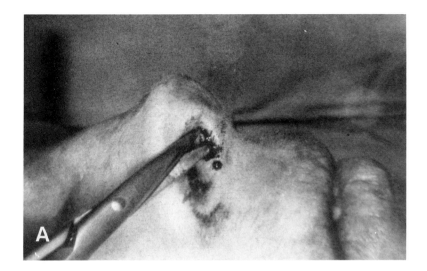

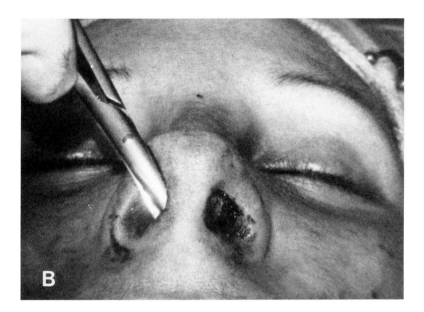

FIGURE 8.   Cartilage autograft as columella strut for nasal tip projection and rotation. Photographs of (A) incision in columella anterior to medial crura; (B) creation of pocket from lobule to premaxilla to accept graft.

own structural components. It is an important concept for surgical correction of difficult tips of any variety. This includes amorphous or thick-skinned tips in both caucasian and noncaucasian patients. It is invaluable in revision surgery, particularly when there is very little alar cartilage left. It can effectively substitute for an entirely absent tip structure (Figure 17A and B). It will also correct asymmetries in the lobule by replacing the existing asymmetric components.

The use of onlay grafts to augment the lobule and increase tip projection produces no change in the columella lobular profile line. A single- or double-layered cartilage graft taken from the septum or concha can be placed above the existing domes. This will increase the height of the nasal tip. These can be inserted through an endonasal or external approach.

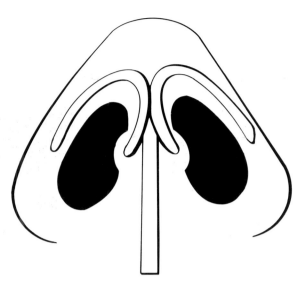

FIGURE 9. Illustration of columella strut augmenting the length of the medial crura.

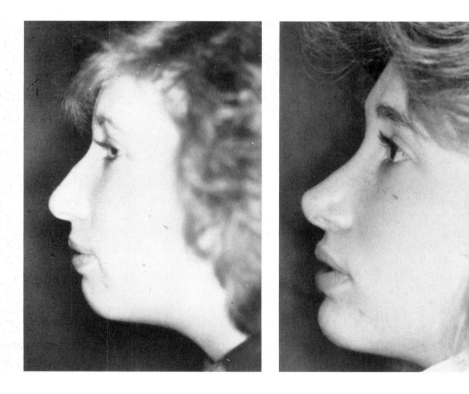

A

B

FIGURE 10. Clinical example of the effects of an intercrural columella strut placed through an external approach. (A) Preoperative lateral view; (B) 2-year postoperative lateral view. Note the elongation of the columella which projects and rotates the lobule. Tip definition improves and an angle is created at the columella-lobule junction.

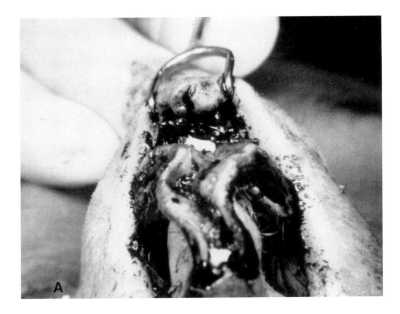

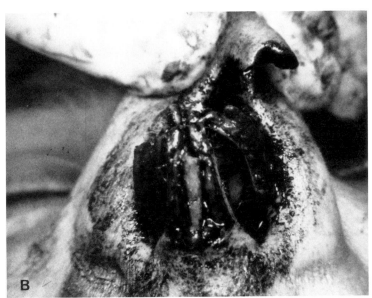

FIGURE 11.   Photographs of (A) twisted medial crura exposed through the external approach; (B) columella strut sutured between medial crura straightening and supporting them.

The external approach is a more accurate method of positioning this as well as any other type of graft. In addition, one can combine this with an intercrural columella strut. This produces a T-shaped graft and serves to fix the position of the underlying support for the onlay graft.

D. PREMAXILLARY GRAFTS

Although the premaxilla is not part of the nose, it is the foundation for nasal tip projection. It forms part of the nasolabial angle which is important in nasal aesthetics. Deficiencies of the premaxillary region contribute to an acute nasolabial angle and a retracted upper lip.

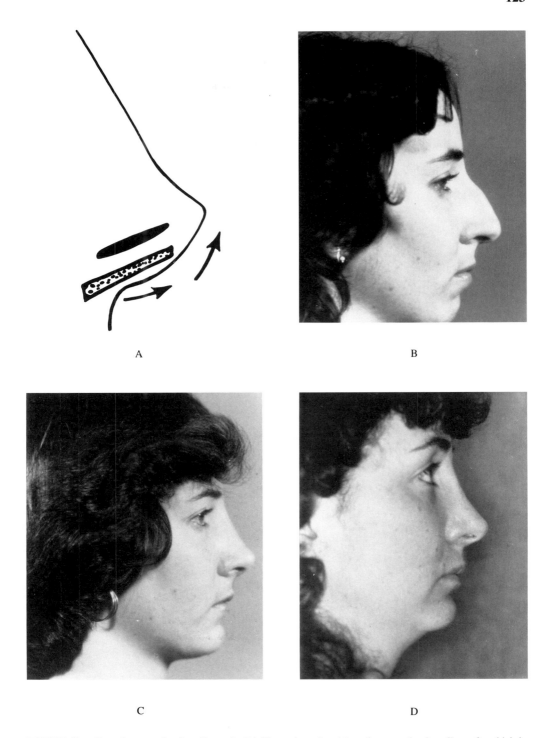

A

B

C

D

FIGURE 12. Use of precrural columella graft. (A) Illustration of position of precrural columella graft, which in addition to projecting and rotating the lobule, recontours the columella and nasolabial angle. (B) preoperative view of patient with poor tip support, short medial crura, and excessive nasal length. (C) A 1-year postoperative view following insertion of precrural columella graft; and (D) 11 years postoperative. Correction is maintained.

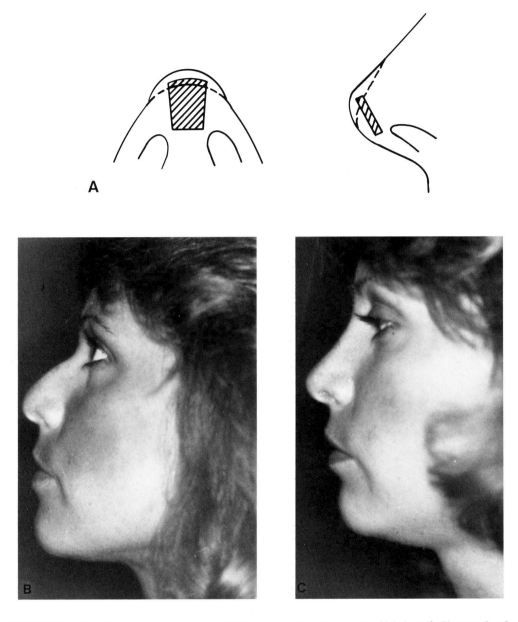

FIGURE 13.   Use of graft confined to lobule. (A) Illustration of ideal placement of lobule graft. Photographs of (B) preoperative view of under-projected and poorly defined tip; (C) 1 year after correction with tip graft increasing tip projection and definition.

Premaxillary deficiency may also contribute to poor columella-tip support resulting in a depressed tip. The premaxilla can be augmented by various means. In the past, multiple small bits of cartilage and/or bone taken from areas removed during rhinoplasty were placed in the premaxilla through an incision in the floor of the nasal vestibule. These produced very little change. In order to produce an appropriate effect, larger grafts are necessary. Conchal cartilage, either layered or rolled, layers of septal cartilage sutured together, and solid segments of rib cartilage are excellent grafts. These grafts can be inserted through the floor of the nasal vestibule or through a sublabial incision (Figure 18A and B). The premaxilla acts more like the rest of the face than the nose as a recipient site for grafting material. Therefore, silastic or other alloplasts can be utilized for premaxillary augmentation without the same fears one encounters in the nose.

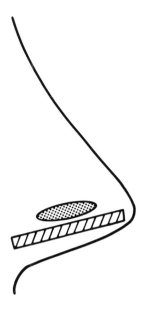

FIGURE 14. Precrural columella-lobule graft (versatile tip replacement graft). Illustration of position of graft which can effectively replace the columella and lobule cartilage components creating
a new tip.

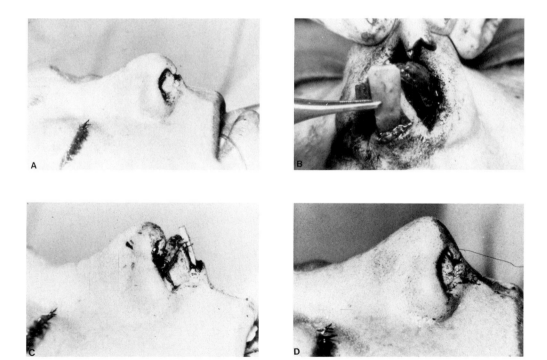

FIGURE 15. Placement of columella-lobule graft. Photographs of (A) tip position prior to graft placement after
an external incision has been made; (B) base view of positioning of graft; (C) lateral view of graft sutured in place
projecting above the dorsal nasal line; (D) skin repositioned and graft in place. Notice increased tip projection as
compared to (A).

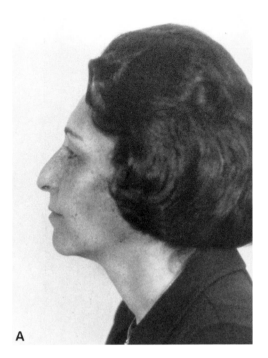
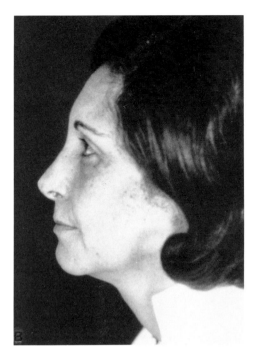

FIGURE 16.   Clinical effect of precrural columella lobule graft. Photographs of (A) preoperative view—short columella and weak lobule structure; (B) 1-year postoperative insertion of columella-lobule graft with resultant increase in columella and lobule length and improved tip projection, definition, and cephalic rotation.

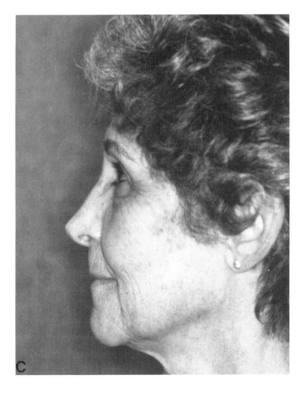

FIGURE 16C.   The same patient 17 years postoperative. Clinical effect is maintained.

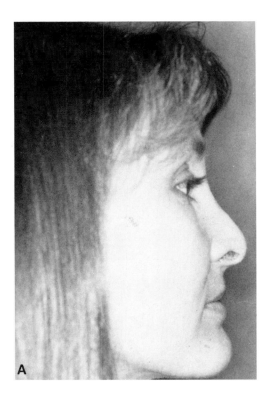 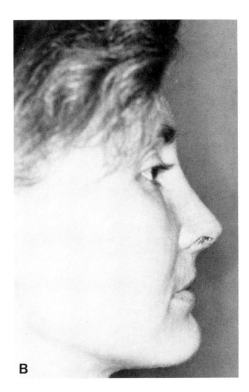

FIGURE 17. Use of columella-lobule graft to correct tip ptosis. Photographs of (A) postoperative tip ptosis with almost complete absence of tip-supporting structure; (B) 2-year postoperative replacement of absent tip structure with columella-lobule septal cartilage autograft.

V. SUMMARY

The lack of immune response, the proven longevity, and the physical and structural characteristics which make cartilage so easy to handle and contour, have made cartilage autografts so desirable. In nasal reconstruction, because of the limited amount of grafting material needed and the easy accessibility of septal and conchal cartilage, autogenous cartilage is the preferred grafting material. In areas where large grafts are needed, such as the chin and cheek, the need to obtain such grafts from the rib, which require significant additional surgery and resultant morbidity, is a deterrent. In addition, the excellent host acceptance to preformed allografts in areas other than the nose have reduced the use of cartilage autografts in these other sites. The surgeon should be familiar with the varied grafting materials available to him in addition to cartilage autografts. In planning and considering the aesthetic improvement of facial features, it is important to incorporate these varied materials in his armamentarium (Figure 18).

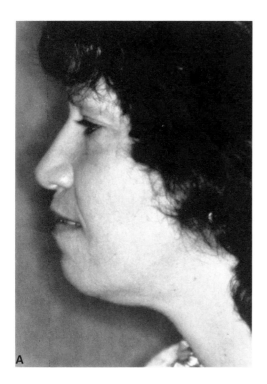
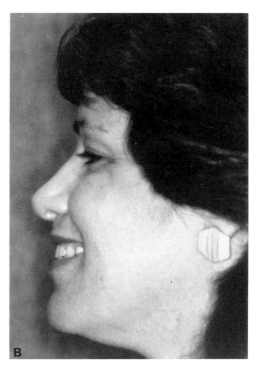

FIGURE 18.   Use of multiple facial grafts. (A) Preoperative view of patient with depressed nasal tip, acute nasolabial angle, receding chin, bimaxillary protrusion, and relatively flat mid-face; (B) 2-year postoperative view of correction with columella strut and premaxillary augmentation with septal cartilage autografts. Mentoplasty and malar augmentation have also been accomplished with prefabricated silastic implants.

REFERENCES

1. **Dingman, R. O.,** Follow-up clinic on costal cartilage homografts preserved by irradiation, *Plast. Reconstr. Surg.,* 50, 516, 1972.
2. **Schuller, J. E., Bardack, J., and Krause, C. J.,** Irradiated homologous costal cartilage for facial contour reconstruction, *Arch. Otolaryngol.,* 103, 12, 1977.
3. **Donald, P. J.,** Cartilge grafting in facial reconstruction with special consideration of irradiated grafts, *Laryngoscope,* 96, 7, 1986.
4. **Muhlbauer, W. D., Schmidt-Tintemann, U., and Glaser, M.,** Long-term behavior of preserved homologous rib cartilage in the correction of saddle nose deformity, *Br. J. Plast. Surg.,* 24, 325, 1971.
5. **Welling, B., Maves, M. D., Schuller, D. E., and Bardach, J.,** Irradiated homologous cartilage grafts, *Arch. Otolaryngol. Head Neck Surg.,* 114, 291, 1988.
6. **Peer, L. A.,** The fate of living and dead cartilage transplanted in humans, *Surg. Gynecol. Obstet.,* 68, 603, 1939.
7. **Dupertuis, S. M.,** Actual growth of young cartilage transplants in rabbits, *Arch. Surg.,* 43, 32, 1941.
8. **Dupertuis, S. M.,** Growth of young human autogenous cartilage grafts, *Plast. Reconstr. Surg.,* 5, 486, 1950.
9. **Peer, L. A., Ihalia, I. S., and Bernhard, W. G.,** Further studies on the growth of rabbit ear cartilage graft, *Br. J. Plast. Surg.,* 19, 105, 1966.
10. **Meijer, R. and Walia, I. S.,** Preserved cartilage to fill facial bone defects, *Biomaterials in Reconstructive Surgery,* L. R. Rubin, Ed., C. V. Mosby, St. Louis, 1983, 509.
11. **Peer, L. A.,** Experimental observations on the growth of young human cartilage grafts, *Plast. Reconstr. Surg.,* 1, 108, 1946.
12. **Davis, W. B. and Gibson, T.,** Absorption of autogenous cartilage grafts in man, *Br. J. Plast. Surg.,* 24, 405, 1971.

13. **Davis, W. B. and Gibson, T.,** Absorption of autogenous cartilage grafts in man, *Br. J. Plast. Surg.,* 24, 405, 1971.
14. **Fry, H. J. H.,** Interlocked stresses in human septal cartilage, *Br. J. Plast. Surg.,* 19, 276, 1966.
15. **Peer, L. A.,** Diced cartilage grafts, *Arch. Otolaryngol.,* 38, 156, 1943.
16. **Gibson, T. and Davis, W. B.,** The distortion of autogenous cartilage. Cartilage grafts: its cause and prevention, *Br. J. Plast. Surg.,* 10, 257, 1958.
17. **Gibson, T. and Davis, W. B.,** A bank of living homograft cartilage: a preliminary report, *Trans. Int. Soc. Plast. Surg.,* 2nd Int. Congr., A. B. Wallace, Ed., Livingstone, Edinburgh, 1960, 452.
18. **Gibson, T.,** Transplantation of cartilage, *Reconstructive Plastic Surgery,* Vol. 1, 2nd ed., Converse, J. M. and McCarthy, J. G., Eds., W. B. Saunders, Philadelphia, 1977, 301.
19. **Heyner, S.,** The significance of the intercellular matrix in the survival of the cartilage alllografts, *Transplantation,* 8, 666, 1969.
20. **Glasgold, A. I., Glasgold, M. J., and Silver, F. H.,** Cartilage grafts in nasal surgery, *Am. J. Rhinol.,* 3(3), 167, 1989.
21. **Tardy, M. E., Denneny, J., and Fritsch, M.,** The versatile cartilage autograft in reconstruction of the nose and the face, *Laryngoscope,* 95, 523, 1985.
22. **Stark, R. B. and Frileck, S. T.,** Conchal cartilage grafts in augmentation rhinoplasty and orbital floor fractures, *Plast. Reconstr. Surg.,* 43, 591, 1969.
23. **Brent, B.,** The acquired auricular deformity. A systematic approach to its annalysis and reconstruction, *Plast. Reconstr. Surg.,* 59, 475, 1977.
24. **Anderson, J. R.,** New approach to rhinoplasty. A five-year reappraisal, *Arch. Otolaryngol.,* 93, 284, 1971.
25. **Anderson, J. R. and Ries, W. R.,** *Rhinoplasty: Emphasizing the External Approach,* The American Academy of Facial Plastic and Reconstructive Surgery, 1986, 74.
26. **Glasgold, A. I.,** Dynamics of the columella strut, *Am. J. Cosmet. Surg.,* 1(2), 41, 1984.
27. **Sheehan, J. H.,** *Aesthetic Rhinoplasty,* C. V. Mosby, St. Louis, 1978, 230.
28. **Kamer, F. M. and Churukian, M. M.,** Shield graft for the nasal tip, *Arch. Otolryngol.,* 110, 608, 1984.

Chapter 9

CARTILAGE HOMOGRAFTS

Paul J. Donald and Hilary A. Brodie

TABLE OF CONTENTS

I. INTRODUCTION

The deformities of the face arising from congenital disorders, trauma, and the residua of ablative surgery for cancer continue to challenge the reconstructive surgeon. This is even more cogent today than in past decades, when those patients with severe facial trauma used to succumb to their associated injuries, and those with extensive neoplasia were considered inoperable. With modern resuscitative techniques and the development of the trauma team with rapid helicopter transport of the seriously injured patient, many patients with extensive injuries including concomitant devastating maxillofacial trauma survive. Similarly many patients with advanced carcinomata of the head and neck, despite extension to the skull base, pterygoid muscles, and cranial cavity are now resectable due to advances in modern head and neck surgery. The defects left as the result of these resections provide a special reconstructive challenge.

Our society's preoccupation with beauty and a youthful appearance increases the demand for cosmetic surgery, which in many cases requires the use of an implant. The tolerance for minor degrees of graft absorption is much less than in the deformities secondary to trauma and cancer surgery so that precision in graft carving is an essential requirement. The need for graft materials to replace, augment, or enhance the deficient areas in the visage of these patients steadily increases. Unfortunately, no grafts completely satisfy all the criteria of a perfect implant.

A substance that is totally compatible with the host tissues, resisting infection being molded, shaped or carved with facility, and resisting absorption, continues to elude us. Many surgeons, frustrated in their use of biological materials, have resorted to alloplastic grafts. Methylmethacrylate, silicone rubber, Proplast, and bioglass, to name a few, all share the common property of nonabsorption. This is clearly a distinct advantage over biological materials. However, the problems of infection and graft extrusion have influenced many surgeons to turn away from alloplasts and resume the use of tissue.

Cartilage satisfies many of the parameters of an ideal onlay graft. It is easy to carve, antigenically relatively inert, and firm, yet not rock hard. It can be procured in abundance either from the patient, or as a homograft taken from another individual during routine surgery, or from the autopsy table and stored for future use. In addition to fresh cartilage and cartilage maintained in sterile saline or antibiotic solutions, various preservatives have been introduced to enhance the storage and sterility, and also to produce subtle alterations in the cartilage matrix to reduce its absorptive potential.

In the history of plastic and reconstructive surgery of the face, it is curious that cartilage grafting is a relatively recent event. Bert,[1] in 1865, was the first individual to transplant cartilage in animals. However, the first recorded autogenous rib cartilage in humans was not implanted until 1900.[2] When one considers that nasal reconstruction was initially described in the classical Indian surgical textbook, the *Sushruta Samhita,*[3] printed around 600 B.C., it is interesting that with the development of reconstructive rhinoplasty through the centuries, attention was devoted mainly to restoring cutaneous integrity. Considerations of skeletal support, much more difficult to attain, have been only relatively recent. Strictly speaking, the *Sushruta Samhita* actually describes the first cartilage graft in the form of a composite graft. It describes the replacement of the amputated nose, a common punishment of the time, for women found in adultery.

The first serious interest in the biology of grafted cartilage did not begin until the 1930s. Peer,[4] in 1939, showed that the chondrocytes of transplanted cartilage remain viable in the host and that the matrix remains unchanged and maintained by these cells. He also showed that in some grafts, absorption took place and the cartilage was replaced by fibrous tissue. Moreover, these early studies by Peer and later by Gibson showed there was little difference in absorption between autologous or heterologous grafts. Peer's observation of absorption, the greatest disadvantage of this material, resulted in loss of interest in cartilage grafts. As a result of this pioneering work,[5,6] research in cartilage implant biology fell into obscurity for many decades.

A basic understanding of the biology of cartilage and its dynamics when implanted is essential for the reconstructive surgeon, so that he may exploit those factors that will best advantage the grafts potential.

II. STRUCTURE AND MORPHOLOGY

Cartilage is a whitish to very light blue homogenous elastic rubbery tissue found at various sites throughout the body. Caplan in his enlightening treatise on cartilage describes four histologically and morphologically distinct types based on both location and function (Figure 1). They are: (1) morphologic, (2) fibrocartilage, (3) articular, and (4) elastic hyaline. Nasal and auricular cartilage, typical of the morphological type, have a fixed "genetically sculpted"[7] configuration that imparts the shapes and convolutions we recognize as characteristic of the pinna and nasal tip. Fibrocartilage is found in the intervertebral disks and has the toughness and resilience necessary for the work required of the spinal column. Articular cartilage is found in the joints of the extremities. It acts as a stress risor and must possess the ability to repeatedly rebound from compressive forces, as well as have some degree of flow to allow one bone to slip over another. Finally, elastic (hyaline) cartilage is found principally at the costochondral junction. Its physical properties allow it to stretch with the expansion of the thoracic cage. The differences between the cartilage types are determined by their differing molecular structures. The most commonly used cartilage used in reconstructive surgery is elastic or hyaline cartilage from the thoracic cage. In many instances, therefore, an elastic type cartilage is called upon to replace a morphologic one. This usually requires carving the elastic cartilage in an attempt to mimic the genetically determined configuration of the morphologic one, an often difficult undertaking. Moreover, the reconstructive effort is dependent upon the carved cartilage maintaining its new shape, as well as its size.

All cartilage is essentially composed of three main elements: cells, matrix, and bound water. The cartilage cell, the chondrocyte, is responsible for secreting the matrix portion of this tissue and is integral in maintaining its viability. The matrix is composed of two main constituents, the proteoglycan matrix and a specific collagen that is almost exclusively found in cartilage. The proteoglycan is a complex molecule composed of a protein core with numerous carbohydrate side chains made up of glycosaminoglycans. The protein core with the attached side chains are arranged along a strand of hyaluronic acid. The collagen and proteoglycan are polymerized into a gigantic convoluted macromolecule whose molecular configuration allows it to trap varying amounts of water and imparts the characteristic properties of resiliency and elasticity.

A. THE CHONDROCYTE

The mesenchymal precartilage cells of the embryo are biochemically and ultrastructurally identical to all other mesenchymal cells.[8] The presence in the nucleus of chondrogenic DNA[9] directs the cell to differentiate and produce the proteoglycan matrix and the type II collagen characteristic of cartilage. The *chondrogenic DNA* may be "switched on" by the presence of bone morphogenic protein (BMP).[10] Indeed, Nathanson and Hay[11] have shown that BMP can induce both fibroblasts and myoblasts to form cartilage. The chondrocyte is a large cell with abundant cytoplasm. It possesses a large nucleus and extensive Golgi apparatus (Figure 2). The plasma membrane has projections that are the result of the exchange of vacuoles from the cytoplasm with the matrix.[12] Matrix vesicles may be the terminal portions of these projections. Matrix vesicles are small membrane-bound structures that occasionally contain

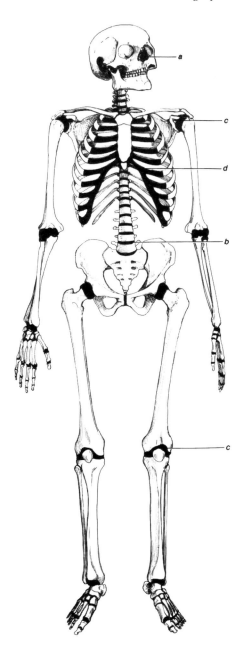

FIGURE 1.   Diagrammatic representation of the varieties of cartilage throughout the body: (a) morphologic cartilage; (b) fibrocartilage; (c) articular cartilage; (d) hyaline or elastic cartilage. (Adapted from Caplan, A. I., *Sci. Am.*, 251, 85, 1984. With permission.)

ribosomes and provide the sites of the earliest calcification in epiphyseal cartilage. Because of their ability to concentrate Ca^{2+} they may provide the nuclei for hydroxyapatite growth.

The distinctive feature of the chondrocyte is its ability to produce matrix. This property is dependent upon at least two known sets of molecular events. First there must be no fibronectin coating the cell. Fibronectin is a high molecular weight glycoprotein that is a major component of the cell surface of fibroblasts. This material must be cleared from the

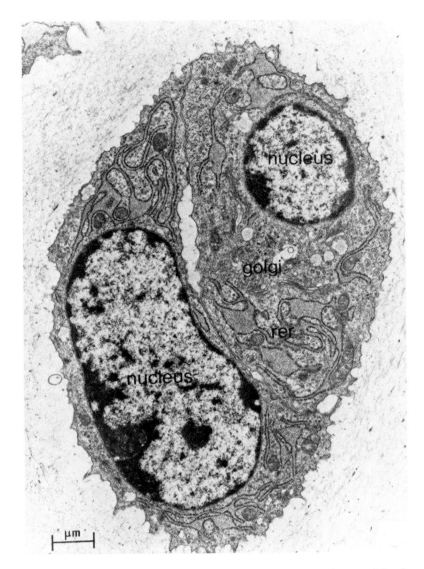

FIGURE 2. These two chondrocytes have recently divided. Note large nuclei and abundant rough endoplasmic reticulum (rer). Newly synthesized matrix is seen between the cells (original magnification × 12,600). (From Sheldon, H., *Cartilage, Vol. 1, Structure, Function and Biochemistry,* Academic Press, New York, 1983, 97. With permission.)

chondroblast's cell surface before matrix synthesis can begin.[13-18] Additionally, there must be the presence of sulfonated proteoglycans in the cell's immediate environment before this activity can occur. If, for instance, chondrocytes are suspended in cell culture free of matrix components, the cell will produce type I rather than the type II collagen idiosyncratic to cartilage; demonstrating the necessity of this component in the chondrocyte's environment.[8,19-22]

The lacunae around each chondrocyte seen in standard light microscopic and ultrastructural preparations do not represent shrinkage artifacts. They are spaces filled with soluble early polymerizing matrix material. This material does not stain with standard staining techniques but can be demonstrated with special preparations.[12] On ultrastructural examination, the matrix of hyaline cartilage is characterized by both deeply staining granules measuring 20 to 70 μm in diameter that represent the proteoglycan component, as well as thin unbanded or slightly banded fibrils representing the collagen.

B. THE MATRIX

The proteoglycan molecule is comprised of a central repeating strand of the disaccharide, hyaluronic acid. Projecting from this central spine are proteins called "core proteins" that are among the largest proteins synthesized by any cell. Each protein moiety weighs in the range of 250,000 to 300,000 G mol wt. The core protein at one end rolls itself into a globule weighing approximately 90,000 G mol wt that is the point of attachment to the hyaluronic acid spine (Figure 3). From each core protein projects a number of polysaccharides. These form a linkage at a point that contains either serine or threonine. The polysaccharides linked to the protein core are the N-linked oligosaccharides, the O-linked oligosaccharides and two larger polysaccharides. These form a linkage at a point that contains either serine or threonine. The polysaccharides linked to the protein core are the N-linked oligosaccharides, the O-linked oligosaccharides and two larger polysaccharides: keratin sulfate and chondroitin sulfate. Overall, a hyaluronic spine can have as many as 100 core proteins attached. Each of these in turn have about 50 keratan sulfate and 100 chondroitin sulfate chains appended. The total weight of this monomer is in the range of 1.5 to 2.5 million, and the molecule once polymerized produces a resultant macromolecule that may weight in the tens of millions.[7]

The synthesis of matrix undergoes six steps.[12] First, the chondrocyte must take up precursor materials, especially those rich in sulfates. Next the protein core material that will project from the hyaluronic acid spine is synthesized. This takes place in the rough endoplasmic reticulum. The glycosaminoglycans that will affix to the core proteins are built in the smooth endoplasmic reticulum. The fourth step involves the final sulfonation of the glycosaminoglycans and their assembly onto the core proteins. This occurs in the Golgi apparatus of the chondrocyte. Golgi vacuoles now carry the monomer proteoglycan and secrete it into the pericellular space in the lacunae of the cartilage. Final maturation and polymerization occurs within the extracellular space and the matrix beyond.

Once the proteoglycan is secreted into the matrix and fully polymerized, this massive molecule can bind large volumes of water many times its own weight. The water is bound by electrostatic forces brought about by the extreme electronegativity of the glycosaminoglycans. The relative positivity of the oxygen end of the water molecule encourages clusters of H_2O molecules to arrange themselves in layers throughout this macromolecule. The ability of these layers of bound water to slide over one another is one of the principal mechanisms producing the resiliency of cartilage. In addition, water is held in the lacunae of cartilage much in the same way that a sponge does.

The water functions not only in contributing to resiliency but is also essential to the nutrition of cartilage. Cartilage has no blood vessels, and nutrients need to diffuse through the matrix. This is done by the migration of shifting of water layers during the process of compression. During this process, water molecules are squeezed and pushed into new positions, while the negatively charged glycosamine molecules are pressed together. Their forces of electronegativity act to repel each other, thus making further compression more difficult, and thereby increasing the elastic resistance with each additional compressive load. The atrophy and thinning of cartilage seen in immobilization and disuse may be accounted for by the diminished nutritional supply brought about by the lack of compressive forces causing this vital shifting and motion of water layers. This may also in part explain the absorption of hyaline cartilage grafts when used as onlays in areas of relative immobility. The success of morphologic cartilage implantation in the nose, for instance, relative to hyaline cartilage grafts from rib may be due to the diminished requirement of the former for this form of nutrition.

The final component of cartilage is collagen. It comprises 10% of the wet weight and 40 to 50% of the dry weight of cartilage.[12] As already mentioned, the molecular structure of the collagen of cartilage is unique and produced only by the chondrocyte. Morphologically

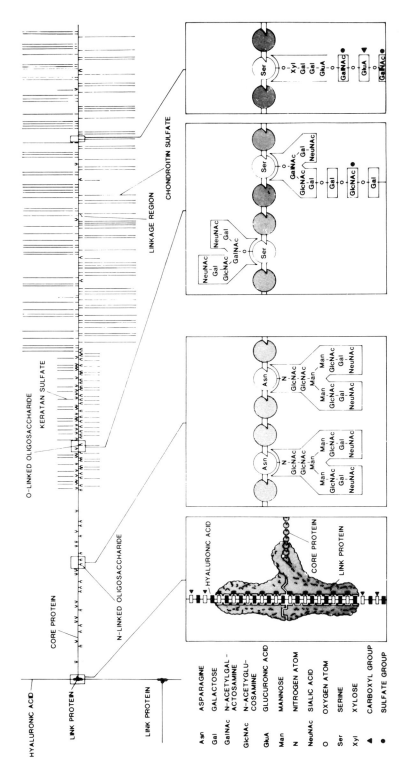

FIGURE 3. Molecular structure of proteoglycan. Note central strand or spine of hyaluronic acid. Projecting from it are so-called "core proteins". These have in turn attached various polysaccharides, notably keratan sulfate and chondroitin sulfate, that give it a characteristic test-tube brush appearance. (Adapted from Caplan, A. I., *Sci. Am.*, 251, 90, 1984. With permission.)

similar precursor cells that are destined to make bone or other connective tissue make type I collagen. Chondral collagen is called type II and, other than in cartilage, is found in small amounts only in notochord, chick corneal epithelium, and neural retina.[8] Any mesenchymal or other primitive precursor cells that make type II collagen will be destined to become chondrocytes. Chondral collagen is comprised of only α_1 chains and their hydroxylysine content is four to five times greater than that of type I collagen.[23] The collagen fibers are very difficult to chemically extract and appear to be tightly complexed to the proteoglycans.

The distribution of collagen fibers and bound water determine the type of cartilage. For example, elastic and reticulin fibers, as well as a dense concentration of collagen fibers are characteristic of the annulus fibrosis of the fibrocartilage of the intervertebral disk.

III. INTERNAL ELASTIC FORCE

The two major cartilage types used for grafting are morphologic and hyaline. Morphologic cartilage possesses the curious quality of "genetic sculpting." When excised completely or in part for implantation at a different site, it maintains its shape indefinitely. This structuring that is so deeply ingrained in its basic molecular configuration was fascinatingly demonstrated in experiments done by De Palma et al.,[24] and Thomas.[25] These workers injected papain into rabbit ears and then attempted to deform them by external pressure. Once the deforming force was removed, the ears sprang back to their original configurations. A similar clinical situation was reported by Robbins,[26] in a man with a hematoma of the auricle that had dissolved a considerable amount of the auricular concha. After evacuation of the blood, the surviving chondrocytes of the anterior and posterior perichondrial leaves regenerated new cartilage of the original configuration. He postulates, as does Gibson,[27] that this is the result of a preprogramming phenomenon of the chondrocyte.

Hyaline cartilage has a system of "interlocking stresses" inherent in its molecular structure and configuration. In 1958, Gibson and Davis first demonstrated this phenomenon in costal cartilage.[28] Eight years later, Fry showed the same thing in nasal septal cartilage that became manifest following either trauma or surgery.[29] There is a balance of internal elastic forces that resist deformation in the intact state on compression and will return the cartilage to its original configuration when the compression and subsequent deformation have been relieved. This property seems to be the responsibility of the protein core and the glycosamine side chains. They produce areas of compression alternating with corresponding areas of tension within the cartilage (Figure 4). Parallel lines of force are also aligned throughout the periphery of the cartilage and these counteract the effects of these internal forces.[30] Once a cartilage block is cut, the stress forces on that side are relieved and no longer counteract the forces on the opposite side of the graft. The result is warping of the implant. Unless carving is such that all of these forces can be released and neutralized, a distorted graft is the result. It takes about 30 min after carving for the distortion process to be complete. An alternative method of graft carving that will avoid this distorting influence is shaving only scant amounts from the periphery of the graft such that these outer restraining forces are not unfettered. According to Gibson,[27] this property of interlocking stresses is maintained by the chondrocytes and is lost when the cell dies. He feels this is the reason for the absence of this property in preserved grafts.

Elasticity of cartilage on the other hand may be a reflection, at least some degree, of collagen crossbonding within the matrix. The elastic modulus for a number of graft preservation techniques has been compared to Glasgold et al.[27a] In our laboratory, we have compared the elastic modulus of cartilage grafts irradiated at different intensities.

Grafts were exposed in dosages from 4 to 10 million rad. Strips of varying thickness were tested on an Instron apparatus, where the stress exerted by the impacting cross-head was plotted against the displacement of the cartilage. A stress-strain relationship could then

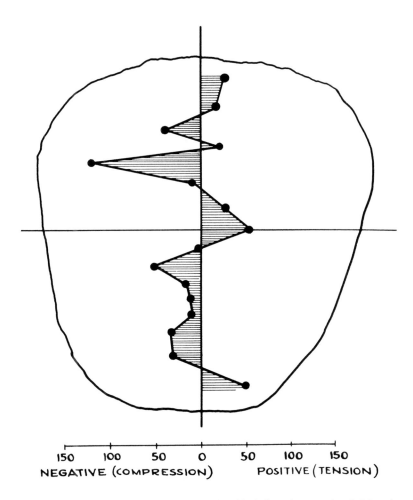

FIGURE 4.   Cross section of a human cartilage block from the costochondral junction illustrating an engineering analysis of the alternating compression and stresses exerted within the graft. (From Gibson, T., *Br. Med. Bull.*, 21, 153, 1965. With permission.)

be established and the elastic modulus calculated. Early data suggests no consistent change in elastic modulus with increasing doses of graft irradiation.

IV. GRAFT ABSORPTION AND ANTIGENICITY

A. ABSORPTION

The ultimate survival of cartilage grafts in the shape, size, and form in which they were initially implanted is hotly contested. Mikelsen[31] expressed surprise at his Western colleagues' findings that cartilage grafts tend to have variable absorption. He reported only three instances of absorption in 1,819 preserved allografts of frozen cartilage he implanted. He placed grafts that had been kept at 3°C to 6°C and that had been stored for no longer than two months. There is good evidence that chondrocytes can survive freezing for this length of time.[31,32] The importance of viable chondrocytes in maintaining the health of the graft is summarized by the categorical statement of Elves that " . . . a certain method of producing cartilage 'resorption' is to kill the cells."[33] However, despite the viability of the chondrocytes, freshly implanted autogenous grafts undergo some degree of absorption as well. Davis and Gibson[34] clearly demonstrated this with autogenous diced costal cartilage prepared in the method described by Peer.[35]

Research into the mechanisms of absorption has revealed a number of factors responsible for this process, some of which can be controlled to a degree in the clinical situation. It has become apparent that chondrocytes are not replaced during the life of an individual.[36] Unlike bone, little remodeling of cartilage takes place in the normal state. The ability of cartilage to regenerate is questionable, however, some evidence that hyaline cartilage will repair and grow after injury has been shown.[37,38] Farkas[39] has shown that 8% of carved autografts of costal cartilage implanted in children for auricular reconstruction grew along with the child.

Cartilage responds to injury in the following way. Initially, there is a loss of proteoglycans in the area adjacent to the site of injury. Some attempt at repair is evidenced by the appearance of metachromasia in the histological staining of the proteoglycans of the matrix in this region, indicating the appearance of more basophilic immature ground substance. In addition, this is evidenced by an increased cellular uptake of sulfur,[40] indicating enhanced chondrocyte activity. Only a scant replenishment of this element occurs, however, and reversal of only mild injury is possible. The chondrocytes along the line of the injury die and there is little replicative response to the cells adjacent to them. The chondrocytes, residing close to the injury that survive, demonstrate an increase in collagen synthesis. However, collagen is destroyed by proteinases that are now much more effective because the collagen fibrils have been laid bare by the loss of their glycosaminoglycan covering.[41] The responsible enzymes are believed to be metalloproteinases that split proteoglycans,[40,42,43] as well as collagenase and neutrophil elastase[44] that attack collagen. Catabolins are a group of messenger-like factors that are secreted by synovium and macrophages and influence chondrocytes to destroy the matrix.[45-48] This would be a factor only in autogenous grafts or allografts containing viable chondrocytes, as these factors have no direct influence on the cartilage itself. Lymphokines are secreted from T cells, especially those of thymic origin.[49] There is some evidence that they are involved in cartilage absorption, especially in inflamed joints,[49,50] but they probably play only a negligible role in grafted cartilage. These factors cause decrease in both glycosaminoglycan and protein synthesis, as well as a minor role in cartilage catabolism.[51] Despite these destructive processes following cartilage damage, it is remarkable that there is very little change in the configuration of the original injury even 6 to 12 months after the traumatic event.

Hyaline cartilage in its normal residence is highly resistant to absorption. Under the usual circumstances of everyday activity, the cartilage resists invasion by vascular tissue. If, however, there is rigid immobilization of the part, vascular invasion occurs. This normal resistance to vascular invasion is thought to be due to the cationic nature of some low molecular weight proteins in the cartilage matrix that act as proteinase inhibitors.[52] Immobilization impedes the normal process of nutrition brought about by molecular water layer shifts during repeated compression and the cartilage tends to increase its water content and decrease its proteoglycan.[33] An interesting paradox exists concerning articular cartilage's need for repeated pressure and compressive loads. If immobilization occurs, absorption ensues. If excessive compressive loads are imposed, absorption occurs. However, a period of continuous compression followed by immobilization will result in some cartilage regeneration.[33]

B. ANTIGENICITY

Earlier work has suggested that cartilage enjoys some sort of immunologic privilege. The proteoglycan component of the matrix was considered immunologically inert. The collagen was deemed nonreactive because of its molecular similarity and ubiquity not only among, but between, species. The chondrocytes were shielded in their lacunae by a matrix that was a barrier to immunologically active cells and a filter to "immunologic messages". Although the present state of knowledge concerning the immunology of cartilage establishes it as a weak antigen, its immunological reactivity in transplantation, as in the case of implantable collagen,[53] another heretofore considered weak antigen, can no longer be disregarded. Chondrocytes have been shown to possess tissue specific antigenic sites.[54-57] Elves[58] has definitively established that these antigenic sites are of the major H system. Although the proteoglycan of the matrix forms an effective barrier to the access of the chondrocyte to immunologically competent cells and humoral antibodies, once a cartilage graft is carved, the chondrocytes adjacent to the implantation site become exposed to these influences.

The type II collagen of the matrix has three antigenically active loci. The most potent are the telopeptides of the C and N terminal portions of the triple helical chain. These portions of the chain do not carry the characteristic glycine in every third position as is seen in the remainder of the triple helix. These antigens are under control of the major genetic histocompatibility locus H-2 and the antibodies are of the T cell dependent type.[59] They are also species specific. Because type II collagen is distinct from the more ubiquitous type I and is characteristically comprised of the three α_1 chains, the actual triple helix itself is antigenic. A third immunologically active site is a central region α chain.[33]

The proteoglycan molecule *in vitro* demonstrates at least two antigenic sites, both located in the protein core of the molecule. One is species common and the other species specific. In the *in vivo* state, the protein core is shielded by the glycosaminoglycans and is likely immunologically inert. However, once cartilage is damaged or cut, as in the case of a carved graft, the protein core may be exposed and become antigenically active.

In cartilage destruction, the presence of immunologically stimulated macrophages play an important role in cartilage absorption. Additionally, lymphocytes are usually seen in abundance surrounding the absorption site. Craigmyle used a second set reaction to show the acquisition of immunity to allografts of cartilage in rabbits.[59-61] Elves[62,63] has demonstrated cytotoxic antibodies in sheep receiving articular cartilage allografts, which appeared months after implantation. Conflicting results have been presented concerning demonstration of H-2 and non-H-2 system antigens to allogenic grafts in mice.[33]

The immunologic destructive process involves three sets of factors: lymphocytes, antibodies, and lymphokines. Lymphocytes can be tissue destructive in themselves in the form of killer cells, or they can be mediators of the immune response. The lymphocytes isolated from their target cell, the chondrocyte, by the matrix may be active when the cartilage is damaged or cut. Heyner[64] has shown that when chondrocytes were stripped of their matrix and implanted in an allogenic host, they were destroyed, and lymphocytes were in abundance at the site of the implantation. The role of antibody antigen complexes in intact cartilage is unclear. The heaviest molecular weight that can penetrate the matrix is about 68,000[65] and most immunoglobulins are in the range of about 120,000. Any process, however, that will result in matrix depletion can increase permeability and increase access of the chondrocyte to immune complexes. Lymphokines are small immunoglobulin molecules produced by lymphocytes after antigenic activation. They may recruit other lymphocytes into the reaction against an implant, activate macrophages, and even be directly cytotoxic themselves. The molecular size is sufficiently small to diffuse across the matrix and damage the chondrocyte.

In summary, it should be stated that many of the immunologic properties of the three major components of cartilage have been determined *in vitro*. The *in vivo* situation is somewhat different but it is clear that cartilage is mildly antigenic. Destructive disease processes, trauma, and the carving of a cartilage graft, however, do result in exposure of these antigenic sites, and may thus engender an immunologic reaction of variable degree.

V. METHODS OF GRAFT PRESERVATION

The numbers of ways in which to preserve cartilage are legion, varying from simple cold storage in saline, antiseptic, or antibiotic solutions to freeze-drying and irradiation. The methods have the goals of maintaining sterility of the graft and hopefully rendering changes that will result in stability of the graft at the implant site, reducing or eliminating absorption.

Storage of cartilage in cold saline, antibiotic solutions, or freezing preserves the viability of the chondrocytes for a variable length of time. The advantages of preserving the cell with its matrix maintenance and producing potential may be outweighed by its antibody-stimulating potential. However, a dead cell likely retains some antigenic potential as well; the significance of which is uncertain. The life span of the cell in storage is uncertain, although claimed to be as long as two months when the graft is frozen.

The second goal of cartilage preservation is that of producing some degree of graft stability. That is to say the loss of the tendency to deform or warp on carving, or after implantation, and the acquisition of resistance to absorption. Clearly most preservation methods remove the tendency of the graft to warp at the time of carving. However, they do not entirely eliminate that tendency once the graft has been implanted for some time at the donor site. The problem of absorption is highly variable and difficult to predict.

A. MERTHIOLATE™

Most of the earlier research work on the survival of preserved grafts was done on those stored in saline or frozen, and on grafts preserved in Merthiolate™. Merthiolate™ preservation has been commonly used for many years and absorption has been considered to be slight and subsequent graft calcification common.[27,66] In my experience in implantation in dog and sheep, with up to four years follow-up prior to sacrifice, all Merthiolate™ grafts had absorption that varied from slight to complete.[67] Merthiolate™ is unfortunately not a good antiseptic, and prolonged storage often results in an infected graft. Prolonged storage also produces softening of the implant making subsequent carving difficult. In our own animal experiments, sixteen Merthiolate™ stored grafts were implanted as onlays on the faces of sheep and dogs. Three of the surviving Merthiolate™ grafts showed evidence of viable chondrocytes. Since the graft was initially dead tissue, it is remarkable that host chondrocytes now inhabit the graft. These cells are presumably the products of the differentiation of pleuripotential mesenchymal cells near the periphery of the graft. Another interesting phenomenon is that of ossification. Such ossification was described by Muhlbauer et al.[66] in Merthiolate™ preserved costal chondral grafts used in the augmentation of saddle nose deformities.

Four of the grafts in the experiment were almost completely ossified and anchored securely in their recipient beds (Figure 5). This was found in both dog and sheep. Two irradiated grafts had 10% and 5% ossification, respectively. This was evidenced by bone spicules and some small centers of ossification. Three of the Merthiolate™ stored grafts implanted in sheep were excised along with their implantation sites. They showed a uniform histological picture. Although on gross inspection, the grafts appeared to be ossified to the graft site; histologically, a layer of fibrous tissue separated the graft from the underlying bone (Figure 6). The outer layers of cartilage of each graft were rich in basophilic proteoglycans and had an extensive territorial matrix (Figure 7). The lacunae were filled with histologically normal appearing chondrocytes. Light microscopy with vital staining was used to test chondrocyte viability. Under the shell of new cartilage, degenerating cartilage was being replaced by amorphous osteoid islands and circular tubules of compact bone with apparent marrow cavities (Figure 8). The cartilage in this central portion of the graft has lacunae containing what appear to be viable chondrocytes. The cartilage, however, appears to be breaking up into globules, and phagocytes are obvious at these sites. Mature appearing osteocytes are obvious in the organized bone.

B. CIALITE™

Cialite™ (sodium 2(ethylmercurimercapto)-benzoxazole-5-carboxylate) has been used in Europe for at least 25 years.[68,69] It is chemically closely related to Merthiolate™ which is ethyl(2-mercaptobenzoate-S). McGlynn and Sharpe[70] reported in 1981 on 67 Cialite stored

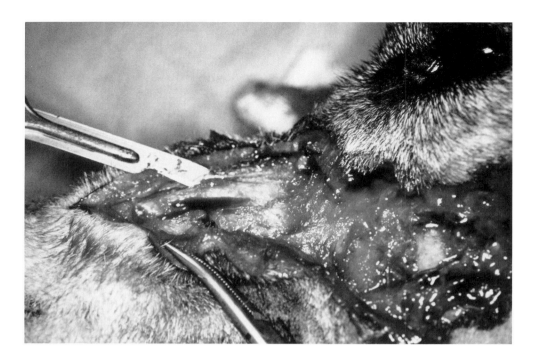

FIGURE 5. Dog #1 showing Merthiolate™ stored implant firmly embedded in bone of snout. (From Donald, P. J., *Laryngoscope*, 96(7), 798, 1986. With permission.)

grafts used in nasal augmentation. A "good result" was obtained in 81% of cases and a poor result (either infection, extrusion, or marked absorption resulting in the reappearance of the original deformity) in 19%. Calcification of the graft was common and associated with a low absorption rate.

C. LYOPHILIZATION

Lyophilized cartilage grafting is used extensively in Europe. Sailer[85] in his exhaustive treatise on this method shows the advantages he has found in his experience. Lyophilization is the technique of freeze-drying where a biological substance is frozen and the water removed by the process of sublimation in a vacuum. The dried material is vacuum packed and stored. The cartilage is harvested from the costochondral junction, stripped of muscle and other soft tissue while preserving the perichondrium. It is stored in a sterile salt solution until sterilized. Sterilization is done just prior to freeze-drying by immersing the cartilage in a 1% solution of β-propiolactone solution at 37°C for 2 to 3 h. The cartilage pieces are rinsed twice for 2 h in a buffered solution. An alternative to this sterilization method is gas sterilization. The cartilage blocks are placed in thin glass tubes in a freezer at -70°C for 30 min. Once frozen, the drying process occurs in a dryer at -40°C for 36 h. The residual moisture is about 5%. The dried material is stored in vacuum packed metal containers. Reconstitution of the material is done by placing the lyophilized blocks in distilled water containing one million U of penicillin and 2 g of distilled water. The rehydration process takes a minimum of two h, and longer for larger pieces. This preservation method not surprisingly causes cell death to the chondrocytes. Kiseleva[71] and Watkins[72] quote an infection rate of 9.4% for implanted autologous cartilage while Sailer,[73] in his review of reports concerning allogenic cartilage grafts, quotes an infection rate of 1 to 6.2%. In his lyophilized grafts he had an initial incidence of 2.6% infected grafts in 265 implants but only 1.7% in his subsequent series of 173 grafts.

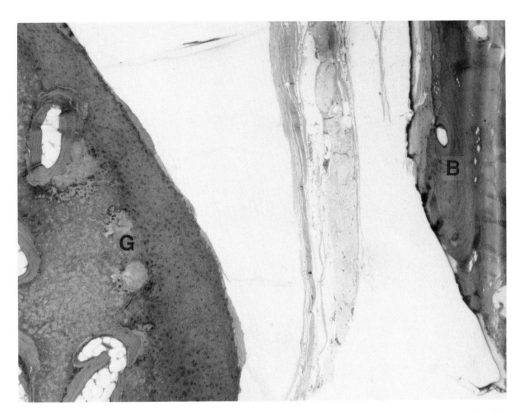

FIGURE 6.   Photomicrograph of graft M3 from Dog #1 showing Merthiolate stored graft (G) and its interface with bone of recipient bed (B). Note heavy layer of compact fibrous tissue between graft and recipient site (HĒ, original magnification ×220). (From Donald, P. J., *Laryngoscope,* 96(7), 798, 1986. With permission.)

Extensive testing in the Macaque monkey using 207 lyophilized grafts on various sites of the maxillofacial skeleton was done. There were no infections. The subperiosteal grafts were fixed to bone by fibrous tissue at 23 d and there was osseous union at 50 d. Curiously there was little difference between xenografts and homografts in this experiment. Some scalloping of the underlying bone was seen similarly to the experience in our experiments. In those grafts harvested up to 50 d postimplantation, no implant absorption was seen. Sixty-three of sixty-six grafts were fixed after 240 to 260 d of implantation. Although the external contour over the grafts appeared unchanged, significant graft absorption was noticed once the grafts were directly inspected. The xenografts had more absorption than the homografts. He feels that the absorption is not extensive enough to warrant even overcorrecting the defect.

Although the experience with processed xenograft cartilage in man has been poor,[28,30,74,75] Ersek et al.[76] have recently reported very favorable results with chemically treated bovine cartilage implants. Of 40 implants, 36 survive unaltered for periods of 1 to 4 years.

In order to investigate the frequency, variety, and the success of cartilage grafting among the otolaryngologic community, a study was conducted in 1980-1981 by Donald and Col[77] under the direction of the AAO (The American Academy of Otolaryngology-Head and Neck Surgery). A questionnaire was mailed to every member of the Academy and the surgeon was asked which methods of cartilage preservation he or she used, how many large implants (blocks >1 cm in diameter) were inserted annually, as well as what the infection and extrusion incidence was, and finally, what the absorption rate was.

Unfortunately only 211 physicians responded, and their measure of graft absorption was purely by clinical impression rather than direct scientific measurement. Given these limi-

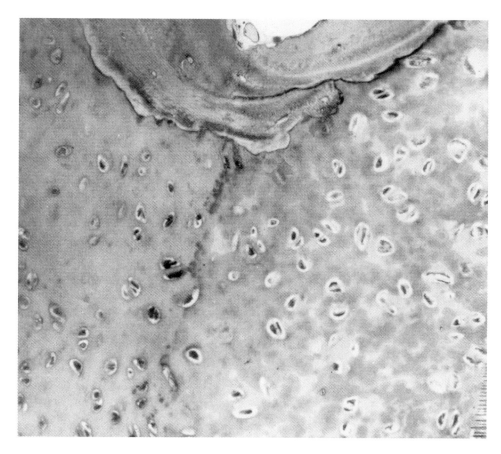

FIGURE 7. Photomicrograph of M3 from Dog #1 showing outer layer of cartilage with viable chondrocytes in a matrix rich in immature proteoglycans. (From Donald, P. J., *Laryngoscope,* 96(7), 799, 1986. With permission.)

tations, the study did however give an impression of the overall success rate, especially when comparing preserved to autologous grafts.

The study showed that low absorption of cartilage grafts was seen most commonly when autologous rather than preserved grafts were used. More physicians had less absorption, and therefore, persistence of grafts of greater size when they used fresh autogenous cartilage compared to when they used the preserved. Figure 9 is a computer-produced analysis comparing the mean absorption percentage experience with preserved cartilage when contrasted with the absorption experienced by those same surgeons, when they implanted autogenous cartilage. The only preservation method that produced less absorption than autogenous cartilage is irradiation. This was statistically significant to the $p < 0.01$ level. The most common methods of preservation were alcohol and Merthiolate™. Although only three physicians implanted formalin preserved grafts, there appeared to be little difference in absorption between this method and the absorption of autologous grafts. However, the numbers of grafts used were small.

VI. IRRADIATED CARTILAGE

In 1972, Dr. Januz Bardach moved from his post as Chairman of the Department of Plastic Surgery, University of Lodz, Poland, to assume the post of Head of the Section of Plastic Surgery and Craniofacial Anomalies, in the Department of Otolaryngology and Maxillofacial Surgery, University of Iowa. He brought with him a 25-year experience in the

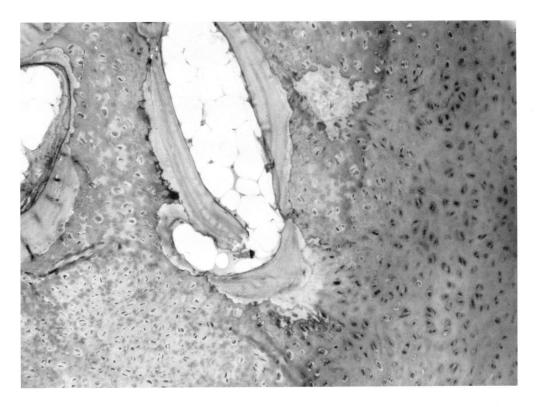

FIGURE 8.   Photomicrograph of graft M3 from Dog #1 near central portion of the graft. Note degenerating cartilage being replaced by islands of osteoid and tubules of compact bone with central marrow cavities (Lees' methylene blue, original magnification × 220). (From Donald, P. J., *Laryngoscope*, 96(7), 800, 1986. With permission.)

ABSORPTION BY METHOD CONTROLLED BY AUTOGRAPH

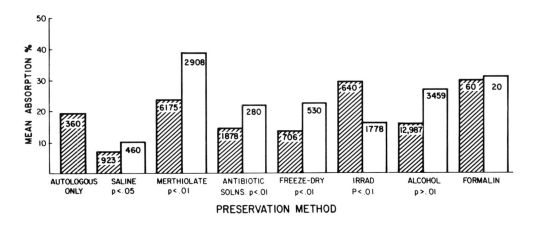

FIGURE 9.   Histogram portraying mean cartilage absorption rate for each method of cartilage graft preservation. Mean absorption rate of each method is compared with that of autologous grafts experienced by same group of surgeons. (From Donald, P. J. and Col, A., *Otolaryngol. Head Neck Surg.*, 90, 89, 1982. With permission.)

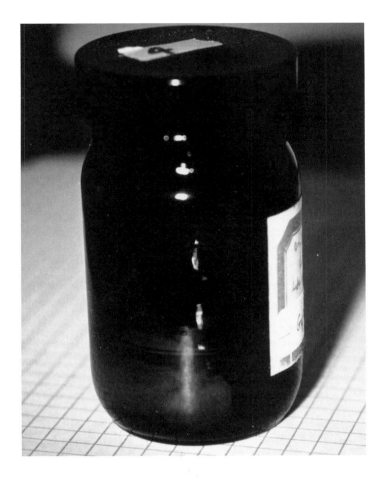

FIGURE 10.   Irradiated cartilage. Notice how radiation has darkened the glass container.

use of irradiated cartilage grafts for reconstructive surgery of the face. Because of his favorable experience, he introduced this technique into the therapeutic regimen at the University of Iowa. As successive groups of residents passed through the program, the technique gained in popularity and became more widely used.

Based on the experience of Bardach et al.[78] we have developed the following technique. Cartilage from the costochondral junction of ribs 4 or 5 to rib number 7 is harvested from cadaver donors who under the age of 35, did not die with cancer or infection and were HIV and hepatitis negative. Young donors are preferred because of the lack of ossification of the cartilage. The cartilage is obtained under clean technique and stored in sterile lactated Ringer's solution or normal saline in a refrigerator. Individual pieces of appropriate length for implantation are placed in glass jars, covered with lactated Ringer's solution and secured with an air tight lid (Figure 10). The grafts are exposed to 4 million rad of γ-irradiation generated from a CO_1 source. At the completion of the irradiation, the bottles are stored at room temperature. The shelf life of the implant is at least two years.

The irradiation changes the color of the glass to a dark brown. The cartilage also darkens somewhat in color. The seal on the bottle is broken only at the time of operation. The irradiation sterilizes the graft but once the seal is broken, the graft becomes potentially contaminated. Portions of unused graft or grafts thought initially to be needed but subsequently remained unused should be discarded. Once the recipient bed is prepared, the graft is carved, keeping in mind the size and three-dimensional configuration desired.

TABLE 1
Amount of Graft Absorption

Classification	Estimated absorption	No. of grafts	Duration of follow-up
Minimal	0—25%	9	7
Moderate	50—75%	24	8
Complete	100%	29	10

From Wellings, D. B., Maves, M. D., Schuller, D. E., and Bardach, J., *Arch. Otolaryngol. Head Neck Surg.*, 114, 291, 1988. With permission.

The recipient bed should be made only large enough to accommodate the graft. This is especially true for the nasal dorsum as there is a tendency for the graft to slip into an unfavorable position if the pocket is made too large. The pocket should be dry. Subperiosteal or extraperiosteal placement may be chosen.

Grafts can be harvested in sizes from 1 to 10 or 12 cm in length and then carved to the size and shape desired. Tissue banks charge about $100/cm of graft length. Numerous tissue banks around the country now have irradiated cartilage grafts available for sale to surgeons. In California, the Northern California Transplant Bank in Palo Alto and the U.C.D. Lion's Eye and Tissue Bank in Sacramento are examples.

The graft is initially carved in a size that is overlarge. A larger graft can be made smaller but the converse is obviously not so. Gradual paring and shaping and repeated insertion is done to ensure precise size and shape. Carving of irradiated cartilage is very simple, the material resembling the consistency of firm soap but without the brittleness. Small areas of ossification if present do impart some brittleness, and care needs to be taken in those circumstances. However, carving is very easy with a #15 or #10 scalpel blade.

Anchoring sutures are rarely used. Temporary transcutaneous stay sutures ("Galloway" sutures) are avoided. We have had two retrograde infections of dorsal nasal implants along such suture tracks. Usually the shape and configuration of the pocket provides adequate fixation. Additional immobilization can be obtained by external taping of the skin.

A little edema rapidly results around the implant, and in the early stages, the graft appears to be solidly united to the underlying osseous or cartilaginous tissues. While this remains in some, many patients acquire a degree of graft mobility with time. The grafts become heavily encased in a fibrous tissue capsule. Perhaps some graft absorption within the capsule imparts this mobility.

Dingman and Grabb[78] reported their excellent results both experimentally in dogs and clinically in facial reconstruction in 1960. Similar results by Alichmiewicz[79] in 1964, and then more recently by Schuller et al.,[80] Agris,[81] and a follow-up report by Dingman[82] uniformly lauded the excellent results of this technique. Availability, ease of preparation, carvability, as well as the subsequent lack of infection, extrusion, deformation, and absorption suggested the ideal nature of this method of cartilage preservation. The greatest drawback of all grafts preserved by various techniques, that of absorption, appeared to be obviated by this method.

The single dissenting paper on the lack of absorption of irradiated cartilage grafts came from Wellings et al.[84] He reported on a long term follow-up study on 42 patients whose grafts were done at the University of Iowa. Table 1 shows the amount of absorption and the average duration of follow-up of 65 grafts in these 42 patients. The group of grafts (50%) that were completely resorbed had the longest follow-up. The only criticism that could be leveled at this study is that only 42 patients of the original 105 that had been implanted returned for follow-up. These may represent the greatest number of unsatisfactory results in patients returning for revision. He also stated that in many of these patients the

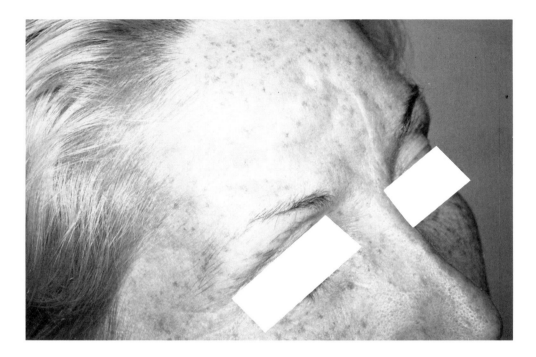

FIGURE 11.   Appearance of forehead one year after recontouring of defect with an irradiated cartilage graft. Most of the graft has absorbed with reappearance of the defect. (From Donald, P. J., *Laryngoscope*, 96(7), 803, 1986. With permission.)

cosmetic correction was maintained, despite even complete graft absorption by replacement with fibrous tissue.

In our implantation studies of irradiated homografts in the sheep and dog, we found a similarly high rate of absorption. These grafts had been left in place from two to six years and at the end of the observation period, total graft absorption was found in 85.7% of implants placed. Indeed, only one of 49 irradiated grafts implanted had any substantial bulk remaining.

This animal experiment did not however, correspond to our own clinical experience. This was especially true when the grafts were not placed under the mimetic musculature of the face. In the animals, all grafts were placed in a subperiosteal pocket under the muscles of facial expression. In our patients, those whose grafts were placed under facial muscles generally had absorption especially when implanted under the frontalis muscle (Figure 11). Those implanted on the chin (Figure 12A and B) or over the malar eminence (Figure 13A and B) had little to no absorption. Virtual uniform success was experienced with implants done over the nasal dorsum. Although some shifting of grafts occasionally occurred, maintenance of projection was preserved. We theorize that the absorption is likely due at least in part to the pressure of this overlying muscle. It is curious that in our studies, 35% of the grafts had what appeared to be a scalloping or depression in the bone at the implantation site.

Other investigators have noted this phenomenon.[37,83,84] Sailer[85] postulates that part of the answer to this phenomenon may be actual bone deposition adjacent to the graft beneath the elevated periosteum under which the graft is placed. This deposition of bone at the periphery of the graft leaves a divot-like configuration in the center of the bed (Figure 14).

The influence of graft shape to the recipient bed may also lead to absorption of both graft and bed. Salthouse and Matlaga[86] have shown that alloplastic grafts with an irregular surface stimulate the cells at the implant site, especially macrophages, to produce higher

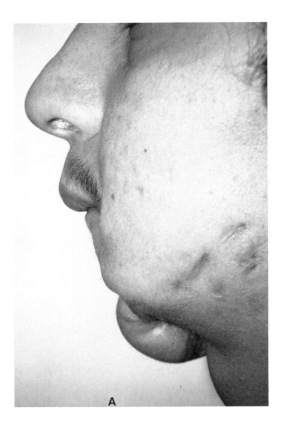 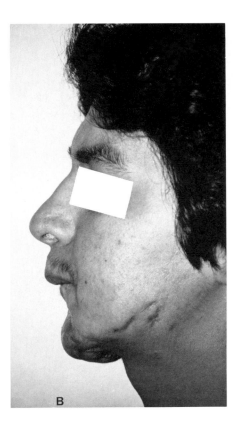

FIGURE 12.   A. Patient following mandibular reconstruction with a deltopectoral flap and rib graft for a gunshot wound of the lower face (preimplantation). B. Irradiated cartilage implant over chin for augmentation following mandibular reconstruction for a gunshot wound of the lower face (four months postimplantation). (From Donald, P. J., *Laryngoscope*, 96(7), 804, 1986. With permission.)

concentrations of lysosomal enzymes. These are produced to a much lesser degree at the interface with a smooth surfaced graft. Whether this phenomenon occurs with the implantation of homologous or autogenous grafts is unclear. It does suggest that a biomechanical mechanism induced by a physical force such as pressure could bring about absorption of both the graft and the tissue at the implantation site. The influence of minimal pressure of an alloplast on bone showing absorption in the ear has been elegantly illustrated by Macri and Chole,[87] and is thought to be brought about by osteoclasts.

The influence of pressure on hyaline cartilage grafts presents paradoxical considerations. It is clear from what has been discussed that continuous alternating compression and relaxation activity is important for cartilage nutrition in its normal site of residence, and that when immobilized, hyaline cartilage tends to resorb. However, the pressure on a graft of such cartilage can induce a destructive process with the appearance of macrophages and lymphocytes exerting the destructive and absorptive influences both on the graft and the implant site. Perhaps the problem resides in the fact that we are attempting to replace morphologic cartilage with hyaline cartilage. Morphologic cartilage such as that of the ear and nose does not become exposed to the rigors of continuous compression and relaxation, while the hyaline cartilage of the knee joint, for instance, has this stress continuously.

At this point in time, our conclusion is that cartilage grafts should not be placed on the face where there will be pressure exerted on it, especially if this is generated by the contracting and relaxing forces of facial musculature.

The significance of subperiosteal vs. extraperiosteal implantation remains unclear. We

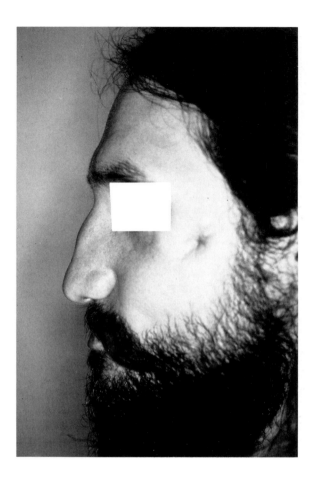

FIGURE 13A.   Patient following gunshot wound to the face with
a depressed zygoma (preoperative).

place our nasal grafts extraperiosteally. The grafts over the frontal sinus area were similarly placed. The grafts for chin augmentation in the cosmetic cases were placed subperiosteally, whereas those larger grafts for augmentation of hemifacial microsomia or deficient chins following mandibular reconstruction, were not. The cosmetic augmentation mentoplasty patients are difficult to assess, as it is well known that even when any chin implant is removed, providing it has resided *in situ* for some months, chin projection is maintained. This is presumably due to the acquisition of fibrous tissue. On the other hand, the reconstructed patients show slow absorption on their grafts of up to 50% of their initial bulk after prolonged residence at the implantation site with some evidence of relapse of chin retrusion.

VII. CONCLUSIONS

A host of homograft cartilage graft preservation methods are available. Unfortunately no technique will prevent the phenomenon of absorption. Irradiated cartilage placed in areas of the face in which the intermittent or continuous pressure of overlying facial mimetic musculature will absorb partially or completely. The nasal dorsum and malar eminence appears to be the most favored site. Further investigation into the biology of these grafts at the molecular level needs to be undertaken to understand and hopefully best take advantage of this preservation technique.

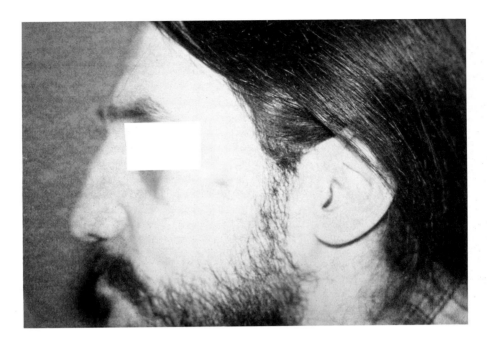

FIGURE 13B.   Irradiated cartilage graft over left malar eminence eight months postimplantation (post-operative). (From Donald, P. J., *Laryngoscope*, 96(7), 803, 1986. With permission.)

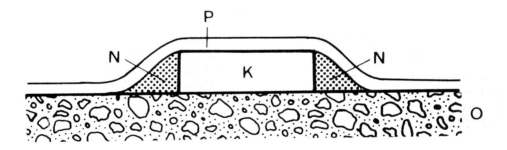

FIGURE 14.   Diagram illustrating the deposition of bone (N) adjacent to an implanted cartilage graft (K) placed in a pocket under periosteum (P). This may account for the appearance of the bony shoulders surrounding a cartilage graft giving a divot-like appearance to the bone of the graft bed. (From Sailer, H. F., *Transplantation of Lyophilized Cartilage in Maxillofacial Surgery: Experimental Foundations and Clinical Success*, S. Karger, New York, 1983, 42. With permission.)

REFERENCES

1. **Bert, P.,** Sur la greffe animale, *C.R. Acad. Sci.,* 51, 587, 1865.
2. **Meijer R. and Walia, I. S.,** Preserved cartilage to fill facial bone defects, in *Biomaterials in Reconstructive Surgery,* Rubin, L. R. Ed., C. V. Mosby, St. Louis, 1983, 509.
3. **Sushruta, S.,** in *Bhishagratma k: An English Translation of the Sushruta Samhita,* based on original sanskrit text, Calcutta, Bose, 1907.
4. **Peer, L. A.,** The fate of living and dead cartilage transplanted in humans, *Surg. Gynecol. Obstet.,* 68, 603, 1939.
5. **Gibson, T., Curran, R. C., and Davis, W. B.,** The survival of living homograft cartilage in man, *Transplant. Bull.,* 4, 105, 1957.
6. **Gibson, T. and Davies, W. B.,** A bank of living homograft cartilage: A preliminary report, in *Transactions of the International Society of Plastic Surgeons,* 2nd Int. Cong., Wallace, A. B., Ed., Livingstone, Edinburgh, 1960,, 452.
7. **Caplan, A. I.,** Cartilage, *Sci. Am.,* 251, 84, 1984.
8. **Kosher, R. A.,** The chondrocyte and chondroblast, in *Cartilage, Vol. 1: Structure, Function and Biochemistry,* Hall, B. K., Ed., Academic Press, New York, 1983, 39.
9. **Urist, M. R.** The origin of cartilage: investigations in quest of chondrogenic DNA, in *Cartilage, Vol. 2: Development, Differentiation and Growth,* Hall, B. K., Ed., Academic Press, New York, 1983, 1.
10. **Hall, B. K.,** Tissue interactions and chondrogenesis, in *Cartilage, Vol. 2: Development, Differentiation and Growth,* Hall, B. K., Ed., Academic Press, New York, 1983, 187.
11. **Nathanson, M. A. and Hay, E. D.,** Analysis of cartilage differentiation from skeletal muscle growing on bone matrix. 1. Ultrastructural aspects, *Dev. Biol.,* 78, 301, 1980.
12. **Sheldon, H.,** Transmissions E.M. of cartilage, in *Cartilage, Vol. 1: Structure, Function and Biochemistry,* Hall, B. K., Ed., Academic Press, New York, 1983, chap. 4.
13. **Yamada, K. M. and Olden, K.,** Fibronectins—Adhesive glycoproteins of cell surface and blood, *Nature (London),* 275, 179, 1978.
14. **Linder, E., Veheri, A., Ruoslahti, E., et al.,** Distribution of fibroblast surface antigen in the developing chick embryo, *J. Exp. Med.,* 142, 41, 1975.
15. **Dessau, W., Sasse, J., Timple, R., et al.,** Synthesis and extracellular deposition of fibronectin in chondrocyte cultures. Response to the removal of extracellular cartilage matrix. *J. Cell. Biol.,* 79, 342, 1978.
16. **Lewis, C. A., Praft, R. M., Pennypacker, J. B., et al.,** Inhibition of limb chondrogenesis *in vitro* by Vitamin A: alterations in cell surface characteristics, *Dev. Biol.,* 64, 31, 1975.
17. **Pennypacker, J. P., Hassell, J. R., Yamada, K. M., et al.,** The influence of an adhesive cell surface protein in chondrogenic expression, *in vitro, Exp. Cell Res.,* 121, 411, 1979.
18. **West, C. M., Lanza, R., Rosenbloom, J., et al.,** Fibronectin alters the phenotypic properties of cultured chick embryochondroblasts, *Cell,* 17, 491, 1979.
19. **Abbot, J. and Holtzer, H.,** The loss of phenotypic traits by differentiated cells. III. The reversible behavior of chondrocytes in primary cultures, *J. Cell Biol.,* 28, 473, 1966.
20. **Coon, H. G.,** Clonal stability and phenotypic expression of chick cartilage cells *in vitro, Proc. Natl. Acad. Sci. U.S.A.,* 55, 66, 1966.
21. **Mayne, R., Vail, M. S., Mayne, P. M., et al.,** Changes in type of collagen synthesized as clones of chick chondrocytes grow and eventually lose division capacity, *Proc. Natl. Acad. Sci. U.S.A.,* 73, 1674, 1976.
22. **Muller, P. H., Lemmer, C., Gay, S., et al.,** Immunochemical and biochemical study of collagen synthesis by chondrocytes in culture, *Exp. Cell Res.,* 108, 47, 1977.
23. **Elves, M. W.,** Newer knowledge of the immunology of bone and cartilage, *Clin. Orthop.,* 120, 232, 1976.
24. **DePalma, R. G., DePalma, M. T., and DeForrest, M.,** Experimental alteration of the shape of rabbit ear cartilage, *J. Surg. Res.,* 4, 2, 1964.
25. **Thomas, L.,** Reversible collapse of rabbit ears after intravenous papain and prevention of recurrence by prostone, *J. Exp. Med.,* 104, 245, 1956.
26. **Robbins, T. H.,** Chondrocyte specialization: a clinical example, *Br. J. Plast. Surg.,* 32, 307, 1979.
27. **Gibson, T.,** Transplantation of cartilage, in *Reconstructive Plastic Surgery,* Converse, J. M. and McCarthy, J. C., Eds., Vol. 1, 2nd Ed., W. B. Saunders, Philadelphia, 1977, 301.
27a. **Glasgold, A. I., et al.,** Mechanical properties of septal cartilage homographs, *Otolaryngol. Head Neck Surg.,* 99(4), 374, 1988.
28. **Gibson, T. and Davis, W. B.,** The distortion of autogenous cartilage grafts: its cause and prevention, *Br. J. Plast. Surg.,* 10, 257, 1958.
29. **Fry, H. J. H.,** Interlocked stresses in human septal cartilage, *Br. J. Plast. Surg.,* 19, 276, 1966.
30. **Fry, H. J. H.,** The healing of cartilage, in *Biological Aspects of Reconstructive Surgery,* Kernahan, D. A. and Vistnes, L. M., Eds., Little, Brown, Boston, 1977, 351.
31. **Mikhelson, N. M.,** Homogenous cartilage in maxillofacial surgery, *Acta Chir. Plast. (Prague),* 4, 3, 1962.

32. **Curran, R. C. and Gibson, T.,** The uptake of labeled sulphate by human cartilage cells and its use as a test of viability, *Proc. R. Soc., London, Ser. B,* 155, 575, 1956.

33. **Elves, M. W.,** Immunology of cartilage, in *Cartilage, Vol. 3: Biomedical Aspects,* Hall, B. K., Ed., Academic Press, New York, 1983, 229.

34. **Davis, W. B. and Gibson, T.,** Absorption of autogenous cartilage grafts in man, *Br. J. Plast. Surg.,* 24, 405, 1971.

35. **Peer, L. A.,** Diced cartilage grafts, *Arch. Otolaryngol.,* 38, 156, 1943.

36. **Albright, J. A. and Misra, R. P.,** Mechanisms of resorption and remodeling of cartilage, in *Cartilage, Vol. 3: Biomedical Aspects,* Hall, B. K., Ed., Academic Press, New York, 1983, 49.

37. **Dupertuis, S. M.,** Actual growth of young cartilage transplants in rabbits, *Arch. Surg.,* 43, 32, 1941.

38. **Peer, L. A., Ihalia, I. S., and Bernhard, W. G.,** Further studies on the growth of rabbit ear cartilage graft, *Br. J. Plast. Surg.,* 19, 105, 1966.

39. **Farkas, L.,** Growth of normal and reconstructed auricles, in *Symposium on reconstruction of the auricle,* Vol. 10, Tanzer, R. C. and Edgerton, M. T., Eds., C. V. Mosby, St. Louis, 1974, 24.

40. **Fessel, J. M. and Chrisman, O. D.,** Enzymatic degradation of chondromucoprotein by cell-free extracts of human cartilage, *Arthritis Rheum.,* 7, 398, 1964.

41. **Quintarelli, B., Dellaro, M. C., Balduini, C., et al.,** The effects of alpha amylase on collagen-proteoglycans and collagen-glycoprotein complexes in connective tissue matrices. *Histochem. J.,* 18, 373, 1969.

42. **Chrisman, O. D.,** Biochemical aspects of degenerative joint disease, *Clin. Orthop.,* 64, 77, 1969.

43. **Dingle, J. T. and Dingle, T. T.,** The site of cartilage matrix degradation, *Biochem. J.,* 190, 431, 1980.

44. **Starkey, P. M., Barrett, A. F., and Burliegh, M. C.,** The degradation of articular cartilage by neutrophil proteinases, *Biochem. Biophys. Acta,* 483, 386, 1977.

45. **Tubb, R. W. and Fell, H. B.,** The effect of synovial tissue on the synthesis of proteoglycan by the articular cartilage of young pigs, *Arthritis Rheum.,* 23, 245, 1980.

46. **Dingle, T. T.,** Catabolin—A cartilage catabolic factor from synovium, *Clin. Orthop.,* 156, 219, 1981.

47. **Ridge, S. C., Oronsky, A. L., and Kerwan, S. S.,** Induction of the synthesis of latent neutral protease in chondrocytes by a factor synthesized by activated macrophages, *Arthritis Rheum.,* 23, 448, 1980.

48. **Deshmukh-Phadke, K., Nanda, S., and Lie, K.,** Macrophage factor that induced neutral protease secretion by normal rabbit chondrocytes, *Eur. J. Biochem.,* 104, 175, 1980.

49. **Van Boxel, J. A. and Paget, S. A.,** Predominantly T-cell infiltrate in hematoid synovial membrane, *N. Engl. J. Med.,* 293, 517, 1975.

50. **Stastny, P., Rosenthal, M., Andres, M., et al.,** Lymphokines in the rheumatoid joint, *Arthritis Rheum.,* 18, 237, 1975.

51. **Herman, J. H., Musgrove, D. S., and Dennis, M. U.,** Phytomitogen induces lymphokine-mediated cartilage proteoglycan degradation, *Arthritis Rheum.,* 20, 922, 1977.

52. **Sargente, N., Kuettner, K. E., Soble, L. W., et al.,** The resistance of certain tissues to invasion. II. Evidence for extractable factors in cartilage which inhibit invasion by vascularized mesenchyme, *Lab. Invest.,* 32, 217, 1975.

53. **Donald, P. J.,** Collagen implants: here today and gone tomorrow?, *Otolaryngol. Head Neck Surg.,* 95, 607, 1986.

54. **Gertzbein, S. D. and Lance, E. M.,** The stimulation of lymphocytes by chondrocytes in mixed cultures, *Clin. Exp. Immunol.,* 24, 102, 1975.

55. **Gertzbein, S. D., Tait, J. H., Devlin, S. R., et al.,** The antigenicity of chondrocytes, *Immunology,* 33, 141, 1977.

56. **Fincham, W. J.,** An Investigation into the Possibility of Humoral Autoantibody Production in Response to Challenge by Allogenic and Synergenic Articular Chondrocytes, M.Tech. thesis, Brunel University, Uxbridge, 1973.

57. **Malseed, Z. M. and Heyner, S.,** Antigenic profile of the rat chondrocyte, *Arthritis Rheum.,* 19, 223, 1976.

58. **Elves, M. W.,** A study of the transplant antigens on chondrocytes from articular cartilage, *J. Bone Jt. Surg.,* 56B, 178, 1974.

59. **Craigmyle, M. B. L.,** Regional lymph node changes induced by cartilage homo and heterografts in the rabbit, *J. Anat.,* 92, 74, 1958.

60. **Craigmyle, M. B. L.,** An autoradiographic and histochemical study of long term cartilage grafts in the rabbit, *J. Anat.,* 92, 467, 1958.

61. **Craigmyle, M. B. L.,** Antigenicity and survival of cartilage homografts, *Nature,* 182, 1248, 1958.

62. **Elves, M. W. and Zervas, J.,** An investigation into the immunogenicity of various components of osteoarticular grafts, *Br. J. Exp. Pathol.,* 55, 344, 1974.

63. **Elves, M. W. and Ford, C. H.,** A study of the humoral immune response to osteoarticular grafts in the sheep, *Clin. Exp. Immunol.,* 177, 497, 1974.

64. **Heyner, S.,** The significance of the intercellular matrix in the survival of the cartilage allografts, *Transplantation,* 8, 666, 1969.

65. **Maroudas, A., Bullough, P., Swanson, S. A. U., et al.,** The permeability of articular cartilage, *J. Bone Jt. Surg.,* 50(B), 166, 1978.

66. **Muhlbauer, W. D., Schmidt-Tintemann, U., and Glaser, M.,** Long term behavior of preserved homologous rib cartilage in the correction of saddle nose deformity, *Br. J. Plast. Surg.,* 24, 325, 1971.

67. **Donald, P. J.,** Cartilage grafting in facial reconstruction with special consideration of irradiated grafts, *Laryngoscope,* 96, 786, 1986.

68. **Betzel, F. and Schilling, H.,** Uber die Biologie, Konsierung und Verpflan zung von Knorpelgewebe Zentbl, Chir, 85, 1170, 1960.

69. **Schmelzle, R.,** Die Verwendung Homologer Gewebekonserven ur Kiefer-Gesichts-Bereich: Hab.-Schr., Tübingen, W. Germany, 1974.

70. **McGlynn, M. J. and Sharpe, D. T.,** Cialite preserved homograft cartilage in nasal augmentation: a long term review, *Br. J. Plast. Surg.,* 34, 53, 1981.

71. **Kiseleva, E. Z.,** Die Anwendung von Fixiertem Leichenknoyel in *der Kiefer - Gesichto Chirurgie Stomatologija,* 1952, 39.

72. **Watkins, A. B. K.,** Twisting of cartilage in saddle nose implants, *Med. J. Aust.,* ii, 43, 1957.

73. **Sailer, H. F.,** Experiences with the use of lyophilized bank cartilage for facial contour correction, *J. Maxillofac. Surg.,* 4, 149, 1976.

74. **Sailer, H. F.,** Gefriergetrockneter Knorpel in der Rekonstruktiven Gesichts chirurgie, *Fortschr Kiefer - Gesichtschir,* 24, 56, 1979.

75. **Peer, L. A.,** *Transplantation of Tissues,* Vol. 1, Williams & Wilkins, Baltimore, 1955, 110.

76. **Ersek, R. A., Rothenberg, P. B., and Denton, D. R.,** Clinical use of an improved processed bovine cartilage for contour defects, *Ann. Plast. Surg.,* 13, 44, 1984.

77. **Donald, P. J. and Col, A.,** Cartilage implantation in head and neck surgery: report of a national survey, *Otolaryngol. Head Neck Surg.,* 90, 85, 1982.

78. **Dingman, R. O. and Grabb, W. C.,** Costal cartilage homografts preserved by irradiation, *Plast. Reconstr. Surg.,* 28, 562, 1960.

79. **Alichmiewicz, A., Bardach, J., Kozlowski, H., et al.,** Research on grafted conserved homogenous cartilage, *Acta Chir. Plat.,* 6, 229, 1964.

80. **Schuller, J. E., Bardach, J., and Krause, C. J.,** Irradiated homologous costal cartilage for facial contour reconstruction, *Arch. Otolaryngol.,* 103, 12, 1977.

81. **Agris, J.,** Personal communication, 1980, as reported in Meijer, R. and Walia, I. S., Preserved cartilage to fill facial bone defects, in *Biomaterials in Plastic Surgery,* Rubin, L. R., Ed., C. V. Mosby, St. Louis, 1983, 509.

82. **Dingman, R. O.,** Follow-up clinic on costal cartilage homografts preserved by irradiation, *Plast. Reconstr. Surg.,* 50, 516, 1972.

83. **Robinson, M. and Thuken, R.,** Bone resorption under plastic chin implants, *J. Oral Surg.,* 27, 116, 1969.

84. **Wellings, D. B., Maves, M. D., Schuller, D. E., Bardach, J.,** Long term results of irradiated homologous cartilage grafts, *Arch. Otolaryngol. Head Neck Surg.,* 114, 291, 1988.

85. **Sailer, H. F.,** Transplantation of lyophilized cartilage in maxillofacial surgery: experimental foundations and clinical success, S. Karger, New York, 1983, 42.

86. **Salthouse, T. N. and Matlaga, B. F.,** Some cellular effects related to implant shape and surface, in *Biomaterial in Plastic Surgery,* Rubin, L. R., Ed., C. V. Mosby, St. Louis, 1983, 40.

87. **Macri, J. and Chole, R. A.,** Bone erosion in experimental cholesteatoma: the effects of implanted barriers, *Otolaryngol. Head Neck Surg.,* 93, 3, 1985.

Chapter 10

BONE GRAFTS IN FACIAL RECONSTRUCTION

Lawrence J. Marentette

TABLE OF CONTENTS

I. INTRODUCTION

Despite the use of alloplastic or cadavaric materials for reconstruction or augmentation of a defect, autogenous bone graft is still considered to be the "gold standard". The results of transplanting fresh osseous tissue are predictable and reliable. Bone grafting and, more specifically, types of graft materials have evolved over the years, from the simple transfer of bony material itself to the recipient site, to the transfer of bone and skin with its own arterial and venous system. There is a wide range of clinical applications of bone grafts in facial plastic and reconstructive surgery.

II. FREE BONE GRAFTS

A. ILIAC CREST

Iliac crest is a popular bone graft in the head and neck as the material of choice for filling defects.[1] Its uses can range from using particulate cancellous marrow packed into a small defect as a filler substance to a large block which can be employed as a grafting material in the reconstruction of mandibular segmental defect. By virtue of its cancellous nature, it allows the rapid ingrowth of blood vessels and soft tissue, thereby ensuring adequate integration with the osseous tissue at the recipient site. Its most common use is in reconstruction of mandibular defects resulting either from trauma or tumor. The defects may range in size from 1 to 2 mm up to a hemimandible. Nonunion of the mandible presents as the persistent mobility at a fracture site. Fibrous tissue has formed between the two ends of the bone and, thus, prevents osseous bridging at the fracture site allowing for the persistent mobility. In some cases, the ends of the bone may be freshened and the scar tissue removed with adequate fixation to allow healing. But, more often than not, there has been some degree of bone resorption at the fracture site. When this occurs, removal of scar tissue and reapproximation of the bone would narrow the dental arch and result in a malocclusion. Therefore, a filler material is needed to bridge the defect in the mandible. In this situation, particulate cancellous bone from the ilium is harvested and the ends of the bone debrided of all soft tissue. Next, intermaxillary fixation is applied to reestablish the patient's premorbid occlusion and the particulate cancellous marrow would then be packed into the fracture site. It is equally important in this situation, not only to provide additional bone at the fracture site, but also to maintain rigid fixation at the site to allow adequate incorporation of the newly transplanted bone graft. This could be accomplished either with intermaxillary fixation or rigid plate stabilization. In the larger mandibular defects where a complete segment of the mandible needs to be reconstructed, iliac crest is harvested as a block of the appropriate size to fit into the recipient site. In the case of a hemimandible, the bone may be harvested in such a way that the contours of the ilium are taken into consideration to allow for curvatures at the angle of the mandible and in the parasymphyseal and symphyseal region. Iliac crest has also been used in orbital surgery in the correction of enophthalmos.[1] Here again, it is harvested as a block of appropriate size and placed along the floor of the orbit, and also at the superior medial and superior lateral aspects of the orbital roof. Although iliac crest has been used as an augmentation material, the resorptive rate, for example as a malar, forehead, or nasal implant, is significant.[2] Iliac crest is harvested by initially making an incision in the skin overlying the anterior portion of the ileum. The incision is made below the level of the ilium, and then the skin is retracted superiorly such that the scar does not override the prominence of the bone, thereby causing discomfort at the waist when wearing pants. The incision is carried down through the skin and subcutaneous tissues, and the skin is then retracted superiorly where the periosteum of the ileum is then incised. Usually the superior rim of the ileum is preserved, and this is cut and hinged medially on the medial periosteum of the ilium. This, then, exposes the cancellous portion of the bone. If particulate iliac crest is needed, a curette can be used to remove the cancellous bone. If, however, a block is needed, then the medial cortex of the ileum is cut, and a chisel is driven down between the lateral cortex and the cancellous interface. In doing so, this preserves the lateral cortex of the ileum, and thus, does not disrupt the gluteal musculature. Care must be taken during the dissection not to injure the lateral femoral cutaneous nerve as meralgia paresthetica would result, which is a severe pain in the distribution of that nerve. Postoperative ambulation is difficult and the patients may be on crutches and a cane for anywhere from 2 to 6 weeks following harvesting of the graft. The degree of incapacitation is usually related to the amount and extent of the bone graft taken.

B. SPLIT RIB

Like iliac crest, split rib grafts have also been a time proven grafting material.[2] Ribs are harvested by making an incision in the inframammary crease on the anterior chest wall. After the incision is carried down through the skin and subcutaneous tissues, the ribs are then identified. This may be the 4th, 5th, or 6th rib. The incision is made through the outer periosteum of the rib extending from the costochondral junction laterally and posteriorly. The extent of dissection and amount of rib taken depends upon the amount of bone needed at the recipient site. After the periosteum has been elevated from the rib, the dissection then carries around the superior and inferior border with care being taken not to injure the intercostal neurovascular bundle. The dissection is then carried along the inner surface of the rib with particular attention being taken to avoid lacerating or incising into the parietal pleura. The rib is then sectioned at the costochondral junction and at a lateral posterior site. The length of this section is dependent upon the amount of graft material required. The morbidity with split rib grafting postoperatively is less than that of iliac crest. However, the most common immediate complication is pneumothorax. This occurs if the parietal pleura has been lacerated, and if this occurs, the pleura needs to be closed and a chest tube may be necessary to maintain the lung in its inflated position. On occasion, if the intercostal nerves are injured during the dissection, a neuroma may persist at the donor site which would present as persistent radiating pain along the distribution of the involved nerve. After the rib is harvested, it is almost completely decorticated (Figure 1) and then split with an osteotome (Figure 2). The decortication offers two advantages. First, it allows the more rapid ingrowth of vessels and soft tissue into the split rib graft, thereby decreasing the chances for postoperative infection and resorption. Secondly, it allows the rib to be bent with the rib bending forceps, thereby allowing the surgeon to custom contour the bone graft to the recipient site (Figure 3). Split rib has been used extensively in the reconstruction of midfacial deformities resulting, for example, from maxillectomy or otomandibular dysostosis. In these cases, the ribs can be contoured to the shape of the maxilla and the zygoma. In cases of reconstruction after maxillectomy, the ribs are used to reconstruct the missing portions of the zygoma, orbital floor, anterior maxilla, alveolar ridge, and palate. In cases of otomandibular dysostosis, the grafts are used in an onlay fashion to augment deficiencies in the zygomatic arch and the zygoma. They are also useful in reconstructing a glenoid fossa when it is absent in these cases. The foundation for the fossa is made from the multilayered rib grafts and lyophilized cartilage can then be placed to act as the gliding surface for the reconstructed mandibular condyle and ramus. Split rib has also been used in mandibular reconstruction. It can be used to replace segmental defects of the mandible, and also as an onlay graft over the alveolar ridge for augmentation of the atrophic edentulous mandible, and also as an adjunct in repair of the atrophic edentulous mandible fracture.[3] There can be significant resorption of split rib grafts when used as augmentation material of the alveolar ridge and, recently, techniques of alveolar ridge osteotomies have become popular, so as to allow the split rib to become an interpositional rather than an onlay graft, thus reducing the amount of long-term resorption.

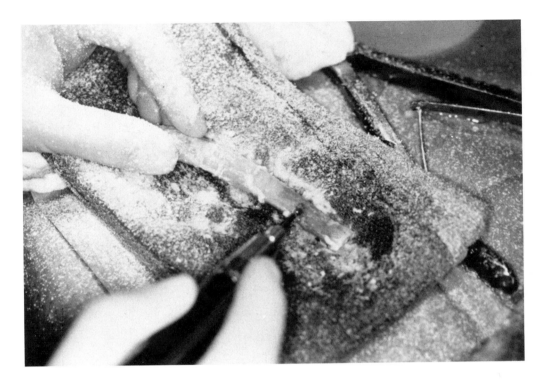

FIGURE 1.   The rib is partially decorticated using a rotary burr. Note the darker color in the area of decortication.

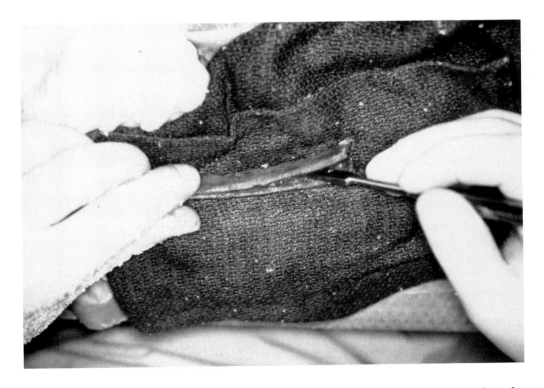

FIGURE 2.   The rib is split with a fine osteotome by hand with care being taken to avoid fracturing the graft.

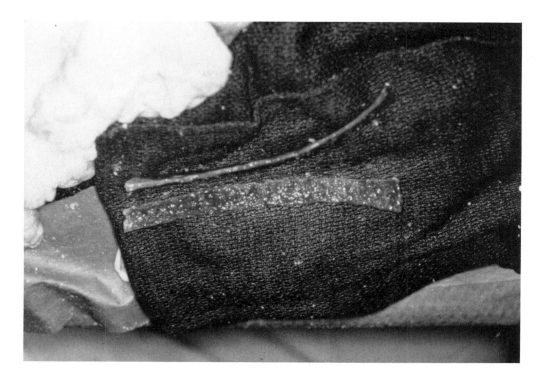

FIGURE 3. The completely split rib can now be bent to fit the contour of the recipient site.

C. CALVARIAL GRAFTS

Calvarial bone grafts have become increasingly popular as a grafting material in max-illofacial surgery.[3] Calvarium is harvested as a partial thickness graft, either removing the outer table only, or the inner table only, thereby maintaining the integrity of the skull and avoiding a full thickness skull defect with its inherent dangers. Inner table calvarial grafts are commonly employed in craniofacial surgery where craniotomy has been done, thereby, allowing access to the inner table of the craniotomy bone flap. Inner table calvarium has the advantage of not leaving a depression in the skull as would result from outer table bone grafting, thereby being more aesthetically pleasing. Outer table grafting is most commonly used when only facial reconstructive surgery is necessary and a craniotomy is not being performed. Outer table harvesting consists of drilling through the outer table into the diploic layer of the skull, and then cutting through the diploic layer leaving the inner table intact. If a coronal incision is employed to gain access to the upper facial skeleton in cases of facial trauma, then the skull is in the operative field. If, however, the bone is being harvested solely for nasal reconstruction, then an incision needs to be made in the scalp in order to gain access to the calvarium. In this case, the incision is made in the hairbearing area of the scalp overlying the right or left parietal bones. The incision is carried down through the scalp, subcutaneous, and galea layers. The periosteum is then incised and reflected. Using a side-cutting burr or an electric driven handpiece, the outer table of the skull is scored to the exact dimension of the required graft material (Figure 4). This is usually a rectangular shape, however, circular or oval defects would require a custom and precise outline to match the defect site. After scoring the bone, the cutting burr is used to further deepen the scored areas circumferentially around the graft site which burrs deeper into the outer table calvarium. When slight bleeding occurs from the bone in the depths of the scored areas, then the diploic layer of the skull has been entered (Figure 5). At this point, deeper cutting into the skull could result in a penetration of the burr to the intercranial cavity and, therefore, circumfer-

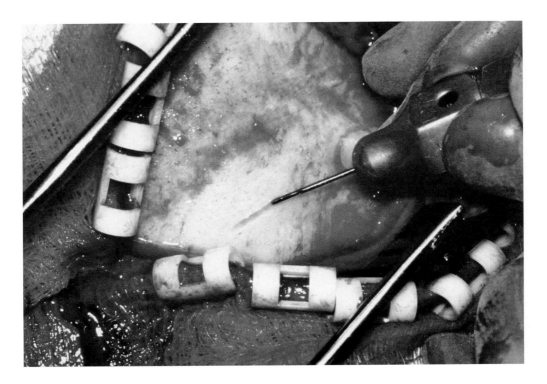

FIGURE 4.   The outer table of the skull is initially scored with a side-cutting burr.

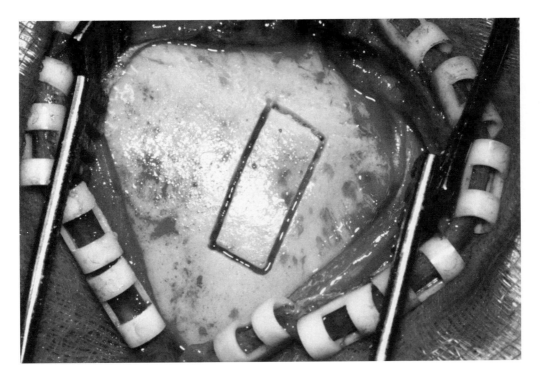

FIGURE 5.   The graft has been completely outlined down into the diploic layer of the skull.

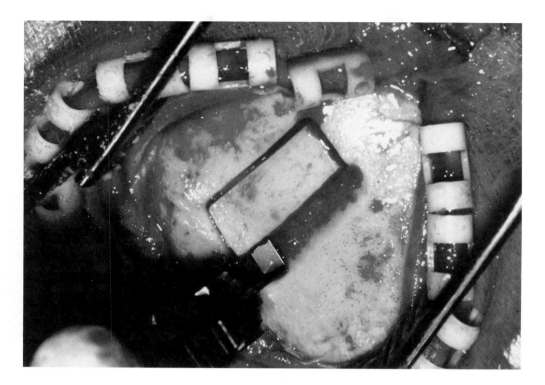

FIGURE 6. After feathering down one edge of the donor site, the right angle saggital saw is being introduced into the diploic layer.

ential drilling is ceased at this point. Next, a round cutting burr is used to feather the bone adjacent to the scored area and on the remaining skull. The burring is not performed on the graft itself. By feathering the edge of the bone, this then allows the surgeon to utilize a right angled sagittal saw blade to cut through the diploic layer. The blade is inserted into the diploic area and then the cuts are made in the diploic layer parallel to the outer and inner table (Figure 6). By utilizing this technique, inadvertent penetration to the cranial cavity itself is extremely remote. Once the diploic cuts have been completed, then the graft is easily removed with forceps and delivered to the recipient site (Figure 7). This has the obvious advantage of eliminating the necessity of doing a craniotomy for harvesting bone graft. Both outer and inner table calvarial bone is of membranous origin, and it has been found clinically to be a material that undergoes minimal resorption. It is of an extremely rigid nature and provides support which is superior to that which can be achieved by split rib. However, by virtue of its rigid nature, the calvarium cannot be bent unless a partial osteotomy is performed which would then weaken the structural support of the graft. Contour corrections are achieved by matching the contour of the calvarial donor site to the contour of the recipient bed.

It is important with any of these free grafting materials to rigidly fix the bone grafts either in the defect site or to the underlying bone. If grafts are movable, soft tissue ingrowth is retarded, thereby allowing more resorption of the graft. However, if the graft material is immobilized either across the defect or to the underlying bone, then capillary and soft tissue ingrowth occurs which reduces the long-term resorption of the graft.

III. OSTEOMYOCUTANEOUS GRAFTS

Resorption of free bone grafts, either partial or complete, has long been recognized as a disadvantage when using these materials. Some hold the opinion that free bone grafts are

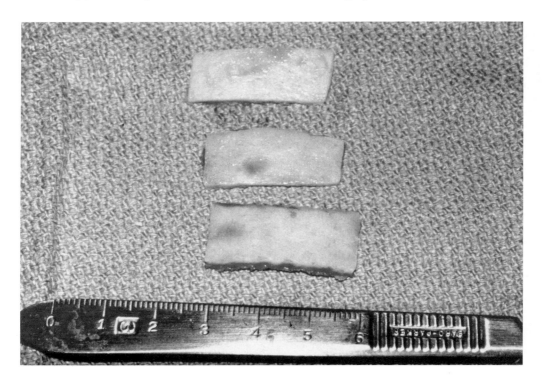

FIGURE 7.   A number of grafts can be harvested conforming to the recipient site.

implants and not true grafts, because the transferred bone cells die prior to adequate vascular ingrowth. From this, the concept evolved of transferring bone grafts with their blood supply in order to maintain the shape of the graft and to prevent obligatory osteoclastic resorption.

A. PECTORALIS MAJOR OSTEOMYOCUTANEOUS FLAP

The pectoralis major myocutaneous flap has become the main stay in the reconstruction of soft tissue defects in the head and neck. Its use can be extended to an osteomyocutaneous flap by harvesting the underlying segment of rib which is attached to periosteum and the overlying origin of the pectoralis major muscle.[4] The blood supply for this osteomyocutaneous flap is based on the thoracoacromial artery. This artery supplies the pectoralis major muscle and it has been shown that perforating vessels exit the surface of the muscle penetrating through the subcutaneous tissues to the skin overlying the muscles. Similarly, it has been reported that the blood supply to the rib is through the overlying periosteum which receives its nutrients from the muscular origin. An incision is made on the anterior chest wall through the skin and subcutaneous tissues running diagonally from the clavicle to the xyphoid process. Skin is usually required with this flap to reconstruct a soft tissue defect of the floor of the mouth. A skin paddle is outlined based on the size of the intraoral defect. The skin and subcutaneous tissues are incised around this skin paddle down to the pectoralis major muscle. The skin is then sutured to the muscle so that shearing of the perforating vessels to the skin will not occur during flap mobilization. The skin is then dissected from the surface of the muscle both laterally and medially, and the entirety of the muscle is outlined. The origin of the muscle is then freed from its underlying attachment to the rib periosteum, except in the area of the rib graft where it must remain intact. The muscle is then dissected free from the chest wall and then rotated with the rib in a superior medial fashion to the oral cavity. The portion of the rib used for the graft should approximate the size and the contour of the mandibular defect. Osteotomies could be performed in a vertical fashion on the underside of the rib for contouring, however, this would weaken the structural support of the graft. Likewise, critical attention must be paid, rigidly fixing the graft in the recipient site. Not only are the forces produced by the masticatory muscles acting at the graft osteosynthesis sites, but also the downward pull of the overlying myocutaneous flap as well. This flap/graft has been used in both lateral and anterior mandibular defects and does carry the advantage of an immediate bony reconstruction following ablative tumor surgery.

B. TRAPEZIUS OSTEOMYOCUTANEOUS FLAP

The trapezius osteomyocutaneous flap has, as well, been advocated for mandibular reconstruction.[5] The trapezius myocutaneous flap can be dissected as a lateral flap or a lower flap. The lateral trapezius myocutaneous flap is based on the occipital artery and the transverse cervical artery and extends from the base of the skull along the superior border of the trapezius out to the shoulder. The lower trapezius myocutaneous flap is based on the transverse cervical artery and is harvested along the back and descending from the base of the skull down towards the inferior border of the trapezius muscle at its origins along the spinous processes of the lateral thoracic vertebrae. The flap may be brought up as a myocutaneous flap, however, it may also include bone from the scapula with periosteum of the bone supplied by nutrient vessels from the overlying trapezius muscle. In this case, the spine of the scapula is the donor site for the bone graft and, as the trapezius myocutaneous flap is elevated, the spine of the scapula is removed, thereby maintaining the musculoperiosteal connection. Up to the 12 cm in length can be obtained from the spine of the scapula and the cortico-cancellous nature of the graft provides rigidity to the reconstructed mandible. It has an advantage over the pectoralis major osteocutaneous flap in that, by virtue of its donor site, the possibility of pneumothorax is eliminated.

C. TEMPORAL COMPOSITE CALVARIAL FLAP

Myo-osseous flaps have become popular for facial reconstruction. The temporal composite calvarial bone flap is a good example of this. Through a coronal approach, the temporalis muscle is exposed. The bone then underlying the temporalis muscle is incised preserving the musculature attachment and the deep temporal artery which provides blood supply to the calvarium. The bone and the muscle are then raised as a unit and then brought forward as a grafting material. This can be used in the maxillectomy reconstruction to obturate a hard palate defect. It can also be used to augment the malar areas where deficiency such as that seen in Treacher-Collins Syndrome is present. This carries with it the advantage of, not only bringing in a vascularized bone graft, but also soft tissue along with it, so that bony and soft tissue augmentation can be performed simultaneously.

IV. MICROVASCULAR FREE BONE GRAFTS

With the advent of microvascular surgery, an entirely new spectrum of bone grafts has emerged as providing viable alternatives to previously described methods. The graft is harvested with its arterial and venous supply, and the vessels are anastomosed to vessels at the recipient site. It is not clear why the pedicle, if it is a free bone graft, could indicate what the vascular pedicle from donor area will be anastomosed to a vascular pedicle at recipient site. The graft with its pedicle can be brought up as an osseous graft or, when in combination with skin paddles, an osteocutaneous graft. Because they have their own blood supply, resorption is minimal with these grafts and they can be placed into a radiated field with a high degree of success. Training in microvascular surgery consists, not only of the anatomical harvesting of the various flaps with their adjacent bone grafts, but also specific training in the microvascular technique of the anastomosis. This involves suturing 1 to 3 mm arteries and veins together using very fine 9 to 0 suture material. The anastomosis is performed with the aid of the operating microscope and very fine microinstrumentation. After the arteries and veins are sutured to similar vessels at the recipient site, clamps previously occluding the vessels are released and the anastomosis checked for any leakage. Postoperatively, temperature and blood supply to the flap is constantly monitored, and if the flap becomes cyanotic or white, or the temperature drops in the skin paddles of the graft flap combination, then the anastomosis is immediately reopened and checked for occlusion either of the arterial side or of the venous side. Proper training in microvascular surgical techniques and a constant practice are required to assure correct arterial and venous anastomosis.

A. SCAPULAR FREE FLAP

The scapular free flap is an osteocutaneous flap based on the circumflex scapular artery. This vessel with its branches supplies the skin overlying the scapula, as well as the bone at the lateral scapular border. This artery divides into two branches, the first supplying skin to the horizontal or scapular flap, and the second to the vertical or parascapular flap. Additional branches supply the periosteum of the lateral border of the scapula. When used as a bone graft, the lateral border of the scapula is harvested which results in a graft of approximately 1.5 × 3.0 cm in thickness and length ranging from 10 to 14 cm. This flap is extremely useful in head and neck cancer reconstruction as it can provide a large amount of bone with its own blood supply and additionally 1 to 2 skin paddles which can be used to resurface large defects in the oral cavity and, in some cases, through-and-through defects also involving the facial skin.

B. RADIAL FREE FOREARM FLAP

The radial free forearm flap utilizes the radius as its donor site.[6] Up to 40% circumference of the radius may be taken and the length available is 10 to 12 cm. This flap is based on the radial artery and vein which supplies the skin of the anterior forearm and through an intermuscular septum, the periosteum of the underlying radius. Because the artery and vein has a fairly lengthy subcutaneous course, the vascular pedicle can be 10 to 12 cm (Figure 8). This is important when the recipient vessels are at a distance from the recipient site of the bone graft. With this flap, the donor site is of the nondominant hand. It is of vital importance that during harvesting of the grafts, as well as the anchorage and anastomotic suturing, that the periosteum remain in contact with the bone. If it should be striped at any point along the bone graft, then the bone is acting as a free rather than a vascularized bone graft. This is important in that a vascularized living bone graft undergoes minimal, if any, resorption, whereas a free bone graft undergoes obligatory osteoclastic resorption and remodeling to some degree as it is replaced with new bone. The bone can be cut to fit the defect. The osteotomy sites are rigidly stabilized and the graft is secured to the mandible. The stabilization is with either plates or screws (Figure 9).

C. ILIAC CREST FREE FLAP

Iliac crest free flap, based on the deep circumflex iliac artery, provides significant amount of cancellous bone, as well as bulk for soft tissue, as well as osseous reconstruction. This vessel has been shown to supply a large area of periosteum over the ilium, thereby providing up to 14 cm in length of free vascularized bone graft. The graft provides approximately 2 to 3 cm in thickness of cancellous bone with a vascularized cortical rim to provide additional support. The cancellous bone provides a good base for which subsequent dental implants can be inserted. The implants are later uncovered and dentures are attached to the implants. However, when used as an osteocutaneous graft, a large amount of soft tissue bulk is

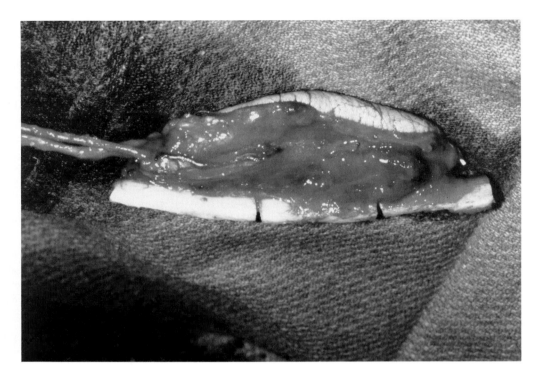

FIGURE 8. The radial free forearm flap has been elevated with two osteotomies made in the bone. The pedicle length can be appreciated as well as the vascular supply to the bone and the overlying skin.

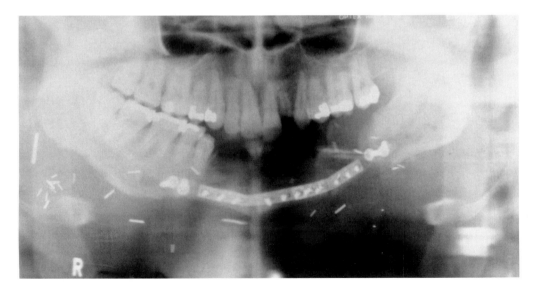

FIGURE 9. The flap has been placed into the recipient mandibular defect. The osteotomies are stabilized with mini-plates and the graft is lag-screwed to the remaining mandibular stumps.

harvested in order to provide adequate blood supply to the skin and to the bone. This bulkiness oftentimes provides an excess of soft tissue when used to reconstruct mandibular defects. These grafts are proving to be extremely reliable even in postradiation patients.

V. SUMMARY

Bone grafting has evolved into a spectrum of techniques ranging from the earliest free particulate cancellous grafts to the present day of microvascular osteocutaneous grafts. In choosing the graft material, it is important for the surgeon to consider the recipient site and what materials have been shown to work best at that site. Also, it is important to consider the surrounding soft tissues at the recipient site, and whether there is scar tissue, induced either by trauma or by radiation. If so, then consideration may be given to bringing in freshly vascularized soft tissue as well as bone.

REFERENCES

1. **Enneking, W. F., Eady, J. L., and Burchardt, H.,** Autogenous cortical bone grafts in the reconstruction of segmental skeletal defects, *J. Bone Jt. Surg.,* 62, 1039, 1980.
2. **Leake, D. L.,** Contouring split ribs for correction of severe mandibular atrophy, *J. Oral Surg.,* 34, 940, 1976.
3. **Powell, N. B. and Riley, R. W.,** Cranial bone grafting in facial aesthetic and reconstructive contouring, *Arch. Otolaryngol.,* 113, 713, 1987.
4. **Cuono, C. B., and Ariyan, S.,** Immediate reconstruction of a composite mandibular defect with a regional osteomusculocutaneous flap, *Plas. Reconstr. Surg.,* 65, 477, 1980.
5. **Balk, S. M., Biller, H. N., Krespi, Y. P., et al.,** The lower trapezius island myocutaneous flaps, *Ann. Plast. Surg.,* 5, 108, 1980.
6. **Song, R., Gao, Y., Song, Y., et al.,** The forearm flap, *Clin. Plast. Surg.,* 9, 21, 1982.

Chapter 11

INDUCED OSTEOGENESIS FOR CRANIOFACIAL RECONSTRUCTION

Dean M. Toriumi and Wayne F. Larrabee

TABLE OF CONTENTS

I. INTRODUCTION

Facial plastic and reconstructive surgeons are constantly searching for the ideal grafting material. Most surgeons prefer to use autogenous bone or cartilage depending on the purpose of the graft. In some cases, harvesting the bone graft is associated with greater morbidity than the primary reconstructive procedure itself. In an effort to avoid this morbidity, some surgeons turned to allogenic demineralized bone that can transform local host cells into bone-forming cells (osteoinduction). This chapter reviews the experimental and clinical evidence demonstrating the osteoinductive properties of demineralized bone. Present theories on the mechanism of bone induction are discussed. Recent research on novel bone inductive factors is reviewed. These newly characterized factors may be used in implants of the future.

II. BONE GRAFTS

In 1821, Phillipe von Walther studied the repair of cranial defects in dogs.[1] These experimental studies sparked the earliest work with calvarial bone grafts. In 1885, Macewen successfully repaired a craniotomy defect with implanted parietal bone chips.[2] Barth studied histologic changes noted during cranial reconstruction, using autogenous bone grafts.[3] When placed in defects in dog skulls, both fresh and dead calvarial bone disks underwent resorption followed by new bone formation. In either case, the bone graft acted as a passive scaffolding through which host bone grew. Barth referred to this process as, "schleichender ersatz" or "creeping substitution". Macewen showed that bone paste produced during burring of bone grafts probably lacked viable osteogenic cells.[4] In 1970, Shehadi found histologic evidence of solid bone healing at 4 months in 80% of skull defects filled with fresh bone paste.[5] With no evidence of viable cells in the bone paste, a question arose about the mechanism of bone formation with the fresh bone powder.

III. THEORY OF INDUCTION

The concept of induction of tissue growth has been defined as the physical-chemical effect which one tissue exerts on another.[6] Urist and McLean[6] transferred 250 samples of various types of motor-skeletal tissue, including several different types of bone grafts to the eye. New bone formation was noted after tissue transfer as a result of induction and/or proliferation of the transplanted tissue. Based on the ability to produce new bone within 10 days of transplantation, the following tissues were thought to possess inherited osteogenic potential:

1. Bone marrow
2. Periosteum from a young growing animal
3. Tissue culture outgrowth of embryonic bone
4. Endosteum and cancellous bone
5. Fibrocartilagenous callus[6]

Weiss described one of the first induction systems in skeletal tissue.[7-9] Weiss transplanted freeze-dried cartilage into salamander limbs and discovered deposits of new cartilage formed adjacent to the graft.[8] Weiss described induction as a mechanism which requires an organic union between donor tissue and host tissue.

Tissue can be tested for osteogenic potential or for its ability to produce bone by:

1. Transfer of donor tissue subcutaneously or to muscle,[10-11] visceral organ,[12] or anterior chamber of the eye [13,14]
2. Tissue transfer to a defect in bone of the host [15-17]
3. Injections of solution or extracts into muscle[18] or a healing fracture [19]

Using these techniques, numerous investigators studied the osteoinductive properties of different tissues, including several different forms of bone grafts.

IV. DEMINERALIZED BONE

Demineralized bone was initially introduced by Nicholas Senn as an antiseptic bone graft taken from ox tibiae to repair canine cranial defects.[20] Senn treated the ox tibiae with "dilute muriatic acid" (HCl) and used the grafts to repair osteomyelitis defects in patients.[20] Several other surgeons found success using demineralized bone by Senn's technique.[21-24] Miller stated that demineralized bone was actually superior to fresh bone grafts.[24] Several other investigators were unable to reproduce Senn's clinical and experimental work, and the use of demineralized bone was abandoned for nearly half a century.[25,26] Ray and Holloway went back to an animal model and showed that demineralized bone closed rat skull defects more rapidly than nondemineralized bone, but they failed to test the bone matrix for inductive activity.[27] In 1961, Sharrard and Collins reported using EDTA-demineralized bone for spinal fusions in three scoliotic children but failed to report follow-up data.[28]

Negative reports predominated the literature until 1965, when Marshall Urist revealed incontrovertible evidence that demineralized bone matrix induced new bone formation in rats and rabbits.[29] Urist reviewed the literature on demineralized bone and discovered that most of the failures occurred when bone was treated with EDTA instead of hydrochloric acid.[30] The EDTA-decalcified bone was ineffective because of the deleterious effects of endogenous neutral proteases. Urist also showed that decalcified dentin induced bone formation when implanted into oral osseous and muscle tissue.[31,32]

Reddi and Huggins studied the osteoinductive capability of demineralized bone powder of uniform particle size.[33] In rats, cartilage, bone, and bone marrow formed in a synchronous and quantitative sequence of events.[33] Alkaline phosphatase activity gradually increases from days 3 to 6 with an explosive rise in enzyme activity on day 7.[33] Initially, local mesenchymal cells migrated towards the bone particles. Then host cells were transformed into chondroblasts by day 5. The ectopic cartilage became vascularized and started to mineralize by day 10, finally being replaced by bone and hematopoietic marrow.[33]

In 1973, Reddi and Huggins demonstrated that size and shape of demineralized bone powder had a profound influence on its osteoinductive properties.[34] An optimal particle size in the range of 74 to 840 μm created a larger yield of cartilage and bone. Fine powders, 44 to 74 μm were rather weak in transformation potency and yielded sporadic and sparse islands of cartilage and bone. This phenomenon is most likely due to the surface area-to-volume ratio of the implanted matrix.[35]

Oxygen tension also had an influence on the temporal sequence of host tissue differentiation. The ingrowth of oxygen-carrying capillaries seemed to induce chondrolysis. In deep regions of the transplants where oxygen tension was low, cartilage was seen first. Other studies have shown that low oxygen tension favored chondrogenesis and higher oxygen tension favored osteogenesis.[36,37]

Collagens and proteoglycans are two major extracellular macromolecules in skeletal and dental bone matrix.[38,39] One of the initial steps in the transformation of host cells into osteoblasts is interaction between collagenous bone matrix and fibroblasts. In 1973, Huggins and Reddi showed that osteogenic potency of collagenous bone matrix was inhibited by heparinized blood plasma by binding to heparin.[40] There is a correlation between the degree of sulfation of various heparin sulfates and their inhibitory effects on collagenous bone matrix.[39] Such findings suggest an interaction between collagenous matrix and anionic components on the cell membrane.

The electrochemical charge of bone matrix is crucial to the osteoinductive capability of demineralized bone.[41] Brief exposure of positively charged rat bone matrix to highly charged electrochemicals resulted in profound but reversible effects on its ability to transform chondroblasts and osteoblasts. Most animal cells have a negative charge due to the presence of N-acetyl-neuramic acid,[42] chondroitin sulfate,[43] and heparin sulfate.[44] Reddi and Huggins postulated that electronegative molecules inhibited transformation by blocking surface-surface interaction between fibroblast and bone matrix.[41] They showed that alteration of electric charge on the surface of bone matrix can reversibly inactivate its bone induction properties.

Investigation of the sequential changes in collagen types that occur during bone formation after transplantation of demineralized bone matrix revealed similarities to other processes of bone growth and repair. In 1977, Reddi et al. showed that type III collagen was present around proliferating mesenchymal cells in contact with implanted bone matrix.[45] This collagen formation is similar to the reported increase in type III collagen in the early phases of wound healing and granulation tissue formation. These early cells may act as progenitor cells that eventually transform into chondroblasts. Type II collagen was associated with chondrogenesis. In conjunction with tissue vascularization, osteogenesis occurred with formation of type I collagen on the surface of type II collagen reactive spicules. These sequential cellular transitions are similar to those seen in bone formation at the epiphyseal plate and site of a healing fracture.[45]

Reddi demonstrated that a proteoglycan specific to cartilage appeared on day 7, gradually dissipated, and was eventually replaced by a smaller proteoglycan on days 11 through 14.[46] The smaller proteoglycan appeared at the same time cartilage resorption began to occur. Ornithine decarboxylase is an important enzyme involved in regulation of polyamine synthesis and cell proliferation. Rath and Reddi showed that the activity of this enzyme peaked on day 3 when the matrix contacts the mesenchymal cells and on day 8 when osteoblasts begin to proliferate.[47] This data suggests that demineralized bone matrix is a local mitogen for connective tissue cells.[48]

V. BONE INDUCTION PRINCIPLE

Marshall Urist introduced the bone induction principle (BIP) as a protein macromolecule in dentin and bone matrix.[49] BIP has the capacity to transform young proliferating, undifferentiated mesenchymal cells of a bony vertebrate into cartilage, bone, or bone marrow cells. The structure of this protein macromolecule is unknown. BIP induces bone formation without transplantation of living cells; however, mode of preparation of the tissue is crucial to its level of activity. Surface or partial decalcification of bone matrix makes BIP activity accessible and retains it in a biologically active form. Complete decalcification renders BIP inactive. In these early studies, new bone formed in 3 to 4 weeks with a good yield of new bone after implantation of 0.6 N HCl surface-decalcified bone matrix.

Once the bone induction system is established, host cells adjacent to the bone matrix become the inducing cells for the next layer of responding cells. Bone induction occurs in two directions: centrifugally to produce lamellar bone and centripetally to produce new bone marrow cells.[49] BIP is somewhat unspecific in that it may produce tissues other than bone, such as cartilage and fibrous or adipose tissue. The actual activity of BIP was thought to be intimately bound to bone collagen and, therefore, very difficult to isolate for bioassay characterization in physical-chemical terms, or sequence analysis.

Millipore chambers filled with decalcified bone matrix and live muscle mesenchymal cells revealed cartilage and bone induction within the chambers and in regions outside the chambers where matrix was contacting opposing tissue just outside the chamber.[50] There was no bone formation in regions around the chambers where host tissues were not in close contact with the decalcified bone matrix. Millipore chambers filled with decalcified bone matrix alone, or live muscle mesenchymal cells alone, did not induce bone formation inside or outside of the chamber. BIP is not freely diffusible and probably moves through adjacent tissues for only short distances, requiring an organic union between host tissue and decalcified bone matrix.

Undecalcified bone grafts undergo resorption and ingrowth of low-density new bone slowly over periods of months to years. Decalcified bone implants rapidly undergo resorption and ingrowth of higher-density new bone in a couple weeks. However, decalcified bone matrix lacks the structural integrity of a fresh nondecalcified bone graft. Furthermore, Urist was unsure of the actual mechanism of osteogenesis with implanted decalcified bone matrix.[49-52]

In 1968, Urist demonstrated induced osteogenesis in ten patients who had intraosseous implants of HCl-demineralized whole human bone matrix.[53] BIP appeared to be a true bone inducing entity, but could not be purified or characterized.

VI. BONE MORPHOGENETIC PROTEIN

Urist identified bone morphogenetic protein (BMP) as a hydrophobic glycoprotein after partially purifying BMP from other proteins using a nondestructive method of differential solubilization to preserve its osteoinductive activity.[54] The BMP activity was thought to be a protein with a 63,000-Da mol wt.[55]

Adult skull trephine defects of specific dimensions are ideal models for animal and clinical research on bone induction because skull bone healing is incomplete.[56-58] Such defects may close in newborn animals but not in adult animals. Urist filled nonhealing 0.8-cm adult rat skull trephine defects with bovine BMP.[59] Trephine defects healed by bony ingrowth from the rim of the defects, and from bony transformation of perivascular mesenchymal cells of the dura mater into chondroid and woven bone. After 3 to 4 weeks, sinusoids formed and the woven bone remodeled into lamellar bone, with blood borne bone marrow cells colonizing the bone, restoring the diploe. The quantity of new bone formation was proportional to the dose of the BMP that was implanted, with trephine defects closing within 4 weeks. BMP was also shown to stimulate DNA synthesis and cell replication in bone and fibroblast cultures, however, the BMP tested was not purified to homogeneity, and the effects could be due to another substance or a combination thereof.[59-61]

BMP only affected DNA synthesis of periosteum and not periosteum-free bone.[62,63] This would be expected in light of the fact that periosteum of bone is rich in undifferentiated cells and fibroblasts, whereas nonperiosteal bone is composed of mature, differentiated osteoblasts.

VII. TRANSFORMING GROWTH FACTOR

Transforming growth factors are characterized by their ability to induce anchorage-independent growth of cells in soft agar cultures.[64-66] TGF-α and TGF-β are two structurally and functionally distinct classes of transforming growth factors. TGF-α is synthesized by retrovirus-transformed rodent cell lines[64] and some human tumor cell lines.[67] TGF-α is a structural analog of epidermal growth factor (EGF), binds to the EGF receptor site stimulating tyrosine-specific phosphorylation and has similar biological activities.[66] The mature 50-amino acid form of TGF-α is cleaved from a 159-amino acid precursor and acts as a potent mitogen of cells of mesenchymal origin.[68]

TGF-β is a disulfide-linked homodimer comprised of two identical 112-amino acid subunits that uses a receptor distinct from either TGF-α or EGF.[69] This potent mitogen is synthesized by a variety of normal and transformed cells in culture,[65] and has been purified from various sources, including blood platelets,[70] kidney,,[71] and placenta.[72] TGF-β has the capacity to induce colony formation of AKR-2B fibroblasts in soft agar,[73] requiring either TGF-α or EGF to stimulate anchorage-independent growth of normal rat kidney (NRK) fibroblasts.[65] Other investigators have described inhibitory effects of TGF-β on both neoplastic and nonneoplastic cell lines in both monolayer and soft agar.[74-76] Furthermore, TGF-β is a strong inhibitor of proliferation in several different primary or secondary cell cultures, including T and B lymphocytes,[77,78] embryo fibroblasts,[79] skeletal muscle,[80] and bronchial epithelium.[81]

Further work with TGF-β led to the identification and purification of two different forms of the factor referred to as TGF-β1 and TGF-β2.[82,83] TGF-β1 was purified from human platelets,[82] and TGF-β2 was produced by the African green monkey kidney cell line as well as other cell lines.[84,85] TGF-β1 and TGF-β2 exhibit approximately 70% amino acid sequence similarity demonstrated by sequence analysis.[83] A third member of the TGF-β family was recently identified, designated as TGF-β3 and found to exhibit 70 to 75% amino acid sequence similarity with TGF-β1 and TGF-β2.[86,87] Recent evidence indicates that there are at least four other molecules with 32 to 38% sequence homology to TGF-β1 and have been found in bone substance.[83]

TGF-β1 and TGF-β2 are functionally identical in most *in vitro* systems; however, in some systems they differ significantly. TGF-β1 and TGF-β2 differ in their effects on hematopoietic progenitor cells,[88] endothelial cell proliferation,[89] and other cell lines.[90]

Seyedin et al. purified and characterized two cartilage-inducing factors (CIF) from bovine demineralized bone.[91] They called these cartilage-inducing factors, CIF-A and CIF-B. CIF-A and CIF-B each induced embryonic rat mesenchymal cells to assume a cartilage morphology in culture and synthesize cartilage-specific proteoglycan and type II collagen. The amino acid compositions of CIF-A and CIF-B are similar but not identical.[91] TGF-β is also abundant in bone and extensive amino acid sequencing revealed that CIF-B and TGF-β are structurally and functionally identical molecules.[92] TGF-β1 is a homolog of CIF-A and TGF-β2 is a homolog of CIF-B.[83]

One of the early studies implicating a role of TGF-β in bone formation involved the observation that culture medium conditioned by viable fetal rat cranial (calvariae) bones contained EGF-dependent, colony-inducing activity of NRK-49F cells in soft agar.[93] TGF-β is highly concentrated in bone extracts with concentrations in excess of 200 μg/kg of tissue.[94] TGF-β levels are also high in platelets; however, bone appears to be the major storage site in the body on the basis of weight.

Centrella et al. studied the effects of TGF-β on cell replication in osteoblast-enriched cell cultures from rat fetal bone by measuring cell number, culture DNA content, and rate of ^{3}H-thymidine incorporation into DNA.[95] They found that the effects of TGF-β on bone cell replication is biphasic with DNA synthesis increasing, peaking, and decreasing with increasing levels of TGF-β. TGF-β has been shown to stimulate DNA synthesis in bone cell populations suggesting that TGF-β has a regulatory function in the process of bone formation.[96-102] When assessing the effect of TGF-β in cell cultures, the effect of TGF-β as well as other factors must be taken into account.[103] In cell cultures, the cells being studied (osteoblasts, osteoclasts, etc.) may be in different stages of development. TGF-β has different effects on cells in different stages of embryonic development. Therefore, the effects of TGF-β on cells in culture can be misleading and must be interpreted cautiously.[104]

The rat ectopic bone formation assay has been used to study the role of TGF-β in bone formation.[105] This *in vivo* assay is well characterized and recapitulates the embryonic development sequence of bone formation.[29] The sequence begins with cartilage formation, followed by hypertrophy and calcification of the cartilage. Then the cartilage matrix is vascularized by hematopoietic cells and endothelial cells. Finally, the cartilage is gradually resorbed and replaced by bone after the appearance of osteoblasts.[105] In cell culture, there are cells in all stages of this continuum, making investigation of bone differentiation *in vitro* very difficult. With the ectopic bone formation assay, there is only one cycle of bone formation in the implant. Furthermore, events take place in a more synchronous fashion throughout the implant. This feature permits major phases of bone formation to be identified using biological parameters (alkaline phosphatase activity, histomorphometry, etc.).[105]

Using the rat ectopic bone formation assay, TGF-β was detected in developing endochondral bone *in vivo*.[106] TGF-β was present in the highest concentration during the implant transition from calcified cartilage to bone. This period corresponds to the time frame in cell culture when osteoblasts are numerous, TGF-β is being produced, and receptors for TGF-β are widely distributed.[95] TGF-β1 and TGF-β2 were present when osteoblasts were developing, and when the transition from calcified cartilage to bone was taking place. The appearance of TGF-β at the time of ossification indicated the importance of TGF-β as a regulator of bone development. TGF-β has been shown to increase the number of differentiated bone cells capable of collagen production.[107]

Specific markers for chondrocytes include formation of types II and X collagen isoforms, elevated alkaline phosphatase activity, and proteoglycan synthesis.[108-111] Proteoglycan has a prominent role in cartilage production and is an important matrix molecule in endochondral bone formation.

High and low affinity binding sites for TGF-β have been detected in cell cultures from a variety of cell models.[112-116] High affinity binding sites have been demonstrated in fetal rats, bovine bone, and rat osteosarcoma cells.[104] Labeling with radioactive TGF-β revealed three discrete TGF-β receptors with M_r 280 kDa, 85 kDa, and 65 kDa in fetal rat osteoblast-enriched cultures.[104] The high molecular weight receptor (280 to 330 kDa) has a high affinity for both TGF-β1 and TGF-β2. The two lower molecular weight receptors exhibit a higher affinity for TGF-β1 than for TGF-β2.

Osteoblast-enriched populations from fetal bone are more sensitive to the mitogenic effects of TGF-β than similar populations from newborns.[104] TGF either had no effect, or inhibits replication in clonal murine osteoblast-like cell lines and rat osteosarcoma cell cultures, which represent a later stage of osteoblast differentiation. These findings suggest that TGF-β acts in the early stages of bone and cartilage development, and tends to increase select cell populations which synthesize bone matrix.

VIII. PURIFIED BONE MORPHOGENETIC PROTEIN

In 1988, Wang et al. purified bone morphogenetic protein (BMP) from guanidium chloride extracts of demineralized bone.[117] This purified BMP[117,118] is not the same as the BMP of Urist.[54] The factor of Wang et al. was purified 300,000-fold, yielding only 40 μg of BMP from 40 kg of bovine bone powder. As little as 50 ng of factor was able to induce cartilage formation; however, the actual amount of active BMP delivered to the site is not known. The activity was characterized as a protein with a molecular weight of about 30 kDa, which yielded proteins of 30, 18, and 16 kDa on reduction. This purified BMP was cloned to further evaluate the activity of each of the three reduced polypeptides of this factor. Wang et al. described the isolation of full-length complementary DNAs (DNAs) encoding the human equivalent of three polypeptides which have been designated BMP-1, BMP-2A, and BMP-3.[117] BMP-1 appears to be unrelated to other known growth factors. BMP-2A and BMP-3 seem to be closely related to proteins of the family of transforming growth factors. Wozney et al. identified the rest of the family of BMP molecules (BMP-1 to BMP-7).[120] Human recombinant BMP-2A has been shown to effectively form bone in several different animal models.[119,120]

IX. OSTEOGENIN

In 1987, Reddi isolated an extracellular matrix-associated, bone-inductive protein known as osteogenin.[122] Purification steps included dissociative extraction of demineralized bone

TABLE 1
Osteoinductive Preparations

Osteoinductive preparation	Activity of highly purified preparation	Recombinant molecule	Activity of recombinant molecule
Transforming growth factor-β	Regulates bone induction	TGF-β 1 or 2	Regulates bone formation
Bone morphogenetic protein[117]	Bone induction	BMP-2A	Bone induction
Osteogenin[122]	Bone induction	BMP-3	Some cartilage formation: no bone-inducing activity
Osteoinductive factor[123]	Bone induction	Osteoglycin	No bone-inducing activity

using 4.0 *M* guanidine hydrochloride followed by affinity chromatography on heparin sepharose, hydroxyapatite chromatography, gel filtration, and C_{18} reverse-phase HPLC. The method is based on the inhibition of the osteoinductive potential of demineralized bone matrix after treatment with heparinized plasma[40] and heparin, possibly binding to active sites in the matrix. In light of this finding, heparin affinity columns were used to purify the bone-inductive protein. The bone-inductive protein was purified >12,000-fold, and the bone inductive activity was associated with three peaks on reverse phase HPLC, indicating microheterogeneity of the factor. Electrophoresis of the fraction with the highest specific activity revealed a diffuse band with a molecular weight of about 22 kDa.

Further investigation of osteogenin revealed that it is the same factor as recombinant BMP-3 which can form cartilage but has not produced any bone as of yet.[121] Analysis revealed that the bone-inducing activity of highly purified, but nonrecombinant osteogenin was probably due to BMP-2A or a combination of BMP molecules present as a contaminating protein.[121]

X. OSTEOINDUCTIVE FACTOR (OIF)

Recently, osteoinductive factor (OIF) was extracted from demineralized bone matrix using guanidine HCl extraction.[123] OIF was isolated and purified using a combination of gel filtration, ion exchange chromatography, and reverse phase HPLC. OIF is a glycoprotein with a molecular weight of 22 to 28 kDa. Using the rat ectopic bone formation assay, highly purified OIF combined with TGF-β1 or TGF-β2 formed bone. OIF by itself did not form bone unless used in much higher concentrations in a site with viable bone-forming cells (periosteum, etc.).

Further investigation of OIF revealed that it does not induce bone formation by itself and the actual bone-inducing activity of the highly purified, nonrecombinant preparation was due to BMP-2A and TGF-β.[120] The molecule that was identified as OIF has been renamed osteoglycin and has no bone-inducing activity. A summary of the present status on these osteoinductive preparations is shown in Table 1.

XI. CLINICAL APPLICATIONS

Fresh autogenous bone or cartilage have been the preferred grafting materials for facial and cranial augmentation or reconstruction. However, donor site morbidity, limited resources, and unpredictable resorption of autogenous bone make it less than ideal as a grafting material. For these reasons, alloplastic (Proplast, Silicone, Supramid, etc.), and allogeneic materials (demineralized bone) have been used.

Alloplastic materials can act as effective implants; however, they will always remain a foreign body, susceptible to movement, erosion, or infection. Advantages of alloplastic materials are the following: unlimited resources, easy molding or shaping of the implants, and relatively little tissue reactivity.

There were great expectations of demineralized bone and its bone inductive properties. However, there are relatively few studies which evaluate the long-term effectiveness of these implants. In 1981, Glowacki et al. used demineralized bone implants for craniofacial reconstruction in 34 patients, 28 with congenital and 6 with acquired defects.[124] In their early follow-up they found rapid union, healing of large defects, avoidance of harvesting procedures, and the potential for an unlimited supply of material. Biopsies performed in several patients revealed bone formation. They felt bone formation occurred via bone induction as opposed to bone conduction. Patients in this study were followed from 4 to 12 months.

Mulliken et al. used demineralized bone in 42 patients with maxillocraniofacial defects.[125] They used demineralized bone implants prepared in three forms: powder, chips, and blocks. Bony healing was evaluated by clinical and roentgenographic examination. Of sites suitable for evaluation, 31 of 35 were clinically healed within 3 months. Resorption of the implant occurred in four patients, three which were corticocancellous demineralized bone, and one that was demineralized bone powder. They felt demineralized bone powder was the most favorable implant, because it exposes the greatest surface area of host tissue to the bone inducing surface of the implant matrix. In this study, length of follow-up was not addressed.

Mulliken found that dense cortical demineralized bone implants used for nasal reconstruction failed to induce enough bone formation to maintain the desired nasal contour.[126,127] Partial (approximately 50%) late resorption of the implants was noted in most of these cases. Mulliken felt this resorption was consistent with laboratory studies demonstrating the importance of maximal inductive surface area for bone transformation.

Ousterhout reviewed 25 patients who underwent reconstruction or augmentation of the craniofacial region with demineralized bone.[128] He had a follow-up period of 6 to 18 months. He found that the amount of bone formed was relative to the surface area available for bone induction. More bone formed when demineralized bone powder was used instead of a solid cortical implant. Compared with the cancellous bone implant, cortical bone offered relatively little surface area for bone induction. When filling a bony defect where the demineralized bone contacted surrounding bone, the implants seemed to work well. When used strictly for augmentation (nasal dorsum, chin, malar region), the implants had a higher degree of resorption. This resorption may be secondary to pressure of the skin overlying the projecting implant.

In our own series, we reviewed 53 patients who underwent primarily dorsal nasal augmentation using demineralized split rib.[129] Most of these patients had saddle nose deformities (congenital or iatrogenic). The patients were evaluated clinically using photographs. Each case was graded according to the percentage of the implant that was resorbed. In most cases, there was approximately 40% to 80% resorption of the implant after a follow-up of 12 to 48 months (Figures 1 and 2). Larger implants demonstrated the greatest degree of implant resorption. Grafts that were sutured together (multiple layer grafts) demonstrated even a greater degree of implant resorption.

The major drawback to using allogenic demineralized bone for augmentation or reconstruction is its high rate of implant resorption. Some degree of implant resorption is likely due to inadequate contact between host tissue and bone inducing implant surface area. This factor is most prevalent with larger or multiple layer demineralized split rib implants. When two pieces of rib are sutured to each other, 50% of the surface area of each implant is rendered ineffective because it is not contacting host tissue. Demineralized bone powder would provide more surface area for bone induction; however, the powder is difficult to work with and cannot provide distinct contour changes.

Another major factor affecting the osteoinductive potential of demineralized bone is the cellular characteristics at the site of implantation. Demineralized bone implants or any osteoinductive implant will induce more bone formation if the implant is placed in a region that has abundant bone-forming cells (periosteum, osteoblasts, etc.). Implantation into muscle

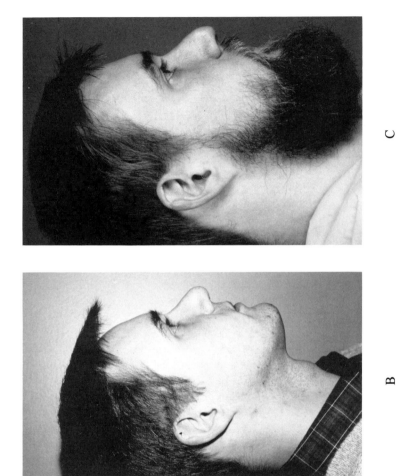

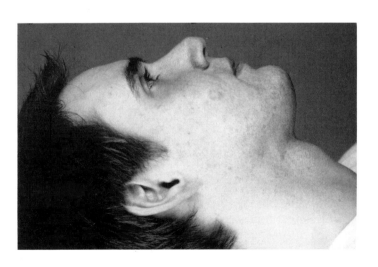

A   B   C

FIGURE 1.   (A) Preoperative lateral view showing severely blunted nasal tip. Demineralized split rib was used as combination nasal dorsum/columellar implant to provide tip support, projection, and definition. The implant was positioned through an open rhinoplasty approach. (B) Postoperative improvement in alar/columellar relationship and dorsal nasal profile 4 months after surgery. (C) Forty-month follow-up revealing severely blunted nasal tip after total resorption of the implant. (From Toriumi, D. et al., *Arch. Otolaryngol. Head Neck Surg.*, 116, 676, 1990. Copyright 1990, Amer. Med. Assoc. With permission.)

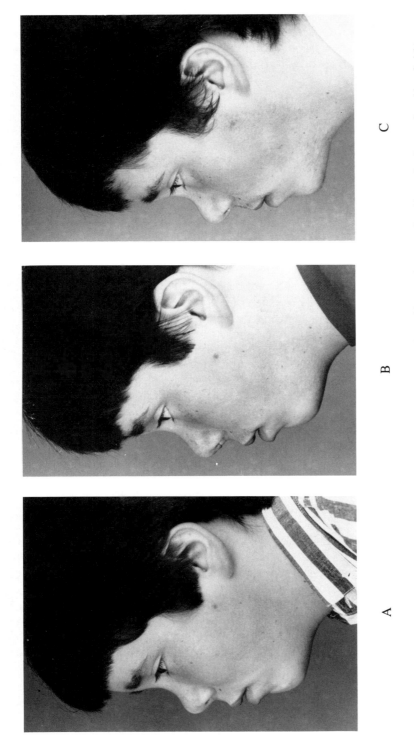

A   B   C

FIGURE 2. (A) Preoperative lateral view showing severe saddle nose deformity in a patient with a previous nasoethmoid complex fracture from blunt facial trauma. (B) Improvement of dorsal nasal profile noted 2 weeks after augmentation of the dorsum was performed with demineralized split rib through an open rhinoplasty approach. (C) Two-year follow-up revealing near complete resorption of the demineralized bone implant. (From Toriumi, D. et al., *Arch. Otolaryngol. Head Neck Surg.*, 116, 676, 1990. Copyright 1990, Amer. Med. Assoc. With permission.)

which is rich in primitive mesenchymal cells may permit transformation of these cells into osteoblasts with subsequent bone formation. However, if demineralized bone is implanted into an area which is not very cellular (scar, areolar tissue, fibrous tissue), chances of osteoinduction are much lower because of the paucity of progenitor cells. Vascularity is also a factor which can influence the osteoinductive potential of demineralized bone implants. A good vascular supply will allow earlier incorporation of the implant and lessen chances of infection. Furthermore, higher oxygen tensions are associated with increased bone formation.[36,37]

In our studies, demineralized bone implants that were used for facial augmentation (dorsal nasal, chin, malar implants) tended to undergo greater degrees of resorption.[129] This is probably due in part to pressure exerted on the implants from the overlying skin or muscle which is already being pushed outward by the implant. This pressure is increased by the facial mimetic musculature. Unless the demineralized bone is rapidly replaced by viable bone-forming cells, the acellular matrix will be resorbed. There also may be some variability in the preparation of the demineralized bone implants even though all of our implants came from the same tissue bank (Mile High Transplant Bank, Denver, CO). One also must consider the possibility of an antigenic response elicited by the host to the cadaver bone despite [60]Cobalt sterilization of the implants. Some investigators have actually looked into attempting to match HLA antibodies between donor and host.

In cases where revision surgery was required because a previous demineralized bone implant resorbed, in most cases biopsy of the residual implant revealed only fibrous tissue. This suggests that there was minimal if any actual bone formation, and the implants essentially acted as a foreign body, ultimately being completely resorbed.

Demineralized bone implants were more successful when used to fill smaller bony defects in the facial skeleton or when implanted next to periosteum or perichondrium. Use of the chips or powdered form of the demineralized bone also appeared to work better than demineralized split rib. Greater success was associated with implantation into a nonstress bearing site where minimal pressure would be applied to the graft. If used in selected cases, demineralized bone can be an effective osteoinductive implant. However, when using this material, the patient should be made aware of the possibility of implant resorption, which may require a secondary operation.

Demineralized bone is not a very effective bone inducing implant because of its limited amount of osteoinductive activity. Its high degree of resorption limits its use to smaller bony defects and cases where demineralized bone powder can be used as a filler. The actual bone inducing activity of demineralized bone most likely represents one of the osteoinductive factors such as TGF-β, BMP-2A, or a combination thereof. However, these factors are present in microgram quantities in demineralized bone limiting the osteoinductive activity of the implants. Many of these factors are similar in structure and activity. Surely they are related in some way. This complex puzzle will not be solved until all of these factors are cloned, expressed, and available for verification of activity of the recombinant molecule.

Once a human recombinant osteoinductive factor like BMP-2A is available in large quantities, the appropriate carrier must be formulated. The carrier must be easy to cut and shape, nonreactive, easy to store, and compatible with the factor. Furthermore, the carrier must resorb in a relatively short period of time so the carrier material can be replaced by new bone formation. If the carrier does not resorb, new bone will add to the volume of the existing carrier material, resulting in enlargement of the implant. A reliable bone-inducing implant should form bone only to the bounds of the initial size of the implant. Control of osteoinductive activity is critical when using such implants in a clinical setting.

XII. FINAL COMMENTS

Although much progress has been made toward isolating and identifying factors that are osteoinductive, the relationship between the multiple factors isolated from bone still remains unclear. Clinical results indicate that demineralized bone is not a very effective bone-inducing implant unless it is used in a fresh bony defect or adjacent to periosteum.

Bone inductive factors carried in a workable vehicle are likely to become the implants of the future. Large scale production of these factors using recombinant DNA methodology is necessary to provide materials for extensive preclinical investigation. Finally, clinical studies will then begin to assess the effectiveness of these bone-inducing implants for craniofacial augmentation or reconstruction.

REFERENCES

1. **Walther, P.,** Wiedereinheilung der bei der Trepanation ausgebohrten Knochenssumcheibe, *J. Chir. Augenh.,* 2, 571, 1821.
2. **Macewen, W.,** Cases illustrative of cerebral surgery. Case of localized encephalitis and leptomeningitis, *Lancet,* 1, 881, 1885.
3. **Barth, F.,** Ueber histologische Befunde nach Knocken-implantationer, *Arch. Klin. Chir.,* 46, 409, 1893.
4. **Macewen, W.,** The growth of bone, in *Observations on Osteogenesis,* James Maclehose and Sons, Glasgow, 1912, 94.
5. **Shehadi, S. I.,** Skull reconstruction with bone dust, *Br. J. Plast. Surg.,* 23, 227, 1970.
6. **Urist, M. R. and McLean, F. C.,** Osteogenetic potency and new bone formation by induction in transplants to the anterior chamber of the eye, *J. Bone Jt. Surg.,* 344, 443, 1952.
7. **Weiss, P.,** *Principles of Development,* Holt, Reinhart & Winston, New York, 1939, 93.
8. **Weiss, P.,** *Differential Growth in the Chemistry and Physiology of Growth,* Parparts, A. K., Ed., Princeton, 1949, 135.
9. **Weiss, P.,** Perspectives in the field of morphogenesis, *Q. Rev. Biol.,* 15, 177, 1950.
10. **DeBruyn, P. P. H.,** Bone formation by fresh and frozen transplants of bone, bone marrow, and periosteum, Hull Anatomical Laboratory, The University of Chicago, *Abstr. Anat. Rec.,* 99, 641, 1947.
11. **Leriche, R. and Policard, A.,** *The Normal and Physiological Physiology of Bone. Its Problems,* Translated by Moore, Sherwood and Key, J. A., C. V. Mosby, St. Louis, 1928.
12. **Pfeiffer, C. A.,** Development of bone from transplanted marrow in mice, *Anat. Rec.,* 102, 225, 1948.
13. **Bisgard, J. D.,** Ossification; influence of mineral constituents of bone, *Arch. Surg.,* 33, 926, 1936.
14. **Dyer, H. M. and Kelly, M. G.,** Cultivation of tumors in the anterior chambers of the eyes of guinea pigs, *J. Natl. Cancer Inst.,* 7, 177, 1946.
15. **Ghormley, R. K. and Stuck, W. G.,** Experimental bone transplantation with special reference to the effect of decalcification, *Arch. Surg.,* 28, 742, 1934.
16. **Gordon, S. D. and Warren, R. F.,** Autogenous diced cartilage transplants to bone: an experimental study, *Ann. Surg.,* 125, 237, 1947.
17. **Reynolds, F. C. and Oliver, D. R.,** Experimental evaluation of homogenous bone grafts, *J. Bone Jt. Surg.,* 32A, 283, 1950.
18. **Heinen, J. H., Jr., Dabbs, G. H., and Mason, H. A.,** The experimental production of ectopic cartilage and bone in the muscles of rabbits, *J. Bone Jt. Surg.,* 31A, 765, 1949.
19. **Levander, G.,** A study of bone regeneration, *Surg. Gynecol. Obstet.,* 67, 705, 1938.
20. **Senn, N.,** On the healing of aseptic bone cavities by implantation of antiseptic decalcified bone, *Am. J. Med. Sci.,* 98, 219, 1889.
21. **Curtis, G. F.,** Cases of bone implantation and transplantation for cysts of tibia, osteomyelitic cavities, and ununited fractures, *Am. J. Med.,* 106, 30, 1890.
22. **Deaver, J. B.,** Secondary bone implantation by a modification of Senn's method, *Med. News (Philadelphia),* 55, 714, 1889.
23. **Mackie, W.,** Clinical observations of the healing of aseptic bone cavities by Senn's method of implantation of antiseptic decalcified bone, *Med. News (Philadelphia),* 57, 202, 1890.
24. **Miller, A. G.,** A case of bone grafting with decalcified bone chips, *Lancet,* 2, 618, 1890.
25. **Barth, A.,** Histologische untersuchungen uber knochen-implantationen, *Beitr. Pathol. Anat.,* 17, 65, 1895.
26. **Schmitt, A.,** Ueber Osteoplastik in klinischer und experimenteller beziehung, *Arch. Klin. Chir.,* 45, 401, 1893.
27. **Ray, R. D. and Holloway, J. A.,** Bone implants: preliminary reports of an experimental study, *J. Bone Jt. Surg.,* 39A, 1119, 1957.

28. **Sharrard, W. J. W. and Collins, D. H.,** The fate of decalcified human bone grafts, *Proc. R. Soc. Med.,* 54, 1101, 1961.

29. **Urist, M. R.,** Bone: formation by autoinduction, *Science,* 150, 893, 1965.

30. **van de Putte, K. A. and Urist, M. R.,** Osteogenesis in the interior of intramuscular implants of decalcified bone matrix, *Clin. Orthop.,* 43, 257, 1965.

31. **Bang, G. and Urist, M. R.,** Bone induction in excavation chambers in matrix of decalcified dentin, *Arch. Surg.,* 94, 781, 1967.

32. **Yeomans, J. D. and Urist, M. R.,** Bone induction by decalcified dentin implanted into oral osseous and muscle tissue, *Arch. Oral Biol.,* 12, 999, 1967.

33. **Reddi, A. H. and Huggins, C. B.,** Biochemical sequences in the transformation of normal fibroblasts in adolescent rats, *Proc. Natl. Acad. Sci. U.S.A.,* 69, 1601, 1972.

34. **Reddi, A. H. and Huggins, C. B.,** Influence of geometry of transplanted tooth and bone on transformation of fibroblasts, *Proc. Soc. Exp. Biol. Med.,* 143, 634, 1973.

35. **Pearson, G. E., Rosin, S., and Deporter, D. A.,** Preliminary observations of the usefulness of a decalcified, freeze-dried, cancellous bone allograft material in periodontal surgery, *J. Periodontol.,* 52, 55, 1981.

36. **Basset, C. A. L.,** Current concepts of bone formation, *J. Bone Jt. Surg.,* 44A, 1217, 1962.

37. **Shaw, J. L. and Basset, C. A. L.,** The effects of varying oxygen concentrations of osteogenesis and embryonic cartilage *in vitro, J. Bone Jt. Surg.,* 49A, 73, 1967.

38. **Matthews, M. B.,** The interaction of proteoglycans and collagen-model systems, in *Chemistry and Molecular Biology of the Intercellular Matrix,* Balazs, E. A., Ed., Academic Press, New York, 1970, 1155.

39. **Reddi, A. H.,** Collagen and cell differentiation, in *Biochemistry of Collagen,* Ramanchandron, G. N. and Reddi, A. H., Eds., Plenum Press, New York, 1976, 449.

40. **Huggins, C. B. and Reddi, A. H.,** Coagulation of blood plasma of guinea pig by the bone matrix, *Proc. Natl. Acad. Sci. U.S.A.,* 70, 929, 1973.

41. **Reddi, A. H. and Huggins, C. B.,** Cyclic electrochemical inactivation and restoration of competence of bone matrix to transform fibroblasts, *Proc. Natl. Acad. Sci. U.S.A.,* 71, 1648, 1974.

42. **Wallach, D. F. H.,** *The Plasma Membrane: Dynamic Perspectives, Genetics and Pathology,* Springer-Verlag, New York, 1972, 115.

43. **Kojima, K. and Yamagasta, T.,** Glycosaminoglycans and electrokinetic behavior of rat ascites hepatoma cells, *Exp. Cell. Res.,* 67, 142, 1971.

44. **Kraemer, P. M.,** Heparan sulfates of cultured cells. I. Membrane associated and cell sap species in Chinese hamster cells, *Biochemistry,* 10, 1437, 1971.

45. **Reddi, A. H., Gay, R., Gay, S., and Miller, E. J.,** Transitions in collagen types during matrix-induced cartilage, bone, and bone marrow formation, *Proc. Natl. Acad. Sci. U.S.A.,* 74, 5589, 1977.

46. **Reddi, A. H., Hascall, V. C., and Hascall, G. K.,** Changes in proteoglycan types during matrix-induced cartilage and bone developments, *J. Biol. Chem.,* 253, 2429, 1978.

47. **Rath, N. C. and Reddi, A. H.,** Changes in ornithine decarboxylase activity during matrix-induced cartilage, bone, and bone marrow differentiation, *Biochem. Biophys. Res. Commun.,* 81, 106, 1978.

48. **Rath, N. C. and Reddi, A. H.,** Collagenous matrix is a local mitogen, *Nature,* 278, 855, 1979.

49. **Urist, M. R., Silverman, B. F., Buring, K., Debuc, F., and Rosenberg, J. M.,** The bone induction principle, *Clin. Orthop.,* 53, 243, 1967.

50. **Buring, K. and Urist, M. R.,** Transfilter bone induction, *Clin. Orthop.,* 54, 235, 1967.

51. **Urist, M. R., Dowell, T. A., Hay, P. H., and Strates, B. S.,** Inductive substrates for bone formation, *Clin. Orthop.,* 59, 59, 1968.

52. **Nogami, H. and Urist, M. R.,** A substratum of bone matrix for differentiation of mesenchymal cells into chondro-osseous tissues *in vitro, Exp. Cell. Res.,* 63, 404, 1970.

53. **Urist, M. R.,** Surface-decalcified allogenic bone (SDAB) implants. *Clin. Orthop.,* 56, 37, 1968.

54. **Urist, M. R., Mikulski, A., and Lietze, A.,** Solubilized and insolubilized bone morphogenetic protein, *Proc. Natl. Acad. Sci. U.S.A.,* 76, 1828, 1979.

55. **Hanamura, H., Higuchi, Y., Nakagawa, M., Iwata, H., Nogami, H., and Urist, M. R.,** Solubilized bone morphogenetic protein (BMP) from mouse osteosarcoma and rat demineralized bone matrix, *Clin. Orthop.,* 148, 281, 1980.

56. **Ray, R. D. and Holloway, J. A.,** Bone implants: preliminary reports of an experimental study, *J. Bone Jt. Surg.,* 39A, 1119, 1957.

57. **Frame, J. W.,** A convenience animal model for testing bone substitute materials, *J. Oral Surg.,* 38, 176, 1980.

58. **Prolo, D. J., Pedrotti, P., Burres, K. P., and Oklund, S.,** Superior osteogenesis in transplanted allogenic canine skull following chemical sterilization, *Clin. Orthop.,* 168, 230, 1982.

59. **Takagi, K. and Urist, M. R.,** The reaction of the dura to bone morphogenetic protein (BMP) in repair of skull defects, *Ann. Surg.,* 196, 100, 1982.

60. **Canalis, E., Peck, W. A., and Raisz, L. G.,** Stimulation of DNA and collagen synthesis by autologous growth factor in cultured fetal rat calvariae, *Science,* 201, 1021, 1980.

61. **Farley, J. R. and Baylink, D. J.,** Purification of a skeletal growth factor from human bone, *Biochemistry,* 21, 3502, 1982.

62. **Canalis, E., Centrella, M., and Urist, M. R.,** Effect of partially purified bone morphogenetic protein on DNA synthesis and cell replication in calvarial and fibroblast cultures, *Clin. Orthop.,* 198, 289, 1985.

63. **Ferguson, D., David, W. L., Urist, M. R., Hurt, W. C., and Allen, E. P.,** Bovine bone morphogenetic (bBMP) fraction-induced repair of craniotomy defects in the rhesus monkey (*Macaca* species), *Clin. Orthop.,* 219, 251, 1987.

64. **DeLarco, J. E., Preston, Y. A., and Todero, G. J.,** Growth factors from murine sarcoma virus-transformed cells, *Proc. Natl. Acad. Sci. U.S.A.,* 75, 4001, 1978.

65. **Roberts, A. B., Anzano, M. A., Lamb, L. C., Smith, J. M., and Sporn, M. B.,** New class of transforming growth factors potentiated by epidermal growth factor: Isolation from non-neoplastic tissues, *Proc. Natl. Acad. Sci. U.S.A.,* 78, 5339, 1981.

66. **Reynolds, S. F., Todaro, G. J., Fryling, G. C., and Stephenson, J. R.,** Human transforming growth factors induce tyrosine phosphorylation of EGF receptors, *Nature,* 292, 259, 1981.

67. **Todaro, G. J., Fryling, C. M., and DeLarco, J. E.,** Transforming growth factor produced by certain human tumor cells: polypeptides that interact with epidermal growth factor, *Proc. Natl. Acad. Sci. U.S.A.,* 77, 5258, 1980.

68. **Derynck, R., Roberts, A. B., Winkler, M. E., Chen, E. Y., and Goeddel, D. V.,** Human transforming growth factor-x: precursor structure and expression in *E. coli, Cell,* 38, 287, 1984.

69. **Frolik, C. A., Wakefield, L. M., Smith, D. M., and Spron, M. B.,** Characterization of a membrane receptor for transforming growth factor type β in normal rat kidney cells, *J. Biol. Chem.,* 260, 10995, 1984.

70. **Childs, C. B., Proper, J. A., Tucker, R. F., and Moses, H. L.,** Serum contains a platelet-derived transforming growth factor, *Proc. Natl. Acad. Sci. U.S.A.,* 79, 5312, 1982.

71. **Roberts, A. B., Anzano, M. A., Meyers, C. A., Wideman, T., Blacher, R., Pan, Y. E., Stein, S., Lehrman, S. R., Smith, T. M., Lamb, L. C., and Sporn, M. B.,** Purification and properties of a type of β transforming growth factor from bovine kidney, *Biochem. J.,* 22, 5692, 1983.

72. **Frolik, C. A., Dart, L. L., Meyers, C. A., Smith, D. M., and Sporn, M. B.,** Purification and initial characterization of a type β transforming growth factor from human placenta, *Proc. Natl. Acad. Sci. U.S.A.,* 80, 3676, 1983.

73. **Tucker, R. F., Volkenant, M. E., Branum, E. L., and Moses, H. L.,** Comparison of intra- and extracellular transforming growth factors from nontransformed and chemically transformed mouse embryo cells, *Cancer Res.,* 43, 1581, 1983.

74. **Tucker, R. F., Shipley, G. D., Moses, H. L., and Holley, R. W.,** Growth inhibitor from BSC-1 cells closely related to platelet type beta transforming growth factor, *Science,* 226, 705, 1984.

75. **Roberts, A. B., Anzano, M. A., Wakefield, L. M., Roche, N. S., Stern, D. E., and Sporn, M. B.,** Type β transforming growth factor: a bifunctional regulator of cell growth, *Proc. Natl. Acad. Sci. U.S.A.,* 82, 119, 1985.

76. **Moses, H. L., Tucker, R. F., Leaf, E. B., Coffey, R. J., Halper, J., and Shipley, G. D.,** Type beta transforming growth factor is a growth stimulator and a growth inhibitor, in *Cancer Cells,* Vol. 3, Feramisco, J., Ozanne, B., and Stiles, C., Eds., Cold Spring Harbor, New York, 1985, 65.

77. **Rook, A. H., Kehrl, J. H., Wakefield, L. M., Roberts, A. B., Sporn, M. B., Burlington, D. B., Lane, H. C., and Fauci, A. S.,** Effects of transforming growth factor β on the functions of natural killer cells: depressed cytologic activity and blunting of interferon responsiveness, *J. Immunol.,* 136, 3916, 1986.

78. **Kehrl, J. H., Roberts, A. B., Wakefield, L. M., Jakowlew, S., Sporn, M. B., and Fanci, A. S.,** Transforming growth factor β is an important immunomodulatory protein for human b lymphocytes, *J. Immunol.,* 137, 3855, 1986.

79. **Anzano, M. A., Roberts, A. B., and Sporn, M. B.,** Anchorage-independent growth of primary rat embryo cells in induced by platelets derived growth factor and inhibited by type-beta transforming growth factor, *J. Cell Physiol.,* 126, 312, 1986.

80. **Allen, R. E. and Boxhorn, L. K.,** Inhibition of skeletal muscle satellite cell differentiation by transforming growth factor-beta, *J. Cell Physiol.,* 133, 567, 1987.

81. **Masui, T., Wakefield, L. M., Lechner, J. F., LaVeck, M. A., Sporn, M. B., and Harris, C. C.,** Type β transforming growth factor is the primary differentiation-inducing serum factor for normal human bronchial cells, *Proc. Natl. Acad. Sci. U.S.A.,* 83, 2438, 1986.

82. **Assoian, R. K. K., Omoriya, A., Meyers, C. A., Miller, D. M., and Sporn, M. B.,** Transforming growth factor-β in human platelets, *J. Biol. Chem.,* 25B, 7155, 1983.

83. **Cheifetz, S., Weatherbee, J. A., Tsang, M. L.-S., Anderson, J. K., Mole, J. E., Lucas, R., Massague, J.,** The transforming growth factor β system, a complex pattern of cross-reactive ligands and receptors, *Cell,* 48, 409, 1987.

84. **Hanks, S. K., Armour, R., Baldwin, J. H., Maldonado, F., Spiess, J., and Holley, R. W.,** Amino acid sequence of the BSC-1 cell growth inhibitor (polyergin) deduced from nucleotide sequence of the cDNA, *Proc. Natl. Acad. Sci. U.S.A.,* 85, 79, 1988.

85. **Ikeda, T., Lioubin, M. N., and Marquardt, H.,** Human transforming growth factor type β2: production by a prostatic adenoncarcinoma cell line, purification, and initial characterization, *Biochemistry,* 26, 2406, 1987.

86. **Ten Dijke, P., Hansen, P., Iwata, K. K., Pieler, C., and Foulkes, J. G.,** Identification of another member of the transforming growth factor type β gene family, *Proc. Natl. Acad. Sci. U.S.A.,* 85, 4715, 1988.

87. **Jakowlew, S. B., Dillart, P. J., Kondaiah, P., Sporn, M. B., and Roberts, A. B.,** Complementary deoxynucleic acid cloning of a novel transforming growth factor-β messenger ribonucleic acid from chick embryo chondrocytes, *Mol. Endocrinol.,* 2, 727, 1988.

88. **Ohta, M., Greenberger, J. S., Anklesaria, P., Bassols, A., and Massague, J.,** Two forms of transforming growth factor-β distinguished by multipotential hematopoietic progenitor cells, *Nature (London),* 329, 539, 1987.

89. **Müller, G., Behrens, J., Nussbaumer, U., Bohlen, P., and Birchmeier, W.,** Inhibitory action of transforming growth factor β on endothelial cells, *Proc. Natl. Acad. Sci. U.S.A.,* 84, 5600, 1987.

90. **van Obberghen-Schilling, E., Roche, N. S., Flanders, K. C., Sporn, M. B., and Roberts, A. B.,** Transforming growth factor β1 positively regulates its own expression in normal and transformed cells, *J. Biol. Chem.,* 263, 7741, 1988.

91. **Seyedin, S. M., Thomas, T. C., Thompson, A. Y., Rosen, D. M., and Piez, K. A.,** Purification and characterization of two cartilage-inducing factors from bovine demineraized bone, *Proc. Natl. Acad. Sci. U.S.A.,* 82, 2267, 1985.

92. **Seyedin, S. M., Segarina, P. R., Rosen, D. M., Thompson, A. Y., Bentz, H., and Graycar, J.,** Cartilage-inducing factor-B is a unique protein structurally and functionally related to transforming growth factor-β, *J. Biol. Chem.,* 262, 1946, 1987.

93. **Centrella, M. and Canalis, E.,** Transforming and nontransforming growth factors are present in medium conditioned by fetal rat calvariae, *Proc. Natl. Acad. Sci. U.S.A.,* 82, 7335, 1985.

94. **Seyedin, S. M., Thompson, A. Y., Bentz, H., Rosen, D. M., McPherson, J. M., Conti, A., Siegel, N. R., Gallupi, G. R., and Piez, K. A.,** Cartilage-inducing factor-A; apparent identity to transforming growth factor-β, *J. Biol. Chem.,* 261, 5693, 1986.

95. **Centrella, M., McCarthy, T. L., and Canalis, E.,** Transforming growth factor β is a bifunctional regulator of replication and collagen synthesis in osteoblast-enriched cell cultures from fetal rat bone, *J. Biol. Chem.,* 262, 2869, 1987.

96. **Centrella, M., Massague, J., and Canalis, E.,** Human platelet-derived transforming growth factor-β stimulates parameters of bone growth in fetal rat calvariae, *Endocrinology,* 119, 2306, 1986.

97. **Robey, P. G., Young, M. F., Flanders, K. C., Roche, N. S., Kondaiah, P., Reddi, A. H., Termine, J. D., Spron, M. B., and Roberts, A. B.,** Osteoblasts synthesize and respond to transforming growth factor-type β (TGF-β) *in vitro, J. Cell. Biol.,* 105, 457, 1987.

98. **Pfieilschifter, J. and Mundy, G. R.,** Modulation of type β transforming growth factor activity in bone cultures by osteotropic hormones, *Proc. Natl. Acad. Sci. U.S.A.,* 84, 2024, 1987.

99. **Guenther, H. L., Cecchini, M. G., Elford, P. R., and Fleisch, H.,** Effects of transforming growth factor type beta upon cell populations grown either in monolayer or semisolid medium, *J. Bone Min. Res.,* 3, 269, 1988.

100. **Pfeilschifter, J., Seyedin, S. M., and Mundy, G. R.,** Transforming growth factor beta inhibits bone resorption in fetal rat long bone cultures, *J. Clin. Invest.,* 82, 680, 1988.

101. **Noda, M. and Rodan, G.,** Type β transforming growth factor inhibits proliferation and expression of alkaline phosphatase in murine osteoblast-like cells, *Biochem. Biophys. Res. Commun.,* 140, 56, 1986.

102. **Pfeilschifter, J., D'Souza, S. M., and Mundy, G. R.,** Effects of transforming growth factor-β on osteoblastic osteosarcoma cells, *Endocrinology,* 121, 212, 1987.

103. **Young, M. F., Robey, P. G., Reddi, A. H., Roberts, A. B., Sporn, M. B., and Termine, J. D.,** TGF-β expression in fetal bovine bone forming cells, *J. Bone Min. Res.,* 1(Suppl. 1), 155, 1986.

104. **Centrella, M., McCarthy, T. L., and Canalis, E.,** Skeletal tissue and transforming growth factor β, *FASEB J.,* 2, 3066, 1988.

105. **Reddi, A. H.,** Cell biology and biochemistry of endochondral bone development, *Collagen Relat. Res.,* 1, 209, 1981.

106. **Carrington, J. L., Roberts, A. B., Flanders, K. C., Roche, N. S., and Reddi, A. H.,** Accumulation, localization, and compartmentation of transforming growth factor β during endochondral bone formation, *J. Cell. Biol.,* 107, 1969, 1988.

107. **Centrella, M., Massague, J., and Canalis, E.,** Human platelet-derived transforming growth factor-β stimulates parameters of bone growth in fetal rat calvariae, *Endocrinology,* 119, 2306, 1986.

108. **McCarthy, T. L., Centrella, M., and Canalis, E.,** Further biochemical and molecular characterization of primary rat parietal bone cell cultures, *J. Bone Miner. Res.,* 3, 401, 1988.

109. **Rosen, D. M., Stempien, S. A., Thompson, A. Y., and Seyedin, S. M.,** Transforming growth factor-beta modulates the expression of osteoblast and chondroblast phenotypes *in vitro, J. Cell Physiol.,* 134, 337, 1988.

110. **Hock, J. M., Centrella, M., and Canalis, E.,** Transforming growth factor beta (TGF-β) stimulates bone matrix apposition and bone cell replication in cultured rat calvariae, abstracted, *Calcif. Tissue Int.,* 42, A32, 1988.

111. **Rossi, P., Karsenty, G., Roberts, A. B., Roche, N. S., Sporn, M. B., and de Crombrugghe, B. A.,** A nuclear factor I binding site mediates the transcriptional activation of a type-I collagen promoter by transforming growth factor-β, *Cell,* 52, 405, 1988.

112. **Oldberg, A., Franzen, A., and Heinegard, D.,** Cloning and sequence analysis of rat bone sialoprotein (osteopontin) cDNA reveals an arg-gly-asp cell-binding sequence, *Proc. Natl. Acad. Sci. U.S.A.,* 83, 8819, 1986.

113. **Segarini, P. R., Roberts, A. B., Rosen, D. M., and Seyedin, S. M.,** Membrane binding characteristics of two forms of transforming growth factor-β, *J. Biol. Chem.,* 262, 14655, 1987.

114. **Cheifetz, S., Weatherbee, J. A., Tsang, M. L. S., Anderson, J. K., Mole, J. E., Lucas, R., and Massague, J.,** The transforming growth factor-β system, a complex pattern of cross-reactive ligands and receptors, *Cell,* 48, 409, 1987.

115. **O'Keefe, R. J., Puzas, J. E., Brand, J. S., and Rosier, R. N.,** Effect of transforming growth factor-β on DNA synthesis by growth plate chondrocytes, modulation by factors present in serum, *Calcif. Tissue Int.,* 43, 352, 1988.

116. **Rizzino, A., Kuszynski, C., Ruff, E., and Tiesman, J.,** Production and utilization of growth factors related to fibroblast growth factor by embryonal carcinoma cells and their differentiated cells, *Dev. Biol.,* 129, 61, 1988.

117. **Wang, E. A., Rosen, V., Cordes, P., Hewick, R. M., Kriz, M. J., Luxenberg, D. P., Sibley, B. S., and Wozney, J. M.,** Purification and characterization of other distinct bone-inducing factors, *Proc. Natl. Acad. Sci. U.S.A.,* 85, 9484, 1988.

118. **Wozney, J. M., Rosen, V., Celeste, A. J., Mitsock, L. M., Whitters, M. J., Kriz, R. W., Hewick, R. M., and Wang, E. A.,** Novel regulators of bone formation: molecular clones and activities, *Science,* 242, 1528, 1988.

119. **Wang, E. A., Rosen, V., D'Alessandro, J. S., Bauduy, M., Cordes, P., Harada, T., Isreal, D. I., Hewick, R. M., Kerns, K. M., La Pan, P., Luxenberg, D. P., McQuaid, D., Moutsatsos, I. K., Nove, J., and Wozney, J. M.,** Recombinant human bone morphogenetic protein induces bone formation, *Proc. Natl. Acad. Sci. U.S.A.,* 87, 2220, 1990.

120. **Wozney, J. M.,** Bone morphogenetic proteins, *Prog. Growth Factors,* 1, 267, 1989.

121. **Celeste, A. J., Ianazzi, J. A., Taylor, R. C., Hewick, R. M., Rosen, V., Wang, E. A., and Wozney, J. M.,** Identification of transforming growth factor-β family members present in bone-inducive protein purified bovine bone, *Proc. Natl. Acad. Sci. U.S.A.,* 87, 9843, 1990.

122. **Sampath, T. K., Muthukumaran N., and Reddi, A. H.,** Isolation of osteogenin, an extracellular matrix-associated, bone-inductive protein, by heparin chromatography, *Proc. Natl. Acad. Sci. U.S.A.,* 84, 7109, 1987.

123. **Bentz, H., Nathan, R., Rosen, D., Armstrong, R., Thompson, A., Segarini, P., Mathews, M., Dasch, J., Piez, K., and Seyedin, S.,** Purification of an osteoinductive factor from bovine demineralized bone, abstracted, *J. Cell Biol.,* 107, 162A, 1989.

124. **Glowacki, J., Kaban, L. B., Murray, J. E., Folkman, J., and Mulliken, J. B.,** Application of the biological principle of induced osteogenesis for craniofacial defects, *Lancet,* 1, 959, 1981.

125. **Mulliken, J. B., Glowacki, J., Kaban, L. B., Folkman, J., and Murray, J. E.,** Use of demineralized allogeneic bone implants for the correction of maxillocranial facial deformities, *Ann. Surg.,* 3, 366, 1981.

126. **Mulliken, J. B. and Glowacki, J.,** Induced osteogenesis for repair and construction in the craniofacial region, *Plast. Reconst. Surg.,* 65, 553, 1980.

127. **Mulliken, J. B.,** Induced osteogenesis and craniofacial surgery, in *Craniofacial Surgery,* Caronni, E., Ed., Little, Brown, Boston, 1985, 42.

128. **Ousterhout, D. K.,** Clinical experience in cranial and facial reconstruction with demineralized bone, *Ann. Plast. Surg.,* 15, 367, 1985.

129. **Toriumi, D. M., Larrabee,, W. F., Walike, J. W., Millay, D. J., and Eisele, D. W.,** Demineralized bone: Implant resorption with long-term follow-up, *Arch. Otolaryngol. Head Neck Surg.,* 116, 676, 1990.

Chapter 12

FASCIAL, PERICRANIAL, AND DURAL GRAFTS IN SURGERY OF THE HEAD AND NECK

Hilary A. Brodie and Paul J. Donald

TABLE OF CONTENTS

I. INTRODUCTION

Connective tissue grafts have been used with increasing frequency over the past century. Within the broad scope of connective tissue grafts, fascia, pericranium, and dura have played an important role in head and neck surgery. In general, these grafts are composed of strong fibrous condensed connective tissue with low metabolic demands. Consequently, they provide a strong grafting material without the unwanted bulk of other grafts. The characteristics of these three grafting materials will be discussed including their anatomy, surgical applications, advantages and limitations, and complications.

II. FASCIAL GRAFTS AND FLAPS

Fascia has been used extensively since the turn of the century for multiple applications in surgical reconstruction. Within head and neck surgery, fascial grafts have been utilized in facial cosmetic and reconstructive surgery, otologic surgery, laryngotracheal reconstruction, and combined neurosurgical procedures. The tissue is often used for contouring or filling in limited defects. The most common sources of fascia for these purposes have been fascia lata and temporalis fascia. Historically, fascia lata was used predominantly because of the tensile strength of the graft. More recently, temporalis fascia has been recognized as having many advantages over fascia lata for head and neck surgery. Temporalis fascia is often in the same operative field. It can be harvested under local anesthesia with minimal postoperative morbidity and without leaving a visible scar.[2,45] An additional important application of fascial flaps is to transfer new blood supply to an area. Situations in which this is indicated include: coverage of free cartilage grafts; to provide a bed over exposed bone on which too place a split thickness skin graft; coverage after debridement of osteoradionecrosis.

A. ANATOMY

The fascia lata is the deep fascia of the thigh and gluteal region. It is thickest over the proximal and lateral region and thinnest posteriorly. Posterosuperiorly, the fascia lata is attached to the sacrum and coccyx, laterally to the iliac crest, and anteriorly to the inguinal ligament and to the superior ramus of the pubis. Medially, the fascia lata is attached to the inferior ramus of the pubis and tuberosity of the ischium, and the lower border of the sacrotuborous ligament. It covers the gluteus medius and splits to encapsulate the gluteus maximus. The fascia over the lateral thigh is very thick forming the iliotibial tract (Figure 1). The tensor fascia lata is attached to the iliotibial tract superiorly. Inferiorly, the iliotibial tract attaches to the lateral condyle of the tibia. The fascia lata is attached inferiorly to the exposed bony points around the knee.

The temporalis fascia lies lateral to the temporalis muscle and deep to the galea aponeurotic layer. The superior margin attaches to the superior temporal line. Inferiorly, the fascia splits into two layers as it envelops and attaches to the zygomatic arch (Figure 2). The deep fascia proceeds inferiorly to the attachment of the temporalis on the coronoid process. The relationship of the superficial temporal vessels to the temporalis fascia is important in the utilization of temporalis fascia as a free or vascularly pedicled flap. The superficial temporal vessels pass through the parotid gland and lateral to the zygomatic arch. The superficial temporal artery usually lies posterior to the vein. As the vessels cross the zygomatic arch, they course deep to the auricularis anterior muscle. Above this region, the vessels are quite superficial in the subcutaneous tissue. The superficial temporal artery runs superiorly for 5 cm then divides into anterior and posterior branches. The vessels course in the temporalis fascia for approximately 12 cm above the anterosuperior auriculocephalic attachment, then proceed superficially into the subdermal fat, anastamosing with the sub-

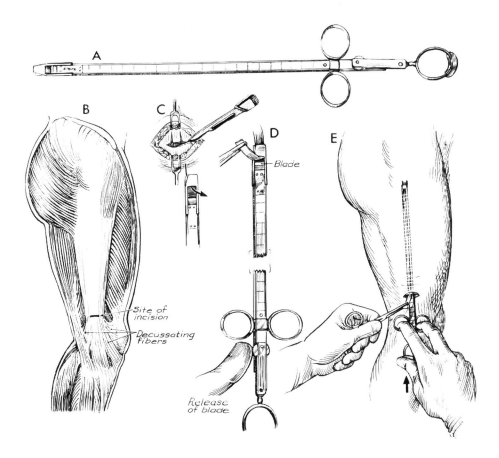

FIGURE 1.   Procuring of a fascia lata graft. (A) A guillotine type stripper. (B) Lateral view of the ileotibial tract portion of the tensor fascia lata; this is the area from which strips are taken for reconstruction. (C) Through an incision low on the lateral thigh, the fascia is cut. (D) The stripper is introduced and the cut fascial edge is grasped with a stout hemostat; the stripper is firmly advanced superiorly until the desired length of fascia is achieved. (E) The fascia is cut at this level and extracted from the wound. (From Converse, J.-M., *Reconstructive Plastic Surgery,* Vol. 1, W. B. Saunders, Philadelphia, 1977, 264. With permission.)

dermal plexus. This is consequently the superior limit of the temporalis fascia flap. Additional blood supply to the temporalis fascia posteriorly is provided from a branch off the occipital artery. The auriculotemporal nerve, which is a sensory branch of the third division of the trigeminal nerve, passes over the posterior root of the zygoma and divides into superficial temporal branches. The nerve is posterior to the superficial temporal vessels as they travel superiorly in the temporalis fascia.

Fascia is a condensation of connective tissue which is of mesodermal origin. It is comprised primarily of type I collagen fibers that are aggregates of striated fibrils 20 to 100 nm in diameter (Figures 3 and 4). The fibers are closely packed and appear as strongly birefringent yellow or red fibers under a polarizing microscope. Type III collagen can also be demonstrated in this tissue. Fibroblasts are interspersed throughout the collagenous matrix. The collagen fibers are arranged in multiple compact sheets. Within each sheet, the fibers tend to parallel one another. The orientation of the direction of the parallel fibers varies between the different sheets. Some of the collagen fibers pass from one layer to the next, resulting in a woven pattern which prevents separation of individual sheets. The resultant tensile strength of this compact interwoven collagenous tissue is approximately 7000 lb/in^2.[19] The strength is measured along the longitudinal axis. In contrast, there is little tensile strength when measured in a transverse direction.

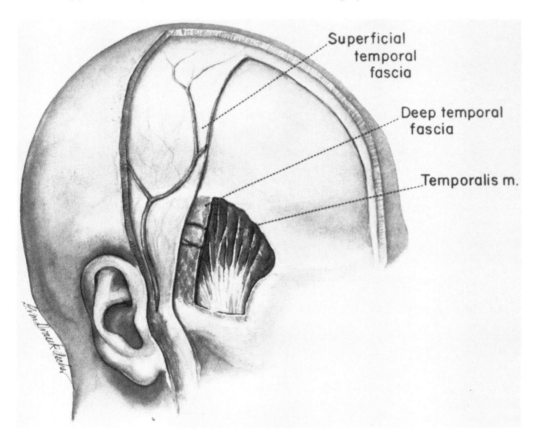

FIGURE 2.   Temporalis fascia illustrating its double layer. (From Abul-Hassan, N. S., von Drasek, A. G., and Acland, R. D., *Plast. Reconstruct. Surg.*, 77, 17, 1986. With permission.)

The fate of fascial grafts has been best studied in the application for tympanoplasties. In these situations, the graft is generally nonviable, secondary to formalin fixation, or having been dried in a fascia press. The success rate in tympanoplasty for viable fascia grafts is similar to results with devitalized fascia grafts. Consequently, the devitalized grafts which are easier to handle are used more frequently in otology. Initially, an inflammatory process occurs with cellular infiltration of primarily lymphocytes. The homograft collagen is gradually resorbed. Histologic studies have confirmed that the homograft attracts host angioblasts, fibroblasts, and epithelial cells.

It is not clear whether the fibroblasts in fascia, grafted in the face, represent the original cells or new cells which have migrated into collagenous matrix of the graft. Regardless of whether the transplanted cells remain viable, the gross morphologic and histologic appearance remains unchanged.[2,19,45] There is, however, some shrinkage in the size of the grafts.

B. CLINICAL APPLICATION

Temporoparietal fascia has been utilized as a graft, rotation flap, or free flap for a multitude of applications. The tissue is easily harvested with a hidden incision line and no donor site defect. There are no functional deficits associated with removal of this fascia. Potential complications associated with obtaining this tissue includes infection, hematoma formation, and injury to the temporal branch of the facial nerve.

Temporoparietal fascia is accessed through a vertical incision in the scalp above the auricle down to the fascia. The incision is beveled in the direction of the hair follicles in order to minimize injury to the roots and consequent alopecia. Superficial fascia which

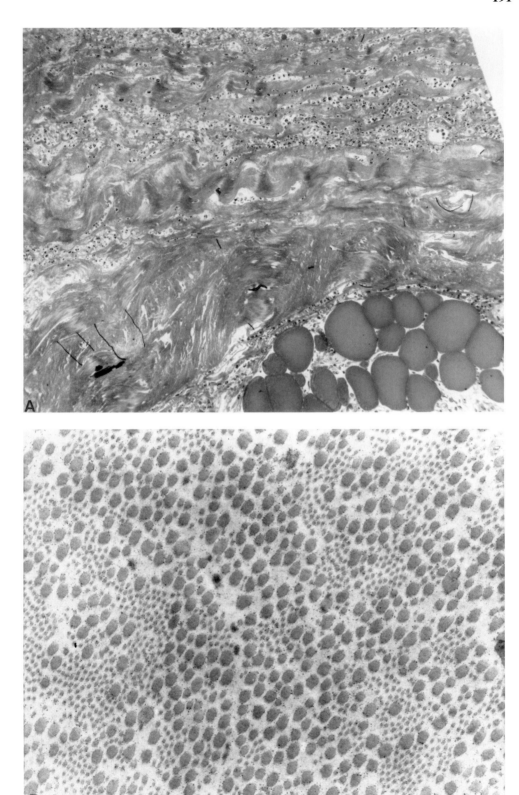

FIGURE 3. Temporalis fascia. (A) Light micrograph of temporalis fascia embedded in epon araldite demonstrating dense collagenous matrix (magnification × 80,000); (B) electron micrograph of temporalis fascia (magnification × 35,000).

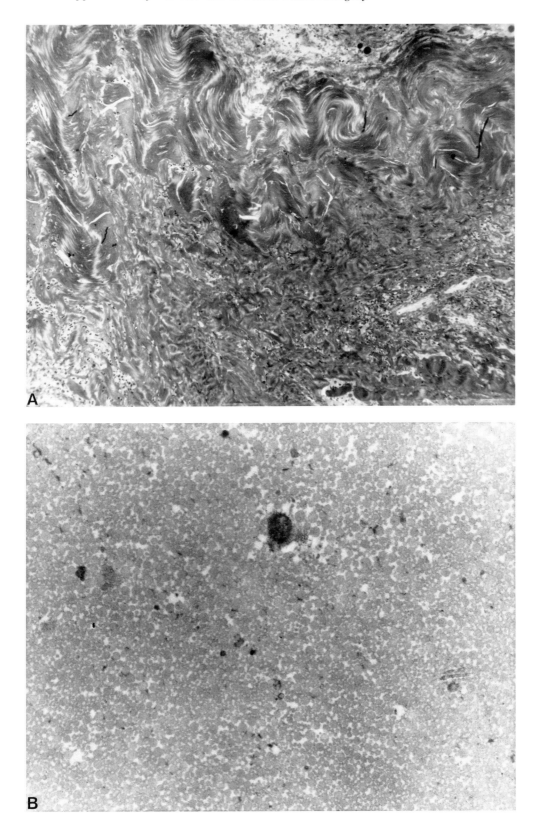

FIGURE 4.   Fascia lata. (A) Light micrograph of fascia lata embedded in epon araldite demonstrating dense collagenous matrix (magnification × 80,000); (B) electron micrograph of fascia lata (magnification × 35,000).

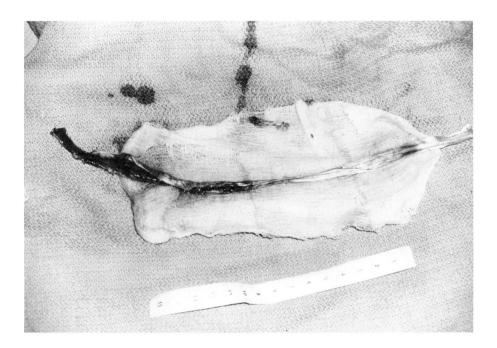

FIGURE 5. Fascia lata strip ready for implantation.

attaches to the zygomatic arch, the deep fascia covering the temporalis muscle, or a combination can be harvested. Superficial fascia elevates easily off the deep fascia with blunt dissection. The superior limit of the dissection is 12 cm above the anterosuperior auriculocephalic attachment where the axial blood supply proceeds superficially into the subdermal plexus. The temporal branch of the facial nerve dictates the anterior limit of the flap. The nerve proceeds $1^1/_2$ cm anterior to the tragus and $1^1/_2$ cm above the zygomatic arch as it angles toward the forehead.

Limited amounts of fascia lata can be harvested through a small incision over the lateral aspect of the thigh. When more substantial amounts of fascia are required, two horizontal incisions can provide the necessary access. A single inferiorly placed incision can be used if the guillotine type stripper is used (Figure 1). Long strips of fascia lata (Figure 5) are obtained with the use of a fascial stripper, thereby avoiding a long incision along the lateral aspect of the thigh. Using this technique, a strip of fascia over the iliotibial band extending from above the knee to the upper thigh can be obtained. A strip 10 to 15 mm in width is harvested. Excision of strips wider than 15 mm is not recommended because this can result in herniation of thigh muscles through the fascia lata.

Transplantation of fascial grafts for various general surgical and orthopedic procedures has been performed since the beginning of the century when McArthur first described the application of a fascial graft in the repair of an inguinal hernia.[43] Fascia lata grafts were shortly thereafter utilized in facial reconstructive surgery. The earliest use was in the treatment of facial paralysis with a fascial sling.[35] Over the past 25 years, the applications for fascia lata and temporalis grafts, in facial reconstructive surgery, has proliferated.

Occasionally, facial reanimation procedures for the rehabilitation of facial nerve palsy are unsuccessful. The surgeon must then resort to some form of suspension procedure in order to restore, at least in part, some resemblance of a normal usage. Dynamic muscular slings are preferable but may require substitution or supplementation by a fascial sling. The patient in Figure 6 had a lateral approach craniofacial resection for a massive recurrent glomus jugulare tumor of the temporal bone with extensive intracranial extension. During

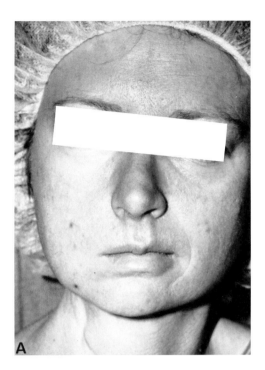 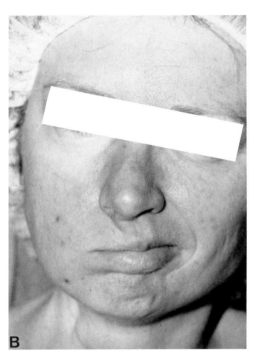

FIGURE 6.   Preoperative photo of patient following skull base resection for large flomus tumor and incomplete return of the hypoglossal to fascial anastomosis. (A) Neutral; (B) with smile.

the procedure, the temporalis muscle was used for middle fossa floor reconstruction. A hypoglossal to VII anastomosis was done to reanimate the face but only the lower main division had any return of function and this was only about 50%. Because of the lack of buccal branch activity, a fascial sling was done from the zygomatic arch to the angle of the mouth (Figure 7A, B, and C). Overcorrection is essential because some degree of relaxation occurs with time (Figure 8). Fascia lata is used for tensile strength and because of the graft length needed. The fascia is sutured to itself around the zygomatic arch and then anchored into strategically placed pockets in the upper lip, angle of the mouth, and lower lip. Bilateral fascial sling surgery is often necessary in patients whose entire lower lip has been denervated because of cancer surgery. Bilateral neck dissections which require bilateral ramus mandibularis resection, because of tumor exigencies, leave a flaccid immobile lower lip. Since it is the essential unit in maintaining oral competence, restoration of normal lower lip position is vital. Slings are sutured bilaterally to the zygomatic arches and knitted subcutaneously with a fascia passer to exit through a short vertical midline incision just below the vermillion-cutaneous border (Figure 9). The lip is hiked up into position and the two strips plicated to one another and the incision closed (Figures 10 and 11).

Temporalis fascia grafts have been used quite successfully in facial contour augmentation to fill defects and cover bony irregularities.[45,26] The grafts can be harvested and transplanted under local anesthesia with minimal associated morbidity. Fascial grafts can provide a smooth contour with minimal surrounding tissue reaction. However, one potential limitation of this graft is its loose consistency, which in certain situations may result in some difficulty in precise placement of the graft. The fascia is implanted through an intranasal or small external incision with special attention to the limits of the recipient pocket. This pocket should match precisely the extent of the defect. Some assistance in graft placement precision is afforded by the use of traction sutures placed at the corners of the graft. These are brought through the skin at the extremities of the implantation pocket and then taped in position for 5 to 7 d.

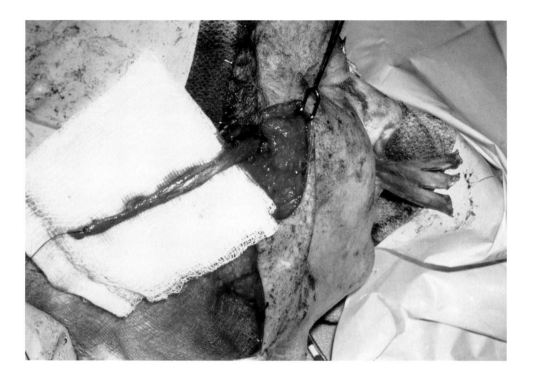

FIGURE 7A.   Fascia graft placed through upper incision and brought out through lip incision.

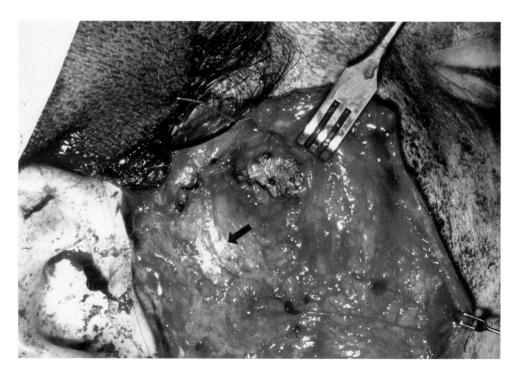

FIGURE 7B.   Fascial sling fixed to zygomatic arch.

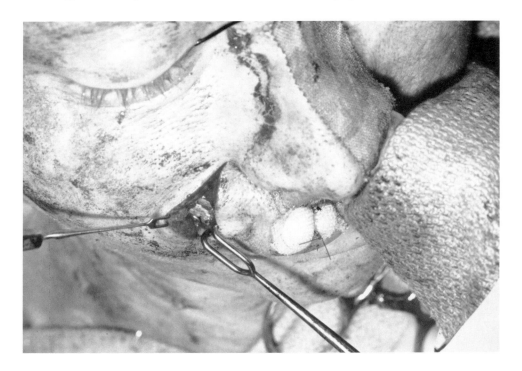

FIGURE 7C.   Fascia inserted into the upper lip almost to midline, at the angle of the mouth, and the later $1/4$ of the upper lip, held in place with tie over bolters.

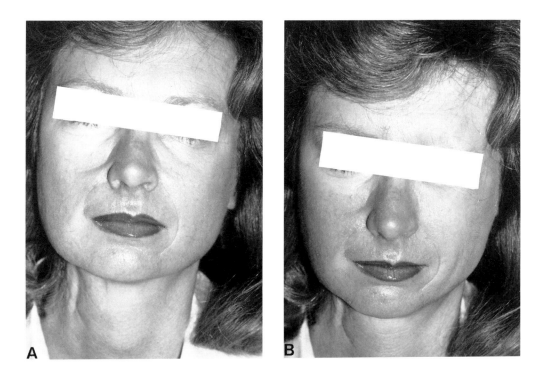

FIGURE 8.   Early postoperative result showing some overcorrection; (A) eyes open; (B) eyes closed.

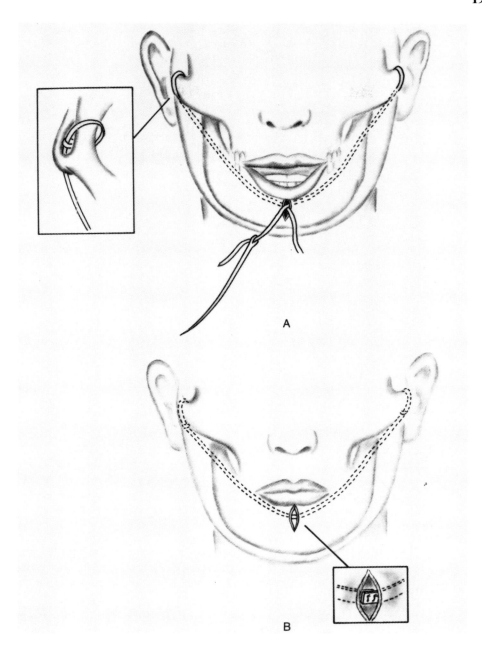

FIGURE 9. (A) Bilateral fascial slings to support lower lip ptosis; (B) note the vertical incision in lower lip through which fascial slips are plicated and the lip cinched in a rostral direction. (From Donald, P. J., *Head and Neck Cancer: Management of the Difficult Case*, W. B. Saunders, Philadelphia, May 1984. With permission.)

The quantity of fascia implanted needs to be overcorrected by 20% to account for the predicted shrinkage.

One of the principal uses of fascial grafts is to efface contour irregularities. This is particularly true in the reconstruction of forehead defects[15] and the placement over irregular areas of the nasal dorsum following rhinoplasty.[10,12,27,36] After hump removal and osteotomy some shattering of bone may occur that can be neither filed nor removed, producing sharp bony protrusions. In the posttraumatic nose even with multiple osteotomies and attempts at

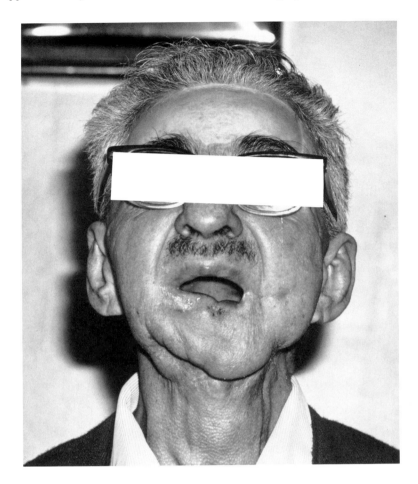

FIGURE 10.   Patient following angle to angle resection of large carcinoma of the oral tongue. Note complete oral incompetence secondary to loss of mandibular support and adynamic lower lip.

straightening, irregular prominences and depressions occur. These can be both filled in and smoothed by the onlay of a fascia graft. Although the open rhinoplasty technique lends itself best to precise placement, grafts can be accurately placed using the closed techniques as well.

In auricular reconstruction, especially when using an alloplastic framework, the surgeon is concerned about graft exposure following even minimal auricular trauma. Overlaying the framework with a fascia graft will provide additional soft tissue covering to the implant. The drawback to this technique is the addition of esthetically undesirable width to the auricle with partial obliteration of some of its fine anatomical details.

Temporalis fascia flaps pedicled on either the superficial temporal or postauricular vessels provides an excellent thin vascular covering for auricular reconstruction.[12,13,66] This technique is especially valuable when severely scarred skin is present from previously unsuccessful operations. The scarred skin can be excised and a split thickness skin graft then placed over the fascial flap.

Temporalis flaps and grafts are also used for repair of craniofacial injuries,[61] eyelid reconstruction,[30] a bed for skin grafting,[12,13,56,65] intraoral grafting,[54] and in the surgical treatment of Frey's syndrome.[8,53,56]

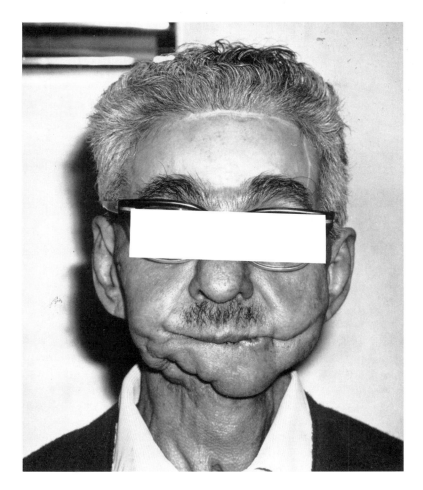

FIGURE 11.   Restoration of oral competence following mandibular reconstruction and fascial slings.

III. PERICRANIAL GRAFTS

The pericranium is a thin connective tissue layer which covers the calvarium. It is an easily obtained tissue which has been used as a free graft, a local rotational flap, and as a free vascularized flap. The pericranium is used to coat, augment, or suspend. Pericranium covers a large surface area and can be harvested without a significant resultant donor defect. The reliable nature of this well-vascularized flap provides surgeons with a flexible tool for head and neck reconstruction.

A. ANATOMY

The scalp is composed of five layers: skin, subcutaneous tissue, galea aponeurosis, subaponeurotic loose areolar tissue, and pericranium (Figure 12). The pericranium extends over the entire calverium and is loosely adherent except at the suture lines where it invaginates. Some authors define pericranium as consisting of the loose areolar tissue and periosteum,[4,49] however, the strict definition limits it to the periosteal layer.

The larger vascular network of the scalp runs predominantly in the subcutaneous layer superficial to the galea aponeurosis. There are multiple perforating vessels extending perpendicularly from the galea aponeurosis to the pericranium.[4,31] Anteriorly, additional blood supply to the interconnecting vasculature of the pericranium is provided by deep divisions

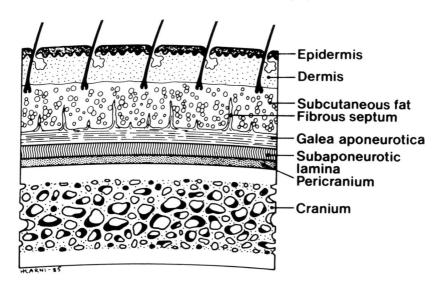

FIGURE 12.   Layers of the scalp. (From Unger, W. P. and Nordstrom, R. E. A., *Hair Transplantation,* 2nd ed., Marcel Dekker, New York, 1987, 43. With permission.)

of the angular, supratrochlear, and supraorbital vessels. Parietal pericranium is further supplied by the deep temporal vessels off the internal maxillary artery and the superficial temporal artery.[4,31] Branches from the occipital and posterior auricular arteries provide additional blood supply to the occipital pericranium. Perforators from the calvarium also contribute to the vasculature to the pericranium.[4]

Histologically, the pericranium is covered by loose fibrillar tissue containing scattered fibroblasts.[29] Deep to the loose fibrillar tissue, the periosteum is denser with increased cellularity and vascularity. The cellular composition of this layer is primarily osteoblastic.[29] The collagen fibers of the periosteum are well organized in a parallel pattern (Figure 13). The thickness of pericranium varies with age. In the younger population the pericranium is thicker with greater vascularity. With aging, the periosteum becomes thinner and less vascular.[4]

Following autogenous free grafting, the pericranium undergoes a variable degree of resorption depending on the site of implantation. This resorption necessitates a 10 to 40% overcorrection when planning for the size of the pericranial graft to be harvested. Despite the resorption, the tissue remains viable. Biopsy of a pericranial autogenous graft, ten months after implantation, revealed viable tissue which resembled scarred pericranium. It has an increased density of collagen fibers which were disorganized but accompanied by normal cellularity for pericranium.

Viable pericranium, as with periosteum harvested from other sites, retains its osteogenic potential. However, the calvarial periosteum has significantly less bone forming capacity, as compared to long bone periosteum, when grafted to skull defects. When pericranium is grafted to a long bone defect, it increases its bone forming capacity fivefold, compared to its potential as an *in situ* flap. There is some question as to whether pericranial grafts may actually decrease the cellularity in calvarial bone grafts when used as adjacent tissue.[49]

B. CLINICAL APPLICATION

Many procedures in which pericranial grafts and flaps can be used, such as craniofacial resections, frontal sinus obliteration, and repair of scalp defects, have by the nature of the operations exposed the pericranium. Pericranial grafts harvested for distant implantation can be accessed through a bicoronal incision. Scalp flaps are elevated in the loose areolar

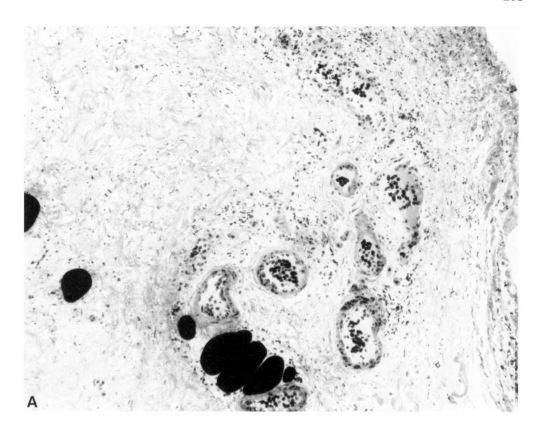

FIGURE 13A. Pericranium.

subgaleal plane. The pericranium is then readily accessible. It is loosely adherent to the skull except at the suture lines and raises easily with a periosteal elevator. Estimation of the size of the graft to be harvested must take into account an overcorrection of 10% to 40% to allow for the subsequent volume loss secondary to surgical edema.[49]

When fashioning a local rotation pericranial flap, the scalp should be elevated in the subperiosteal plane of dissection as opposed to the subgaleal loose areolar layer, as described above. Following elevation of the scalp flap, the design of the pericranial flap is marked out on the undersurface of the flap, leaving as wide a base as possible. Dissection of the pericranium from the galea should be limited to that amount necessary to allow for rotation of the pericranial flap.[4] Limiting the amount of dissection of pericranium from the galea minimizes the reduction in vascular supply from the perforating vessels.

There is minimal donor site morbidity associated with this graft. The bicoronal incision scar is hidden and there is no donor site defect. Once the pericranium is removed, the galea lies against the calvarium. However, this does not typically result in adhesions or other significant complications.[49]

Pericranium has been used in a wide number of reconstructive efforts such as coating of bone grafts,[28,49,71] osteotomy sites,[49] and titanium plates.[49] It is used for augmentation of temples,[49] nasolabial folds,[49] nasofrontal angle,[49] glabellar frown lines,[49] lips,[49] and periorbitally.[49] Utilizations also include: suspensions of upper lip[49] and eyelids;[49,72] support for mucosal flaps; closure of nasal septal perforations;[20,21] frontal sinus obliteration,[63] reconstruction in craniofacial resections;[5,6,33,44,50,64,69] CSF fistula closure;[4,39] reconstruction of traumatic defects of the anterior cranial fossa;[25] repair of complex scalp wounds;[23,11] ear reconstruction;[4] and cleft palate repair.[59,60]

The most common use of pericranium is as a flap for reconstruction, following skull

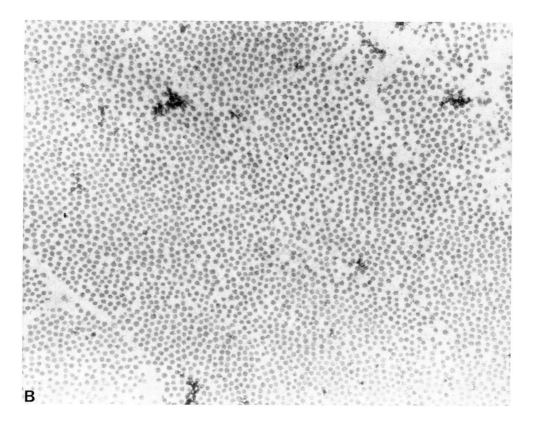

FIGURE 13B.   Light micrograph of pericranium embedded in epon araldite demonstrating loose collaginous matrix (magnification × 80,000). Electron micrograph of pericranium (magnification × 35,000).

base surgery. In these resections, a portion of the floor of the cranium is excised along with the primary tumor and dura, which may be resected as well. The reconstruction demands a stout support for the sutured or rebuilt dura and overlying brain, as well as a vascularized bed for the nutrition of a skin graft or ingrowth of mucosa. During the scalp incision, the elevation is carried superficial to the pericranium. As large as possible a flap of pericranial tissue is elevated, separate from the scalp flap (Figure 14). The pericranial flap is dissected down to the cranial edge over which it is to be infolded. The flap is tucked over the edge of the cranium and placed along the calvarial floor on the intracranial side between dura and bone (Figure 15A and B). Usually the pressure of the overlying brain will hold the flap in place. If not, tissue glue can be applied to stick the flap to bone. A split thickness skin graft can then be packed into place or a cutaneous flap rotated onto the facial side of the defect. Occasionally, the pericranium is left bare and mucosa will overgrow it in about 3 weeks. In previously irradiated cases, a graft or preferably a flap should be used.

Another use of the pericranial flap is to act as a vascularized bed to assist the take of a graft of cartilage on a craniotomy flap, such as illustrated in Figure 16. It may also be used to obliterate a small frontal sinus cavity after mucosal exenteration, following chronic infection or trauma.

IV. DURAL GRAFTS

Dura mater is a bilayer connective tissue which lines the inner surface of the skull and is the outer layer enveloping the brain and spinal cord. Cadaveric human dura has been harvested and used for a wide range of applications over the past 30 years. Although it is

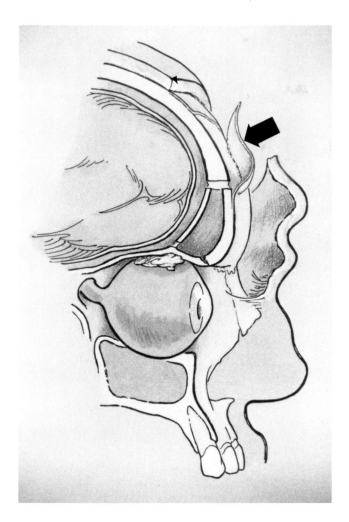

FIGURE 14A.   Diagram of the midsagittal section of head and coronal
scalp flap elevated separately from the pericranial flap. The arrow points
to the pericranial flap.

used primarily in neurosurgical procedures, dural homografts have also been utilized in
otologic, orthopedic, urologic, periodontal, gynecologic, and cardiac surgery. Various methods for sterilization and storage of cadaveric human dura to be used as a homograft have
been employed, including lyophilization, gamma irradiation, chemical dehydration, and
storage in alcohol.

A. ANATOMY

Embryonically, the dura mater covering the brain consists of two layers. In the adult,
these layers are closely joined except at various positions where they separate to enclose
the dural venous sinuses. The dura is a thick inelastic membrane. The outer layer is loosely
adherent to the inner surface of the skull except at suture lines, foramen magnum, and base
of the skull where it is more firmly attached. The outer layer functions as periostium for
the inner surface of the skull, while the inner layer or meningeal layer provides a supportive
membrane to the brain. Reflections of the meningeal layer create dural partitions including
the falx cerebri, falx cerebelli, tentorium cerebelli, and diaphragma sellae which further
support the brain.

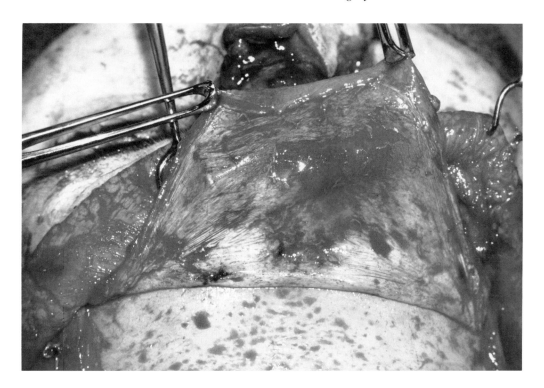

FIGURE 14B.   Photo of a generous pericranial flap.

The blood supply to the dura is quite extensive, originating from the external and internal carotids and the vertebral arteries. The major supply is from the external carotid system which includes terminal branches of the ascending pharyngeal artery, terminal branches of the occipital artery, and the middle and accessory meningeal arteries off of the maxillary artery. The internal carotid arteries supply dura via meningeal branches originating in the cavernous portion of the internal carotid artery and via anterior meningeal branches off of the anterior and posterior ethmoidal arteries.

Histologically, dura mater is comprised of dense laminated sheets of parallel bundles of collagen fibers. These sheets are interconnected with elastin fibers. The endosteal or thicker outer layer of dura is more cellular containing both fibroblasts and osteoblasts. This layer also has greater vascularity. The meningeal or inner layer of dura is thinner containing collagen fibers arranged perpendicularly to the outer layer fibers. The inner layer is lined by flattened mesothelial cells.

Following implantation of this homograft, there is a fibroblastic infiltration of the collagenous framework with associated increased vascularity.[40] The granulation process proceeds from the periphery toward the center of the graft.[47] A lymphocytic infiltrate may also be present. Gradually, the homograft diminishes in size and is replaced by endogenous connective tissue. The replacement tissue is histologically similar to the tissue adjacent to the graft.[9,32,70] The dura mater graft serves as a collagenous connective tissue template into which cell ingrowth from the host tissue can proceed. In addition, when the graft is placed adjacent to mucosal edges, it serves as a scaffold over which the epithelium will grow. Nayot demonstrated that 5 mm^2 lyophilized dura grafts, implanted in the oral mucosa of hamsters, were covered by a thin immature epithelium within 10 d of implantation.[46] One month following implantation, the grafted area appeared normal and was histologically indistinguishable from adjacent tissue. Dura mater grafts do not require early vascularization and are gradually replaced by the adjacent invading connective tissue.[46]

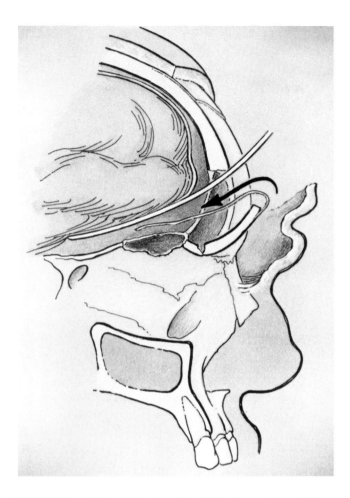

FIGURE 15A. Midsagittal section of head following anterior cranial base resection (note defect in anterior cranial fossa floor). Frontal lobes are retracted and the osteoplastic flap tipped anteriorly. Pericranial flap (arrow) is tucked over the top of the osteoplastic and onto the anterior cranial fossa floor.

Osteogenesis has been reported to occur in animal models within the lyophilized dura mater, but no similar findings have been reported in human recipients.[40]

B. CLINICAL APPLICATION

Clinical experience with homograft dura mater first began in 1958.[16,58,62] Since that time various methods have been used in the preparation and storage of the graft material. Cadaveric dural grafts are usually stored in a lyophilized form and sterilized by gamma irradiation. Dura in this form is available as Lyodura (B. Braun, Melsungen). Lyophilized dura can also be sterilized with ethylene oxide.[51] A second commercially available dural graft, Tutoplast (Lyofil-Pfrimmer, Erlangen), is prepared by treatment with an enzymatic process, dehydrated with an organic solvent, and sterilized with gamma irradiation. Dura mater sterilized by gamma irradiation and stored in 70% ethyl alcohol has also been utilized.

Dura mater homografts have been widely used in the repair of posttraumatic defects, cerebrospinal fluid fistulae, and surgical dural defects, and have produced an acceptably low level of complications.[1,55] MacFarlane[40] reported on the results of implantation of Lyodura in 100 neurosurgical patients. In the overall analysis, 87% were free of compli-

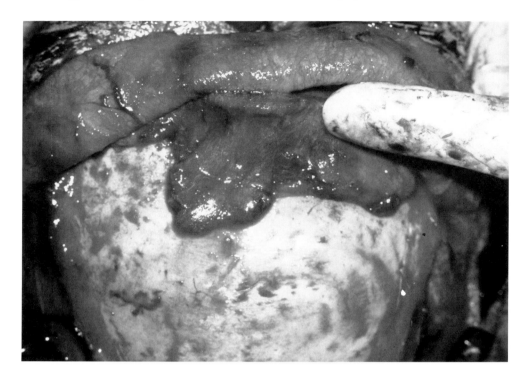

FIGURE 15B. Pericranial flap tucked over the top of an osteoplastic flap and onto the anterior cranial fossa floor.

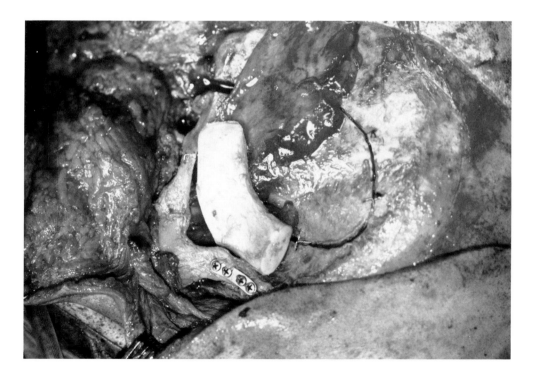

FIGURE 16. Pericranial flap interposed between irradiated cartilage graft and craniotomy flap.

cations. Seven patients had transient CSF leaks and one patient had a persistent CSF leak which required closure. Wound infections occurred in 1% of the patients. There was a 2% incidence of aseptic meningitis and a 2% incidence of bacterial meningitis.

Dural grafts are composed primarily of a collagenous matrix which is relatively hypocellular. Consequently, they have low immunogenic potential. Lyophilization further reduces their antigenicity and facilitates their preservation.[38,48] Despite the reduction in immunogenicity of the graft with lyophilization, dura does maintain some species specific antigenicity. This residual antigenicity has been used to explain an immunologically induced meningitis in a patient who had received a lyophilized dural graft.[34]

Cantore[17] argues for the use of gamma irradiation and storage in 70% ethyl alcohol in place of lyophilization.. They reported on 15 patients reexplored more than 6 months after implantation of, either a lyophilized dural graft, or a dural graft stored in ethyl alcohol. The alcohol stored dura was reportedly better preserved while the lyophilized grafts appeared to be undergoing resorption. Other authors have found good preservation and vascularization of lyophilized dura after implantation for 7 months.[40] Additional advantages of the alcohol stored dura: it is less expensive and can be used immediately without the need to rehydrate the tissue.

All of the above-described methods of sterilization of the dural homografts are quite effective for the normally encountered infectious agents with one exception. The infectious agent responsible for Creutzfeldt-Jacob disease, a rare fatal neurodegenerative disorder, is incompletely inactivated by the common methods for sterilization. The Creutzfeldt-Jacob disease agent is resistant to 10% formaldehyde, 70% alcohol, boiling, ultraviolet radiation, ionizing radiation, and ethylene oxide.[7,14,18,24] There is one isolated reported case in the literature of a patient who developed Creutzfeldt-Jacob disease following implantation of a dura mater graft.[67] Although the homograft is the most likely source for the transmissible agent, this remains unproven. No other patients who received Lyodura from the same lot developed the disease. This example serves to emphasize the necessity of screening donors for evidence of neurologic disease as recommended by the American Association of Tissue Banks.[3] In addition, dura mater grafts should be obtained from patients under the age of 50 and with no history of treatment with human growth hormone derived from pooled cadaver pituitaries, as this would place the donor in a higher risk category.

Dural grafts have been used in a variety of reconstructive efforts such as: periodontal grafting;[9] esophageal replacement,[42] mucogingival grafting;[22,57] vestibuloplasties;[37,41] oral cavity and oronasal fistula repair;[47,52] and reconstruction of the orbital floor.[32] It acts as a filler or nonviable collagenous framework over which epithelial flaps can be placed and eventually become attached to. Its obviously most common use is in the replacement of resected dura. It is well accepted at the recipient site and will often be eventually covered by a skin graft or ingrowth of mucosa. It is best, however, to cover it with a pericranial flap.

REFERENCES

1. **Abbott, W. M. and Dupree, E. L.,** Clinical results of lyophilized human cadaver dura transplantation, *J. Neurosurg.*, 34, 770, 1971.
2. **Aebi, E., Quickert, M. H., and Beard, C.,** Studies on autogenous and homogenous fascia lata, *Eye Ear Nose Throat Mon.*, 50, 45, 1971.
3. American Association of Tissue Banks, Standards for tissue banking, AATB, Arlington, VA, 1984.
4. **Argenta, L. C., Friedman, R. J., Dingman, R. O., and Duus, E. C.,** The versatility of pericranial flaps, *Plast. Reconst. Surg.*, 76, 695, 1985.
5. **Arita, N., Mori, S., Sano, M., Hayakawa, T., Nakao, K., Kanai, N., and Mogami, H.,** Surgical treatment of tumors in the anterior skull base using the transbasal approach, *Neurosurgery*, 24, 379, 1989.

6. **Arnold, H. and Pirsig, W.,** Tumor of the ethmoid with intracranial and intranasal growth, *Neurosurg. Rev.,* 3, 221, 1980.

7. **Asher, D. M., Gibbs, C. J., and Gajdusek, D. C.,** Slow viral infections: safe handling of the agents of subacute spongiform encephalopathies, in *Laboratory Safety: Principles and Practices,* Miller, B. M., Ed., American Society for Microbiology, Washington, D. C., 1986, 57.

8. **Baddour, H. M., Ripley, J. F., Cortez, E. A., McAnear, J. T., Steed, D., and Tilson, H. B.,** Treatment of Frey's syndrome by an interpositional fascia graft: report of case, *J. Oral Surg.,* 38, 778, 1980.

9. **Bartolucci, E. G.,** A clinical evaluation of freeze-dried homologous dura mater as a periodontal free graft material. Study in humans, *J. Periodontol.,* 52, 354, 1981.

10. **Barton, W. L.,** A temporal muscle fascia graft for the traumatic nose, *J. Med. Assoc. Ga.,* 73, 192, 1984.

11. **Bhattacharya, V., Sinha, J. K., and Tripathi, F. M.,** Management of scalp injuries, *J. Trauma,* 22, 698, 1982.

12. **Brent, B., Upton, J., Acland, R. D., Shaw, W. W., Finseth, F. J., Rogers, C., Pearl, R. M., and Hentz, V. R.,** Experience with the temporoparietal fascial free flap, *Plast. Reconstr. Surg.,* 76, 177, 1985.

13. **Brent, B. and Byrd, H. S.,** Secondary ear reconstruction with cartilage grafts covered by axial, random, and free flaps of temporoparietal fascia, *Plast. Reconstr. Surg.,* 72, 141, 1983.

14. **Brown, P., Gibbs, C. J., Amyx, H. L., et al.,** Chemical disinfection of Creutzfeldt-Jakob disease virus, *N Engl. J. Med.,* 306, 1279, 1982.

15. **Byrd, H. S.,** The use of subcutaneous axial fascial flaps in reconstrution of the head, *Ann. Plast. Surg.,* 4, 191, 1980.

16. **Campbell, J. B., Bassett, C. A., and Robertson, J. W.,** Clinical use of freeze-dried human dura mater, *J. Neurosurg.,* 15, 207, 1958.

17. **Cantore, G., Guidetti, B., and Delfini, R.,** Neurosurgical use of human dura mater sterilized by gamma rays and stored in alcohol: long-term results, *J. Neurosurg.,* 66, 93, 1987.

18. Committee on Health Care Issues, Am. Neurol. Assoc., Precautions in handling tissues, fluids, and other contaminated materials from patients with documented or suspected Creutzfeldt-Jakob disease, *Ann. Neurol.,* 19, 75, 1986.

19. **Crawford, J. S.,** Nature of fascia lata and its fate after implantation, *Am. J. Opthalmol.,* 67, 900, 1969.

20. **Fairbanks, D. N.,** Closure of nasal septal perforations, *Arch. Otolaryngol.,* 106, 509, 1980.

21. **Fairbanks, D. N. and Chen, S. C.,** Closure of large nasal septal perforations, *Arch. Otolaryngol.,* 91, 403, 1970.

22. **Filicori, R., and Calandriello, M.,** Introductory note on the use of lyophilized dura mater grafts in mucogingival surgery, *Riv. Italmatol.,* 28, 117, 1973.

23. **Fonseca, J. L.,** Use of pericranial flap in scalp wounds with exposed bone, *Plast. Reconstr. Surg.,* 72, 786, 1983.

24. **Gajdusek, D. C., Gibbs, C. J., Asher, D. M., et al.,** Precautions in medical care of, and in handling materials from, patients with transmissible virus dementia (Creutzfeldt-Jakob disease), *N. Engl. J. Med.,* 297, 1253, 1977.

25. **Gillespie, R. P., Shagets, F. W., and de los Reyes, R. A.,** Temporalis myofascial repair of traumatic defects of the anterior fossa, Technical note, *J. Neurosurg.,* 64, 977, 1986.

26. **Guerrerosantos, J.,** Recontouring of the middle third of the face with onlay cartilage plus free fascia graft, *Ann. Plast. Surg.,* 18, 409, 1987.

27. **Guerrerosantos, J.,** Temporoparietal free fascia grafts in rhinoplasty, *Plast. Reconstr. Surg.,* 74, 465, 1984.

28. **Habal, M. B.,** Aesthetic considerations in the reconstruction of the anophthalmic orbit, *Aesthetic Plast. Surg.,* 11, 229, 1987.

29. **Habal, M. B. and Maniscalco, J. E.,** Observations on the ultrastructure of the pericranium, *Ann. Plast. Surg.,* 6, 103, 1981.

30. **Holt, J. E., Holt, G. R., and van Kirk, M.,** Use of temporalis fascia in eyelid reconstruction, *Ophthalmology,* 91, 89, 1984.

31. **Horowitz, J. H., Persing, J. A., Nichter, L. S., Morgan, R. F., and Edgerton, M. T.,** Galeal-pericranial flaps in head and neck reconstruction. Anatomy and application, *Am. J. Surg.,* 148, 489, 1984.

32. **Iannette, G. and D'Arco, F.,** The use of lyophylized dura in reconstruction of the orbital floor, *J. Maxillofac. Surg.,* 5, 58, 1977.

33. **Johns, M. E., Winn, H. R., McLean, W. C., and Cantrell, R. W.,** Pericranial flap for the closure of defects of craniofacial resection, *Laryngoscope,* 91, 952, 1981.

34. **Johnson, M. H. and Thompson, E. J.,** Freeze-dried cadaveric dural grafts can stimulate a damaging immune response in the host, *Eur. Neurol.,* 20, 445, 1981.

35. **Kirschner, M.,** Ueber Freie Shenen-und Faszientransplantation, *Bietr. Klin. Chir.,* 65, 472, 1909.

36. **Kirschner, R. A.,** Vascular fascial island graft for partial nasal reconstruction utilizing an H flap for forehead repair, *Am. J. Otolaryngol.,* 1, 338, 1980.

37. **Krekeler, G.,** Using lyophilized dura in open vestibuloplasty, *ZWR*, 83, 639, 1974.
38. **Laurentaci, G., Occhiogrosso, M., and Favoino, B.,** *In vitro* inhibition of rat serum complement activity by an extract of lyophilized human dura mater, *J. Neurosurg. Sci.*, 26, 219, 1982.
39. **Loew, F., Pertuiset, B., Chaumier, E. E., and Jaksche, H.,** Traumatic, spontaneous and postoperative CSF rhinorrhea, *Adv. Tech. Stand. Neurosurg.*, 11, 169, 1984.
40. **MacFarlane, M. R. and Symon, L.,** Lyophilized dura mater: experimental implantation and extended clinical neurosurgical use, *J. Neurol. Neurosurg. Psychiatry*, 42, 854, 1979.
41. **Martis, C., Lazaridis, N., Karabouta, I., and Trigonidis, G.,** Free transplantation of lyophilized dura for vestibuloplasty: a clinical and histological study, *J. Oral Surg.*, 37, 646, 1979.
42. **Mattes, P.,** Esophageal replacement with lyophilized dura, *Lanbecks Arch. Chir.*, 343, 93, 1977.
43. **McArthur, L. L.,** Autoplastic sutures in hernia and other diseases. Preliminary report, *JAMA*, 43, 1162, 1901.
44. **Merville, L. C., Diner, P. A., and Blomgren, I.,** Craniofacial trauma, *World J. Surg.*, 13, 419, 1989.
45. **Miller, T. A.,** Temporalis fascia grafts for facial and nasal contour augmentation, *Plast. Reconstr. Surg.*, 81, 524, 1988.
46. **Nayot, C. and Beagrie, G. S.,** An assessment of biocompatibility of lyodura in the oral mucosa of the hamster, *J. Periodontol.*, 49, 181, 1978.
47. **North, A. F., Gould, A. R., and Means, W. R.,** Microfibrillar collagen and dehydrated dura xenografts for the closure of oroparanasal communications, *J. Oral Surg.*, 39, 97, 1981.
48. **Occhiogrosso, M., DeTommasi, A., and Vailati, G.,** Antigenic properties of fresh and lyophilized human dura mater, *J. Neurosurg. Sci.*, 31, 129, 1987.
49. **Powell, N. B. and Riley, R. W.,** Pericranial free grafts in the face, *Arch. Otolaryngol. Head Neck Surg.*, 115, 187, 1989.
50. **Price, J. C., Loury, M., Carson, B., and Johns, M. E.,** The pericranial flap for reconstruction of anterior skull base defects, *Laryngoscope*, 98, 1159, 1988.
51. **Prolo, D. J., Pedrotti, P. W., and White, D. H.,** Ethylene oxide sterilization of bone, dura mater, and fascia lata for human transplantation, *Neurosurgery*, 6, 529, 1980.
52. **Reuther, J. F., Wagner, R., and Braun, B.,** Experimental study on the free transplantation of mucosa and lyophilized dura to the oral cavity, *J. Maxillofac. Surg.*, 6, 64, 1978.
53. **Roark, D. T., Sessions, R. B., and Alford, B. R.,** Frey's syndrome—a technical remedy, *Ann. Otol. Rhinol. Laryngol.*, 84, 734, 1975.
54. **Robinson, K., Stern, K., and Giunta, J.,** Intraoral-mucosal-xenogenous fascial grafting, *Oral Surg. Oral Med. Oral Pathol.*, 42, 14, 1976.
55. **Rosomoff, H. L. and Malinin, T. I.,** Freeze-dried allografts of dura mater—20 years experience, *Transplant Proc.*, VIII (2)Suppl., 1, 133, 1976.
56. **Saad, M. N. and Khoo, C. T.,** Skin graft survival on a fascia lata graft, *Br. J. Plast. Surg.*, 33, 143, 1980.
57. **Schoo, W. H. and Coppes, L.,** Use of palatal mucosa and lyophilized dura to create attached gingiva, *J. Clin. Periodontol.*, 3, 166, 1976.
58. **Sharkey, P. C., Usher, F. C., Robertson, R. C., et al.,** Lyophilized human dura mater as a dural substitute, *J. Neurosurg.*, 15, 192, 1958.
59. **Skoog, T.,** The use of periosteal flaps in the repair of the primary palate, *Cleft Palate J.*, 2, 232, 1965.
60. **Skoog, T.,** The use of periosteum and Surgicel for bone restoration in congenital clefts of the maxilla, *Scand. J. Plast. Reconstr. Surg.*, 1, 113, 1967.
61. **Stanley, R. B., Jr. and Schwartz, M. S.,** Immediate reconstruction of contaminated central craniofacial injuries with free autogenous grafts, *Laryngoscope*, 99, 1011, 1989.
62. **Stern, W. E.,** The surgical application of freeze-dried homologous dura mater, *Surg. Gynecol. Obstet.*, 106, 159, 1958.
63. **Stiernberg, C. M., Bailey, B. J., Calhoun, K. H., and Quinn, F. B.,** Management of invasive frontoethmoidal sinus mucoceles, *Arch. Otolaryngol. Head Neck Surg.*, 112, 1060, 1986.
64. **Stiernberg, C. M., Bailey, B. J., Weiner, R. L., Calhoun, K. H., and Quinn, F. B.,** Reconstruction of the anterior skull base following craniofacial resection, *Arch. Otolaryngol. Head Neck Surg.*, 113, 710, 1987.
65. **Tavis, M. J., Thornton, J. W., Harney, J. H., Woodroof, E. A., Bartlett, R. H.,** Graft adherence to de-epithelialized surfaces: a comparative study, *Ann. Surg.*, 184, 594, 1976.
66. **Tegetmeier, R. E. and Gooding, R. A.,** The use of a fascial flap in ear reconstruction, *Plast. Reconstr. Surg.*, 60, 406, 1977.
67. **Thadani, V., Penar, P. L., Partington, J., Kalb, R., Janssen, R., Schonberger, L. B., Rabkin, C. S., and Prichard, J. W.,** Creutzfeldt-Jakob disease probably acquired from a cadaveric dura mater graft. Case report, *J. Neurosurg.*, 69, 766, 1988.
68. **Wallis, K. A. and Gibson, T.,** Gustatory sweating following parotidectomy: correction by a fascia lata graft, *Br. J. Plast. Surg.*, 31, 68, 1978.

69. **Wetmore, S. J., Suen, J. Y., and Snyderman, N. L.,** Preauricular approach to infratemporal fossa, *Head Neck Surg.,* 9, 93, 1986.

70. **Wirth, C. J. and Jager, M.,** Experimental investigations of primary healing and remodeling of lyophilized connective tissue dependent on the graft bed, *Arch. Orthop. Trauma Surg.,* 96, 105, 1980.

71. **Wolfe, S. A.,** The utility of pericranial flaps, *Ann. Plast. Surg.,* 1, 147, 1978.

72. **Wolfe, S. A.,** Correction of a persistent lower eyelid deformity caused by a displaced orbital floor implant, *Ann. Plast. Surg.,* 2, 448, 1979.

73. **Converse, J.-M.,** *Reconstructive Surgery,* Vol. 1, W. B. Saunders, Philadelphia, 1977, 264.

74. **Abul-Hassan, N. S., von Drasek, A. G., and Acland, R. D.,** Surgical anatomy and blood supply of the fascial layers of the temporal regions, *Plast. Reconstruct. Surg.,* 77, 17, 1986.

75. **Unger, W. P. and Nordstrom, R. E. A.,** *Hair Transplantation,* 2nd ed., Marcel Dekker, New York, 1987, 43.

Part III—Applications of Natural and Synthetic Polymers

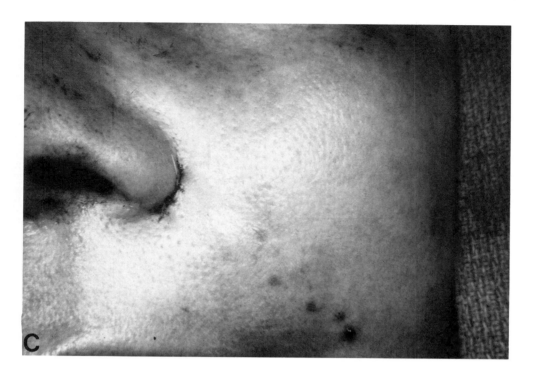

FIGURE 1C.   Immediate postoperative effect. The groove is eliminated.

Chapter 14

INJECTABLE FLUID SILICONE FOR SOFT-TISSUE AUGMENTATION

David S. Orentreich and Norman Orentreich

TABLE OF CONTENTS

I. INTRODUCTION[1-3]

The ideal biocompatible soft-tissue augmentation implant should fulfill certain criteria:

1. Easily obtainable by qualified physicians at reasonable costs
2. Capable of fabrication in the form desired
3. Capable of repeated sterilization and prolonged storage at room temperature
4. Easily implanted
5. Induces a self-limited fibroplastic response
6. Not physically modified by soft tissue
7. Chemically inert
8. Does not cause inflammation or foreign body reaction
9. Does not cause amaurosis when injected into facial skin
10. Nontoxic
11. Noncarcinogenic
12. Nonteratogenic
13. Does not cause allergy or hypersensitivity
14. Capable of resisting mechanical strains
15. Physical consistency of treated tissue similar to normal tissue
16. Long-term persistence of tissue contour restoration
17. Not subject to latent degenerative or calcific changes
18. Persistence in the originally deposited location with minimal or no movement (drift) or absorption, even with movement of the part treated
19. Corrects defect in one treatment

Silicone fluid fulfills the criteria listed above, except for #1, #8, and #19. To our knowledge, no FDA-approved product is currently marketed in the U.S.A. With rare exception, injectable-grade silicone fluid provokes a "foreign-body reaction" only to the desirable extent of producing intentional beneficial fibroplasia and hence soft-tissue augmentation. Finally, liquid silicone's properties and mechanism of action dictate the need for gradual augmentation over multiple sessions.

One additional criterion, that of a substance with low abuse potential, i.e., one that is independent of physician technique, is conspicuous by its absence from the foregoing list. Any device, drug, or surgical instrument—indeed any tool in the physician's armamentarium—has the potential to be used incorrectly. Reading articles describing the use of silicone, while indispensable, is not a substitute for adequate training under the careful supervision of a physician experienced in its proper administration.

In the authors' opinion, injectable-grade (defined below) silicone fluid, administered by the microdroplet serial puncture technique, is presently the safest and most efficacious of all available autogenous and nonautogenous tissue-compatible materials for lifelong dermal and subdermal implantation within the human body.

II. DEFINITIONS AND CHEMISTRY[4-16]

Silicone, a term introduced at the turn of the century by the chemist F. S. Kipping of Nottingham, England, is a generic designation for a family of polymers based on the element silicon (Si). These polymers range from fluids of different viscosities to semisolid (gel) and solid states.

Siloxane is a mnemonic acronym derived from *sil*icon, *ox*ygen, and meth*ane*. Dimethylsiloxane polymers are large molecules of repetitive units $((CH_3)_3SiO-[(CH_3)_2SiO]_x-Si(CH_3)_3)$ with viscosities that are a function of the extent of polymerization designated in the chemical formula by the subscript "x."

Unrefined polydimethylsiloxane fluid of 350 cSt is actually a mixture of polymer molecules of differing lengths, ranging from ten to several hundred repetitive units, and averaging 130.

Industrial or electrical-grade 350 cSt fluid silicone is manufactured by Dow Corning Corporation and is called electrical-grade 200 silicone fluid. In its unpurified state it is unsuitable for any medical purpose. Dow Corning® food-grade 200 silicone fluid (350 cSt) is suitable for human ingestion (simethicone).

A more purified grade known as Dow Corning medical-grade 360 liquid silicone (350 cSt) was developed in the 1960s. Medical-grade 360 fluid is principally used for lubricating suture materials and disposable hypodermic needles and syringes, for coating the inside of containers for medicinals and blood products, and as an emollient (dimethicone) in protective skin lotions. When used for the parenteral purposes above, a small amount of medical-grade silicone is unavoidably implanted in the body. It has been estimated that the average insulin-dependent diabetic subcutaneously injects liquid silicone at the rate of 2 to 5 ml/yr as a consequence of using disposable syringes and needles. Medical-grade silicone fluid was not, however, initially planned or marketed for soft-tissue augmentation, although it was certainly used for this purpose in the United States and other countries. In 1965, Dow Corning Corporation developed a still more highly purified form of liquid silicone to be used for augmenting soft-tissue in clinical investigations authorized by the Food and Drug Administration (FDA). This material, which contained fewer heavy metals, low-chain-length polymers and other impurities, was 350 cSt, sterilized, and labeled MDX 4-4011. The FDA did not have an opportunity to act on the investigational new drug application (NDA), since following its completion and submission, it was withdrawn in 1976 for corporate business reasons. However, the Dow Corning Corporation issued a statement that the study found MDX 4-4011 to be safe and effective for injection.

Due to the ambiguity of the term "medical-grade," the term "injectable-grade" fluid silicone is used by the authors to designate polydimethylsiloxane fluid of known viscosity (350 cSt) that has been filtered and sterilized so as to remove heavy metals, low-chain-length polymers, and other impurities. This refining process produces a chemically pure product, free of particulate matter, and suitable for human soft-tissue implantation and augmentation by the techniques described.

Injectable-grade fluid silicone is clear, colorless, odorless, tasteless, nonvolatile, and has an oily feel. The viscosity of fluid silicone is constant within the range of human body temperature: once injected, silicone fluid does not harden or soften. Fluid silicone is chemically unaltered by prolonged storage at room temperature or by exposure to air, most chemicals, and sunlight. Fluid silicone does not support the growth of microorganisms nor is it altered by them. Silicone fluid can be contaminated by contact with certain rubbers from which it will leach out irritating chemicals, such as agerite alba (monobenzyl ether of hydroquinone). Thermal stability allows repeated steam autoclaving or dry heat sterilization within significant alteration. Silicone should never be gas-sterilized because of its absorptive properties. Steam autoclaving may produce a harmless milky color due to accretion of water. It is not necessary to refrigerate silicone.

The satisfactory results obtained with injectable-grade material and microdroplet techniques of injection (see Sections VII and X) must not, however, be confused with untoward results and complications arising from the use of impure (altered) "silicone fluid," injection of contraindicated sites, and injection of large volumes.

III. BACKGROUND OF CONTROVERSY[17-29,32-37]

Soft-tissue deposition of animal, vegetable, and mineral oils, as well as various acids produces paraffin-like granulomatous responses. This has been found with camphorated oil, cottonseed oil, sesame oil, fish oil, cod liver oil, beeswax, and a melange of similar substances.

One very large clinic in Japan practiced injections of a mixture of silicone and 1% "sweet oil" (olive oil). This "Japanese" or "Sakurai" formula was exported to California, Mexico, South America, and elsewhere, where it was used extensively, especially for breast augmentation in volumes of hundreds to a thousand or more ml per breast.

Additives to silicone fluids, henceforth referred to as "adulterants," are but one factor beclouding the medical use of injectable-grade silicone. Putatively safe and effective materials touted for the augmentation of soft-tissue came to be administered in massive doses by unqualified individuals who injected "secret formulas." The consequences were occasionally disastrous. Well-publicized fiascos were misrepresented as resulting from the use of "silicone."

The single injection of a large volume of liquid paraffin, or any other oil, may result in its migration along tissue cleavage planes of least resistance. This adverse effect was compounded in certain anatomic locations by muscular propulsion of the fluid material. With the introduction of liquid silicone for injection into soft tissues, the already well-recognized physiologic inertness of the pure material often prompted the misguided addition of irritant oils in order to "lock" large volumes of injected silicone into sites of deposition by inducing an inflammatory reaction and subsequent fibrous encapsulation. Such mixtures were often simply referred to as "silicone." Silicone mixed with 1% sesame oil or 1% oleic acid was used in many of the California treatments. Furthermore, large volumes were used to produce immediate complete augmentation since it was not recognized that further delayed augmentation would occur as a result of new collagen synthesis around the silicone.

Nevertheless, apart from complications following injections into breasts or other glandular tissues (the glandular nature being another aspect of unsuitability), to date there is rare evidence of serious, untoward sequelae from properly performed microvolume injections of injectable-grade silicone into other sites.

IV. ANALYSIS OF PUBLISHED PURPORTED SILICONE REACTIONS[22,25,26,33,35-59]

Reviewing the literature on purported silicone reactions reveals several fundamental flaws. Proof is lacking that the complications presented are due to polydimethylsiloxane per se. Condemning silicone as the cause of a serious complication solely on the basis of a patient's verbal history, another physician's report, or the assumed purity of a material obtained from unknown sources is subject to errors of communication.

Common pitfalls in the silicone literature arise from

1.   Authors who report complications especially when observed in patients treated by another physician, and do not themselves independently establish the source, and more importantly, the purity of all silicone used in each patient.
2.   Authors who report adverse reactions to silicone wherein they specifically state that the patients received adulterated material.
3.   Absent or incomplete documentation of the method of skin preparation prior to silicone injection; technique of injection; location; frequency (interval between sessions); and volume of fluid injected.
4.   Failure to perform a pathologic examination of tissues involved by the reaction.
5.   Inadequate analysis for silicone in pathologic tissues (see below for appropriate methods).
6.   Failure to analyze for adulterants in pathologic specimens.
7.   Failure to indicate whether the reaction was associated with any concurrent, systemic, or local infection, such as adjacent furuncle or acute sinusitis.
8.   Failure to attribute the complications to overinjection.
9.   Failure to recognize that sequelae were caused by injecting sites too frequently, e.g., at intervals of 1 to 2 weeks.
10. Failure to recognize that untoward reactions were caused by injection of usually contraindicated sites, such as eyelid rhytids and glandular breasts.
11. Failure to recognize that untoward reactions attributed to silicone were most likely caused by subsequent treatment of the area with other agents; for example, local facial corticosteroid injections, which may have been responsible for the reported "complication" described as dermal and subcutaneous atrophy.

In reviewing the literature of purported reactions to silicone, we found that no cases were substantiated by appropriate, intradermal skin testing to the augmenting material actually used on the patient and a control skin test with injectable-grade silicone. In the past 35 years, we have not encountered a positive skin test reaction to injectable-grade silicone in routine patients, in patients who developed an idiosyncratic reaction (see Section XI.J), or those referred to our practice with alleged silicone reactions. Patients with clinical evidence or a history of allergic reaction to injectable bovine collagen have had intradermal testing to silicone and were negative.

In summary, neglecting to prove that patients with untoward reactions received injectable-grade silicone, or to search for other etiologic factors, propagates the myths surrounding the use of injectable-grade silicone. Failure to distinguish fact from conjecture in the silicone literature creates confusion regarding injectable-grade silicone's safety and efficacy and leads to the drawing of unsupported conclusions.

V. THE CURRENT LEGAL STATUS OF INJECTABLE FLUID SILICONE FOR SOFT-TISSUE AUGMENTATION[25,60-66]

Silicone microdroplet injection therapy is of recognized therapeutic value. Dating back 35 years, this treatment has wide support in the medical literature. Since 1973, subcutaneous injections of filling material (including silicone) have been specifically included in the Physicians' Current Procedural Terminology (CPT, No. 11950 to 11954), a comprehensive listing of medical and surgical procedures prepared and updated annually by the American Medical Association.

Because of the ongoing need for fluid silicone in the treatment of severe facial defects, especially in children, the FDA allowed the Dow Corning study to be continued and the material to be supplied by Dow Corning Corporation to physicians for this purpose. On October 25, 1979, the FDA Bureau of Devices gave written investigational drug evaluation (IDE) approval to the University of California, San Francisco (USCF), Department of Ophthalmology, Dr. Walter Stern, to evaluate the use of 1000 cSt silicone fluid for replacement of the vitreous of the eye as a part of the treatment for vitrectomy. In the early 1980s, the University of California, Los Angeles (UCLA), Department of Ophthalmology, Dr. Steven Ryan, joined the original sponsor (UCSF) and the investigation became a joint study. Liquid silicone of various grades has been used for many years for purposes other than soft-tissue augmentation, as stated in Section II.

The Food, Drug and Cosmetic Act permits physicians to use, for therapeutic purposes, medical devices made to a physician's order (custom devices) and intended to meet the special needs of his or her practice. In the circumstances of an individual physician's medical practice, the use of fluid silicone complies with these provisions of the Food, Drug and Cosmetic Act. Since Dow Corning Corporation's studies, no pharmaceutical company has filed for FDA approval for the sale in interstate commerce of fluid silicone for soft-tissue augmentation.

VI. TISSUE RESPONSE TO DEPOSITIONS OF MICROVOLUMES (MECHANISM OF ACTION)[8,14,22,32,67-74]

Soft-tissue inflammatory cell reaction to depositions of small volumes of fluid silicone (equal to or less than 0.1 ml) is slight when injections are properly administered in single treatments. Injectable-grade silicone elicits less physiologic reactivity than almost any other foreign material, although in a strict and desirable sense, it is not absolutely biologically inert. The combination of puncture with a needle and deposition of silicone results in early migration of polymorphonuclear leukocytes to the area, followed in several days by a moderate infiltrate composed mainly of small round cells. The infiltrate largely dissipates in about 6 months. Slight phagocytic activity is evident even later by the presence of macrophages and giant cells in limited numbers, which do not proliferate or agglomerate into gross granulomatous nodules.

At first, small globules of fluid silicone deposited at the dermal-subcutaneous interface displace connective tissue bundles and thus are surrounded by pseudocapsules of preexistent collagen. Later, a microscopically observable thin-walled collagen capsule forms around the tiny globules of silicone. Deposition of initially large or cumulatively large volumes produces many "honeycomb" cysts lined by opaque and thicker capsules.

The eventual tissue response to silicone is thus fibroplastic, resulting in increased collagen deposition localized to the immediate surrounding area. The production of collagen by fibroblasts coupled with the mass displacement of dermal connective tissue by the silicone microdroplets corrects the soft-tissue defect. This new collagen formation is self limited and does not become extensive even with deposition of large volumes, provided that lymphatics

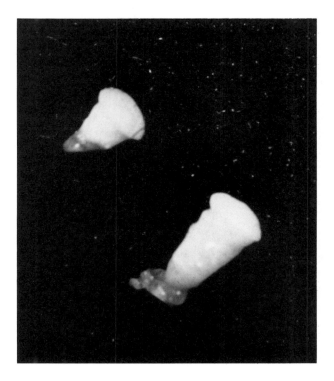

FIGURE 1. A site on the medial aspect of an arm was injected with 0.2 ml of injectable-grade silicone. One year later, this site and an untreated adjacent site were punch excised. Collagen augmentation in the treated site (specimen on the right) is obvious.

and blood vessels have not been compressed. Optimal augmentation is facilitated by the limited, rather constant, and predictable degree of collagen synthesis that results from the injections of silicone fluid microdroplets (0.005 to 0.01 ml) using the serial puncture technique (discussed below) (Figure 1). Unlike silicone, the injection of other liquid materials for soft-tissue augmentation has resulted in extensive fibrosis.

Antibodies to injectable-grade silicone have never been demonstrated and true adjuvant disease has never been provoked.

VII. INDICATIONS AND VOLUME REQUIREMENTS

When using the microdroplet serial puncture technique, each needle puncture and injection deposits between 0.005 and 0.01 ml of injectable-grade fluid silicone (a "microdroplet"). The average single treatment session for a middle-aged individual with facial rhytids requires between 0.50 and 0.75 ml of silicone fluid. Injection of this volume entails between 50 and 150 individual needle punctures and usually suffices to treat the neck, labial commissure grooves, nasolabial creases, malar grooves, crow's feet, frown lines, and forehead lines.

Treatment sessions are usually repeated at intervals of 1 month or longer until the desired degree of augmentation is achieved. This interval allows time for new collagen to develop around the silicone microdroplets and is necessary to achieve the desired effect without overcorrection. The number of sessions will depend on the degree of dermal atrophy and the individual's fibroplastic response.

Depositing silicone at different depths in the skin may produce either desirable or undesirable effects (Figure 2). Excess intradermal injection of silicone into skin of normal

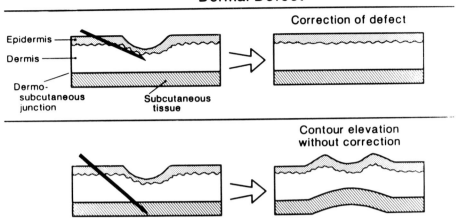

FIGURE 2A.   Surface remodeling demonstrated by augmentation with relatively superficial (i.e., intradermal) injection of fluid silicone.

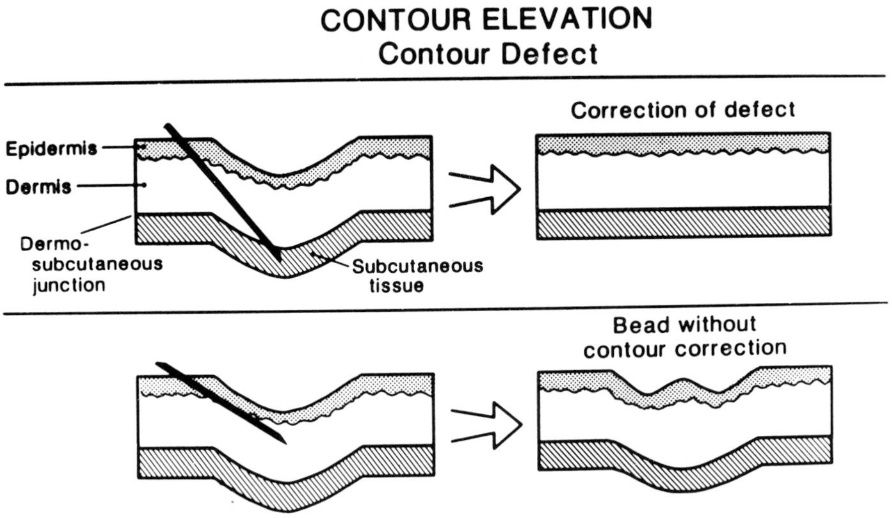

FIGURE 2B.   Contour elevation demonstrated by subdermal injection of fluid silicone.

thickness will usually produce a "beading" effect (Figure 2B), especially when the skin overlies bone (i.e., forehead). Visible beading is to be avoided (see section XI.G). However, certain scars and rhytids lack dermal thickness; in these circumstances, controlled intradermal injection is preferable and produces the precise desired augmentation (microelevation). If silicone was injected at the deeper dermal-subcutaneous interface under these same defects, a less optimal correction would usually result (Figure 2A). We apply the term *surface remodeling* to augmentation by the relatively superficial (i.e., intradermal) injection of fluid silicone expressly to obtain a smoother skin surface (Figure 2A). Examples of surface remodeling are augmentation of certain depressed acne scars and chicken pox scars. Surface characteristics of scar tissue, such as hyper- or hypopigmentation, telangiectasia, and adnexal pore size, are usually unaffected by silicone augmentation.

Conversely, with contour depressions and rhytids, where an epidermis and dermis of approximately normal thickness lie upon subcutaneous tissue of less than desirable depth, it is preferable to deposit the silicone just below the dermis. Intradermal injection in these cases may produce undesirable beading. This type of augmentation is called *contour elevation:* subdermal injections of fluid silicone that alter facial contours but minimally change surface skin topography (Figure 2B). Examples of contour elevation are augmentation of nasolabial creases, malar grooves, and zygomatic arches.

A. SCARS[27,75-78]

Fluid silicone may be injected to lift depressed scars that result from various causes, provided they are not bound down by strong fibrous adhesions. Attempted elevation of an unyielding, bound-down scar, such as the "ice pick" scars of acne vulgaris and some varicella scars, will force silicone fluid into distensible surrounding skin and produce a "doughnut effect," making the depression still more pronounced. Ice pick scars are best treated by other methods (i.e., punch excision with or without full-thickness autologous skin grafting). The broad distensible atrophic scars that are the aftermath of acne, neurotic and psychopathic excoriations, adventitious trauma, varicella, microbial infection, scarring dermatoses, conventional surgery, and skin grafting can effectively be raised to normal skin-surface level. For a depression of about 1 cm^3, a total volume of approximately 0.5 ml of silicone injected in about five repeated treatments (0.1 ml per treatment) usually suffices.

In order to determine whether a scar will respond satisfactorily to silicone augmentation, the physician may employ one or both of the following techniques. A scar that is distensible by manual stretching of the scar borders, or is corrected by a test injection of a sterile physiologic saline or lidocaine solution, will usually respond satisfactorily to silicone augmentation.

B. RHYTIDS[22,51,79]

For age-associated furrows or sunken contours of the face, small to moderate total volumes injected beneath the depressions (up to a few milliliters per region administered over successive treatments) suffice for optimal cosmetic correction (Figure 3). For furrows on the forehead and depressions in skin closely stretched over bony or cartilaginous prominences, smaller volumes per session and cumulatively are effective. Small volumes are also effective for the vertical and oblique "frown lines" in the glabella region. The amount injected in the glabella needs to be controlled to avoid a general fullness that may develop in the area. Nasolabial creases are particularly amenable (Figure 4), however, care must be taken not to inject laterally into cheek tissue that is already relatively full. Doing so would cause further protrusion of the nasolabial fold (Figure 3) and accentuation of the nasolabial crease (see Section XI.G for treatment). Sunken facial contours on the upper cheeks, such as the malar groove, depressed planes in the mid-cheek area, and facial eminences (brow, molar, including zygomatic arch, and angle of the mandible) can be effectively augmented.

C. PERIORBITAL AREA AND EYELIDS[54]

Some cosmetic improvement may be achieved in periorbital crow's feet-type rhytids. Care must be taken to inject very small quantities of fluid silicone. The silicone tattooing technique is commonly used for most of these superficial wrinkles (see Section X).

Eyelid rhytids are usually better treated with blepharoplasty and resurfacing techniques such as chemical peel or dermabrasion rather than soft-tissue replacement. On the other hand, localized atrophy of eyelid skin caused by traumatic scarring or linear scleroderma has been successfully corrected with microdroplet injections of silicone fluid.

The infraorbital groove, which contributes to dark "circles" under the eyes, may be augmented by injectable-grade silicone fluid, totaling approximately 0.025 to 0.05 ml per side per session. The injection is best made with an acute skin-to-needle angle to avoid needle contact with the infraorbital rim.

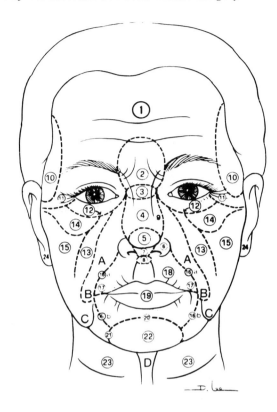

RHYTIDS:
1   FOREHEAD FURROWS
2   GLABELLA "FROWN LINES" (VERTICAL & OBLIQUE)
3   RADIX (HORIZONTAL) FURROWS
4   DORSUM OF NOSE
5   TIP OF NOSE
6   ALA NASI
7   COLUMELLA
8   COLUMELLA/LABIAL JUNCTION
9   LATERAL NASAL WALL
10 TEMPLE
11 PERIORBITAL ("CROW'S FEET") CREASES
12 INFRA-ORBITAL GROOVE (DARK "CIRCLE" UNDER THE EYE)
13 MALAR GROOVE
14 MALAR EMINENCE (INCLUDING ZYGOMATIC ARCH)
15 CHEEK
16a UPPER NASOLABIAL (CHEEK-LIP) CREASE
16b LOWER NASOLABIAL (CHEEK-LIP) CREASE
17 LABIAL COMMISSURE GROOVE
18 LIPS (PERIORAL RADIAL CREASES)
19 VERMILION
20 LABIOMENTAL CREASE
21 CHIN-CHEEK GROOVE
22 CHIN
23 NECK
24 EARLOBE
REDUNDANCIES:
A   NASOLABIAL FOLD
B   CHEEK POUCH
C   JOWLS
D   DEW-LAP (WATTLES)

FIGURE 3.   Facial topography. Numbered regions are amenable to injectable-grade silicone augmentation. Redundancies (indicated by letters) are to be avoided.

D. EARLOBES

Earlobes often become thin and wrinkled with chronologic and photoaging. A lifetime of adornment with earrings and the attendant traction may contribute to the earlobe's degeneration. The lobes can be made fuller and more functional with fluid silicone injections totaling approximately 0.05 ml per earlobe per session. Several sessions are usually required.

E. MOUTH[62,80]

Cosmetic improvement may be achieved in circumoral radial creases and the labial commissure groove.

The lips can be made fuller by injecting small amounts of silicone fluid into or just inside of the vermilion. Small total volumes are used at each session since even minor changes in contour may impart a significant change in perceived appearance.

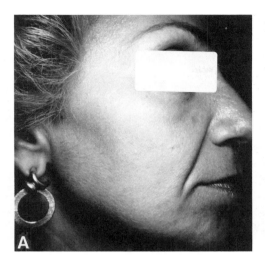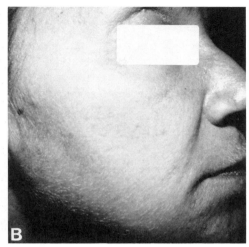

FIGURE 4. (A) Nasolabial creases before treatment. (B) Improvement in appearance after 21 injection sessions with injectable-grade silicone over 30 months.

F. NOSE[1,81]

Depressed defects of the dorsum of the nose, such as saddle-nose deformity, minor degrees of nasal asymmetry, and defects of the nasal tip or ala nasi rim following rhinoplasty or trauma may be cosmetically improved by the introduction of microdroplets of fluid silicone.

G. CHIN[22]

The injection of fluid silicone has a limited but useful role in augmentation of the chin for correction of minor degrees of asymmetry, microgenia, and for optimization of chin contour after alloplastic (e.g., Silastic®) implantation. The chin-lip and chin-cheek grooves may also be improved.

H. NECK

The horizontal rhytids on the sides of the neck respond well to silicone-induced collagen augmentation. Rhytidectomy is best for correction of redundant skin and vertical skin folds (dew-lap). Silicone augmentation is also useful for correcting the contour deformity that results when an excessive amount of fat is removed from the submental area by liposuction or rhytidectomy.

I. CONTOURING[14,22,82-89]

Relatively large cumulative volumes are required for extensive, deeply depressed contours of the face or other parts. Such depressions, especially in the face, may be associated with alveolar bone resorption following rejected dental implants or other dental problems. They may also result from surgery or trauma, especially in the nasal, orbital, or zygomatic regions; or from various conditions of congenital, hereditary, and unknown causes that are responsible for atrophy, dystrophy, or underdevelopment of tissue.

Restoration of facial contour has been achieved in hemifacial atrophy (Romberg's disease, linear scleroderma, or coup de sabre). Augmentation should proceed gradually over many sessions at intervals of 1 month or more. The serial puncture microdroplet injection technique is used to reduce the possibility of ''drift'' and overcorrection, since the cumulative volume injected may be considerable. The total volume required usually varies between 10 and 50 ml, but as much as 97 ml was injected into a woman over a 9 year period, commencing at age 16. The total quantity recommended per treatment session of the affected side ranges from 0.5 to 2 ml. Migration of fluid has not occurred when these procedures are followed.

Larger volumes of fluid silicone may be required for restoration of facial contour in progressive lipodystrophy because of bilateral involvement.

Trunk deformities amenable to correction by silicone are pectus excavatum of minor degree, subclavicular depression caused by congenital absence of the pectoralis major muscle, depression in the abdominal wall caused by partial absence or secondary (neurotrophic) atrophy of the rectus abdominus muscle, and indentations secondary to trauma, surgery, atrophodermas, necrobiosis lipoidica, and localized scleroderma.

In all cases of body contouring the silicone is injected subcutaneously and not into the muscle.

J. PODIATRY[90-96]

Injections of silicone in the foot have been used to provide a subdermal cushion between digital and plantar bony prominences and intractably painful corns, calluses, and scar tissue. Silicone implantation is also useful for the treatment of healed, chronically recurring, neuropathic ulcers and for local areas of pain in the absence of keratotic formation. Silicone improves these conditions by reducing friction and pressure.

K. DECUBITUS ULCERS

Any skin area exposed to chronic pressure can eventually break down and ulcerate due to diminished vascularity. Patients prone to these conditions include the chronically bedridden or wheelchair-bound, and those with amputation stumps who wear a prosthesis. Treatment for pressure and decubitus ulcers is best started before the earliest skin signs of chronic pressure become visible over a bony prominence. We are unaware of any published study on the treatment of decubiti by this method — the above information is based on personal experience.

VIII. PREPARATION OF PATIENTS[97]

Before treatment begins it is essential, as with any cosmetic procedure, to review with the patient the indications and expected results, the material's mechanism of action, techniques of injection, expected sequelae and possible adverse side effects, as well as the limitations of silicone injections. It is explained that silicone replaces lost tissue and does not resurface damaged skin or redrape redundant areas. Silicone corrects previous loss of collagen but cannot prevent future loss caused by further aging, actinic damage, facial expression mannerisms, or scarring. Therefore, maintenance injections for certain rhytid-prone areas at 6 to 12 month intervals may be helpful.

In selecting and accepting patients for treatment such factors as their motivations, preconceived expectations, uncertainties, and general psychological makeup should be taken into account. Photographs taken before treatment are desirable. Patients are made aware of pretreatment facial redundancies and bulges due to dermatochalasis and subcutaneous localized lipomatous accumulations, such as cheek pouches, jowls, and dew-laps (Figure 3). We do not recommend administering silicone to patients who refuse pretreatment photographs.

As a test procedure to judge the probable outcome of soft-tissue augmentation or whether a scar will yield to elevation, infiltration with a lidocaine solution may be performed. This procedure is especially useful when one is assessing the suitability of silicone augmentation for correction of nasal deformities. If success is judged to be likely, silicone may then be injected with the advantage of local anesthesia. Sedation before injection is rarely required for adults, but may be needed for children undergoing treatment for a deformity such as hemifacial atrophy.

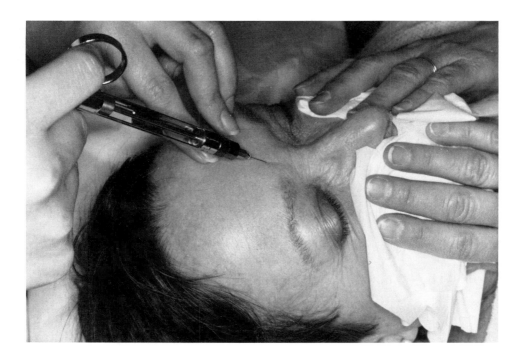

FIGURE 5. Technique of injecting an area on the face. Patient applies pressure to recently injected sites to prevent or minimize bruising.

Alternative augmentation procedures may be discussed with the patient prior to use of silicone injections.

As with most other transdermal injections, there is a minimal risk of infection after microdroplet administration of injectable-grade silicone; aseptic precautions are followed as with any injection procedure. The skin is first thoroughly cleansed to remove cosmetic material or any other residue. Otherwise, makeup, dirt, etc., can be inadvertently tattooed into the skin and may cause foreign body reactions that are mistakenly attributed to the silicone. For evaluation and marking of the prospective treatment sites, the patient is usually placed in a sitting position and the lighting adjusted to allow optimal visualization of the cosmetic defects. The areas to be augmented are marked with a cotton-tipped applicator dipped into an antimicrobial dye. Povidone-iodine 10% solution serves the dual role of topical antiseptic microbicide and visible dye. In general, no sequelae is observed from the injection of silicone fluid through skin marked with povidone-iodine solution. Rarely, a patient may be allergic to povidone-iodine solution, and another dye can be substituted (e.g., metaphen or merthiolate). Depending on personal preference, the patient may be injected in a supported sitting position or first repositioned to recumbency (Figure 5). Occasionally, it is advantageous to inject the patient in other positions that accentuate a defect's appearance.

IX. INSTRUMENTATION[25]

Injectable-grade fluid silicone is stored in glass bottles with glass or teflon-coated bottle caps. The silicone fluid should not come into contact with rubber, dust, lint, fingerprints, etc., as these may provoke foreign body reactions.

The syringes used should be of the long tuberculin type to allow accurate control of amounts injected and to provide mechanical power for the propulsion of viscous fluids.

A modified 0.25 ml syringe for injection of viscous fluid (Figure 5) has been developed by one of the authors (N. Orentreich, U.S. Patent 4,664,655).

The authors use a disposable 30-gauge hypodermic needle with metal hub and specially designed extra large flanges to ensure a firm grip when inserted and locked into the Luer-Lok tip. (Solo Pak®, MPL, Inc., 1820 West Roscoe Street, Chicago, IL 60657; Catalog No. P63230 Metal Hub Special).

X. TECHNIQUES OF INJECTION[1,20,22,26,27,30,33,51,62,63,66,71,82,98]

Three principal methods have been advocated for the injection of liquid silicone: the fanning technique, whereby the subcutaneous course of injection parallels the skin surface; the microdroplet serial puncture technique, whereby a fine needle is directed at an angle to the skin surface and the multiple subdermal depositions of silicone are spaced 2 to 10 mm apart; and the tattooing technique, whereby the needle is stabbed rapidly into and out of the skin with near constant digital pressure upon the plunger.

The characteristics of the soft-tissue defect (its shape, depth, and size) may suggest the use of one or a combination of these methods.

After years of comparison, however, the authors do not recommend the fanning technique and advise that it be used with utmost caution because of its tendency to produce pooling of the silicone in the injection tract.

With the preferred microdroplet serial puncture technique, partial local anesthesia may be obtained by spraying ethyl chloride or freon refrigerant onto the skin just prior to injection. Generally, adults require no topical anesthesia. The application of cold packs also achieves partial analgesia but the pressure and moisture may obscure the cutaneous defects and applied markings. The vermillion may be anesthetized using topical mucuous membrane anesthetics containing either lidocaine or benzocaine. For those patients with a low tolerance for the discomfort of silicone injections, the use of nitrous oxide inhalation analgesia may be helpful.

The needle is inserted into the skin at intervals 2 to 10 mm apart at the appropriate angle for optimal penetration and deposition. The angle of insertion may vary; more oblique (approaching perpendicular) for greater depth or more acute (approaching parallel to the skin) for superficial deposition. Superficial deposition is indicated when treating skin that overlies bony, vital, and vascular structures. A microdroplet of fluid silicone (0.005 to 0.01 ml) is deposited at the appropriate depth upon each insertion of the needle. When using a 30-gauge needle and the microdroplet serial puncture technique, it is not necessary or practical to aspirate prior to injection. When incidentally injected into a blood vessel, the silicone microdroplets act as an anticoagulant and are otherwise well tolerated.

In contradistinction to bovine collagen injections, the intentional production of a slight overcorrection immediately after injection of silicone is to be avoided. The defect should be undercorrected, with gradual augmentation induced over several sessions.

To prevent ecchymosis, direct pressure is promptly applied to the injected areas by fingers and hands (Figure 5). There is no need to seal puncture sites with collodion or a 6—0 nylon suture. An important advantage of the microdroplet serial puncture technique is that it minimizes the chance of embolism.

For fine work, especially on the face, the deposition of many tiny silicone droplets by the microdroplet serial puncture technique is superior to the bulkier deposition of silicone by the fanning technique. Since fibroplasia and augmentation occur at the surface of silicone droplets, the amount of new collagen formed will be directly proportional to the surface area of the injected silicone implant. A given volume of silicone dispersed into many small droplets (serial puncture technique) provides a larger total surface area for collagen synthesis than would the same volume divided into fewer but larger globules (fanning technique). Microdroplet injection also effectively eliminates migration by stimulating a collagen capsule that holds the silicone at the site of implantation.

Intervals between sessions are usually 1 month in the early phases of treatment to a given area. Intervals longer than 1 month pose no problem however, both physician and patient must be aware that augmentation will proceed at a slower rate. As the defects improve, intervals of 1 to 6 months or more are appropriate. Treatments given less than 1 month apart are permissible if different areas are treated. When a patient is unable to return for the next treatment session for 6 months or longer, and it is estimated that they will require approximately six or more treatment sessions to achieve optimal soft-tissue augmentation, two sessions at intervals of one week or less may be performed during the early stages of treatment.

The silicone tattooing technique is performed by rapidly and repeatedly inserting the 30-gauge needle at 1 to 3 mm intervals into the dermal or superficial subcutaneous layers while near constant or intermittent pressure is maintained on the syringe plunger. Silicone is thus expelled during both insertion and withdrawal of the needle. However, due to the speed of injection and short time the needle is in the skin, minute quantities of silicone (less than 0.005 ml) are actually deposited with each puncture. This technique requires a high degree of manual dexterity and is best practiced after one has achieved facility with the microdroplet serial puncture technique. It may be suitable for treatment of fine rhytids, such as crow's feet and some forehead and horizontal neck creases. Beading is somewhat more likely to occur with this technique.

When rapid augmentation with larger volumes was performed in order to produce instant gratification, a variety of dispersal techniques were attempted. The authors, however, do not apply massage, snap a tongue depressor against the skin, or apply a hand-held vibrating machine to disperse silicone after injection since these methods are imprecise and may unnecessarily traumatize facial tissues. The injection of microdroplets at each puncture site obviates the need for dispersion by other techniques.

XI. ADVERSE REACTIONS AND PRECAUTIONS

A. PAIN

Some pain occurs with needle insertion but is not related to the silicone. Discomfort may be minimized by using the finest needles feasible (30 gauge) and by local or inhalation anesthetics.

B. EDEMA[99]

Edema results from the trauma of needle insertion and usually resolves within several hours to days. Since it may produce temporary correction of defects, judgment of cosmetic improvement should be made after both the edema resolves and collagen synthesis takes place. A transitory papular urticarial reaction is occasionally seen at the sites of needle puncture within minutes of injection (dermographism).

C. ECCHYMOSIS

If ecchymosis occurs, it is usually mild and related to needle puncture, needle gauge, thinness or looseness of the skin, and the surface anticoagulant property of silicone. Bruising is more prominent in areas with a dense vascular network. It is advisable for patients to avoid the use of aspirin for 7 days prior to treatment. The application of firm pressure reduces the incidence and extent of ecchymosis and prevents loss of fluid through the needle track puncture site. Patients may apply makeup to camouflage bruises immediately after treatment.

D. ERYTHEMA[12,20,25,89]

Slight to moderate transient erythema may appear immediately after injection. The triple response of Lewis (wheal and flare) reaction may be more pronounced in patients with dermographism and a tendency toward contact or pressure urticaria. It usually persists for a few hours and may be masked with makeup. Persistent erythema of an injected area may result if the injection of silicone has been made too superficially (i.e., intradermally) or with adulterated "silicone". Persistent erythema may be diminished by topical application of anti-inflammatory adrenocorticosteroid preparations or intradermal injection of triamcinolone acetonide 1 to 2.5 mg/ml in 0.05 to 0.10 ml aliquots.

E. DYSCHROMIA[25,84]

The injection of silicone has been reported on rare occasion to cause a brownish-yellow discoloration of the skin. This is probably caused by either very superficial intradermal deposition or injection of adulterated "silicone." A bluish tinge may result from superficial deposition of fluid silicone in thin (translucent) skin, such as striae, atrophic acne scars, and some varicella scars.

It is important to carefully document preexisting pigmentation in the form of written records and photographs and to inform patients of the rare pigmentary changes associated with treatment.

F. TEXTURE AND SENSATION[22,99]

The texture of soft-tissue containing evenly dispersed microdroplets of fluid silicone is very natural. The patient does not experience any unnatural sensation or sensitivity to touch in such locations. Larger cumulative amounts of silicone, as may be required to correct hemifacial atrophy, may impart a slight rubbery consistency on palpation. In light of the overall cosmetic improvement, this change is usually acceptable to the patient. It may occasionally revert to a natural texture given sufficient time. Injection of fluid silicone in greatly excessive amounts or, purportedly, too superficially in the dermis has been known to cause stretching of the skin and blockage of lymphatics. Brawny fullness or a peau d'orange texture may result.

G. OVERCORRECTION[22,50,100]

Overcorrection at a particular silicone implantation site may occur if an excessive quantity is injected at one time or cumulatively over several sessions. Attempting to satisfy a patient's desire for instant gratification by injecting large volumes violates a fundamental principle of injectable silicone therapy.

The term "beading" is used to describe small (1 to 5 mm) firm papules which form at individual sites of needle insertion. They are usually skin-colored but may be slightly erythematous or brownish-yellow. These beads are the result of collagen deposition around superficially implanted microdroplets; they are not granulomas. They may occur when attempting either surface remodeling or contour elevation (Figure 2). Beading is most common on the forehead where skin tightly overlies bone. A few patients develop "beading" at augmentation sites even after all precautions have been followed. In some cases the effect is temporary and the papulation subsides spontaneously during the ensuing months.

Overcorrection of deeper tissues while attempting contour elevation is very uncommon when the serial puncture microdroplet technique is used with intervals of 1 month or more between treatment sessions. It usually takes the form of a somewhat diffuse swelling of the treated area.

Beading and overcorrection of deeper tissues are amenable to intralesional injections of anti-inflammatory corticosteroid, usually triamcinolone acetonide (1.0 to 5.0 mg/ml with approximately 0.1 ml injected per cm^3 of elevated tissue). Microelectrodesiccation, and, if necessary, dermabrasion or tangential shave-excision surgery are also effective for "beading."

Although experience is limited, the use of suction-assisted lipectomy to treat excessively augmented tissues injected with unknown fluid implant materials, adulterated silicone, or even injectable-grade silicone may be worthwhile in selected cases.

H. EMBOLISM[1,31,33,101-105]

Care is taken to avoid intravascular injection of fluid silicone. This precaution applies to injection of any material that is immiscible in blood or of a particle size that may cause embolism. It applies as well to soluble preparations such as local anesthetic agents containing epinephrine, which may cause vasospasm ("functional embolism").

The authors have never observed or encountered any reports of ophthalmic symptoms after injectable-grade silicone injection into facial skin using the microdroplet serial puncture technique. This may be a result of silcone's fluid nature and its anticoagulant properties.

I. GRANULOMATOUS REACTIONS[33,35,36,42,44,45,48,51]

Granulomatous inflammatory reactions to injected "silicone" have been called "siliconomas," a misnomer since silicone itself cannot become a tumor ("-oma"). Furthermore, cells that phagocytize silicone (macrophages) do not multiply in a tumorous fashion. Reports of granulomatous reactions to "silicone" fall into several etiologic categories: cases of overinjection, injection into contraindicated sites, injection of adulterated material, and injection of substances of unknown chemical composition. The authors have not experienced granulomatous reactions with injectable-grade silicone administered by the microdroplet serial puncture technique.

J. IDIOSYNCRATIC REACTIONS TO INJECTABLE-GRADE SILICONE[39]

These rare, local, isolated, inflammatory reactions are characterized by a well-demarcated area of swelling with or without erythema. They occur with an approximate incidence of 1:5,000 to 10,000 treatment sessions in our practice. These reactions may appear months or years after injection and involve one, or rarely several, of the many areas treated. They are frequently preceded by an infection such as acute sinusitis, a furuncle, otitis media, or dental abscess. Patients have a negative intradermal skin test to injectable-grade fluid silicone. The reactions respond within days to weeks to intralesional corticosteroid injections and oral antibiotics; treatment is repeated monthly until final resolution. After a negative intradermal skin test and resolution of the idiosyncratic reaction, the authors have performed further silicone augmentation on some of these patients without recurrence. When a biopsy is performed, the histopathologic specimen usually shows a nonspecific chronic inflammatory reaction. One explanation for these idiosyncratic reactions is that tissues infiltrated with a nonviable material, such as fluid silicone, may rarely act as a nidus for infection. Infectious organisms may come in contact with silicone infiltrated tissues by local extension or via the circulation. Another possibility is that silicone, although pure when injected, is capable of absorbing some chemicals present in the living tissues. If the partition coefficient of a particular chemical allows it to concentrate in the silicone, it may provoke a reaction.

Such rare complications should not be a valid reason to deny the benefits of silicone treatment to patients.

K. DRIFT[36,106-109]

Drifting of silicone liquid (or any other injectable implant for that matter) will occur when large volumes (several to 1000 ml) are injected into a single site, such as the breast or leg. Distant migration of silicone gel from ruptured breast implants has also been reported. These large volumes, which cannot be contained by the receiving tissues, are propelled in a cephalad or caudad direction by gravity, muscle action, and external pressure along tissue planes of least resistance.

Silicone has erroneously been held responsible when areas of naturally occurring redundant facial tissue develop concomitantly with silicone injections administered over time. These areas usually correspond to typical bulges seen with chronologic and photoaging, such as the nasolabial folds, cheek pouches, the jawline jowls, and dew-laps (Figure 3). In some instances these bulges existed prior to silicone treatment but were not noticed by the patient and physician. Increased attention to appearance leads to closer scrutiny of the face by both patient and doctor. General dissatisfaction with an aged appearance causes the patient and occasionally the physician to incorrectly blame the problem on silicone "drift." Examination of pretreatment photographs will usually dispel this misconception.

Finally, gravitational or dependent drift of silicone has been putatively reported to occur months to years after injection. This type of "drift" is difficult to reconcile with the laws of physics since the specific gravity of silicone is less than that of water. Silicone liquid floats on water. Since the specific gravity of human soft tissue is even greater than that of water, silicone fluid would migrate or drift, if indeed it did, upward in a cephalad direction. The authors have never observed the presence of silicone liquid in relatively cephalad locations, months or even years after it was injected into caudal areas, nor are we aware of such published reports.

The microdroplet injection technique effectively eliminates "migration" by stimulating a collagen capsule that holds the silicone at the site of implantation. Only the most fibrotic bound down tissues, e.g., ice-pick acne and certain varicella scars, etc., are not distensible enough to contain microdroplets of injected fluid silicone.

L. CONNECTIVE TISSUE DISEASE[58,59,110-112]

The occurrence of connective tissue diseases, including human adjuvant disease, has been reported after augmentation mammoplasty by the injection of foreign substances such as paraffin, processed petrolatum, adulterated silicone or mixtures of these. Scleroderma, has been reported in women after silicone gel bag augmentation mammoplasty; however, no cause and effect relationship was established. The incidence of scleroderma in women with breast augmentation has been calculated to be the same as that for nonaugmented women. To our knowledge, there have been no cases or reports of connective-tissue disease subsequent to, or as a consequence of, patients who have received only injectable-grade silicone fluid therapy.

The authors have successfully augmented atrophy at the sites of linear scleroderma (coup de sabre) in about 20 patients over the past 30 years with no untoward effect. Furthermore, we have not seen any increased evidence of scleroderma in our large group of patients treated over 35 years with injectable-grade silicone injections.

XII. RELATIVE AND ABSOLUTE CONTRAINDICATIONS

A. BREASTS[18,29,34,113-118]

Injection of fluid silicone into glandular breast tissue is absolutely contraindicated. The great majority of severe complications attributed to fluid "silicone" involved injection into breast tissue and the use, in most cases, of large volumes of adulterated material. The injection of massive quantities of any augmenting material, even medical-grade silicone, into breast parenchyma may be capable of causing compression of fat with release of fatty acids, fat atrophy, and granulomatous or inflammatory reactions. Additional complications encountered after injection of material into breasts, such as lymphedema, peau d'orange, infection and ulceration, could be related to factors other than the inherent nonreactivity of tissues to fluid silicone. Foremost among these factors are mechanical compression of tissue and blockage of lymphatic channels.

Aside from the unlikelihood of improving breast appearance, fluid injection mammoplasty interferes with clinical, mammographic, and other known methods to detect neoplastic breast masses. Nevertheless, in humans beings there is no known causal relation between the injection of silicone into the breasts and breast cancer.

We have injected atrophic cutaneous defects in skin overlying breasts with beneficial results and long-term safety.

B. EYELIDS

Except in special circumstances, such as atrophic traumatic scars and linear scleroderma (coup de sabre), eyelid tissue is usually unsuitable for augmentation because of its thinness, overdistensibility, and tendency for discoloration. This does not ordinarily include the infra-orbital groove.

C. VASCULAR ABNORMALITIES[62]

As a precaution against embolism, fluid silicone should not be injected where arterio-venous communications may have resulted from surgery or trauma. Injections are also best avoided in areas of lymphostasis.

D. BOUND-DOWN SCARS[30]

Depressed scars that are tightly bound down by fibrotic adhesions (nondistensible), especially the "ice pick" scars of acne vulgaris and some varicella scars, resist elevation. Overzealous attempts to inject beneath such scars may result in collarette elevation of surrounding skin ("doughnut effect"), thus exaggerating the depressions.

E. FIBROCYSTIC LESIONS[98]

Cavities of cysts should not be filled with silicone, but the depressed distensible scars that remain after spontaneous or surgical resolution of epidermal or inflammatory cysts may be elevated by microdroplet injection of silicone.

F. EXPECTATION OF PERFECT TRANSFORMATION[97]

Facial rhytids and deep furrows often correspond to underlying fibromuscular attachments of skin to fascia. Injectable-grade silicone augmentation generally produces satisfactory cosmetic improvement.

However, soft-tissue augmentation with liquid silicone does not substitute for rhytidec-tomy or liposuction, which redrapes redundant skin and removes excess fat; dermabrasion or chemical peel, which resurfaces by abrading or peeling away wrinkled, scarred, or actinically damaged skin; and full-thickness punch autografting, which replaces defective skin, such as "ice pick" scars.

The physician will occasionally encounter patients with unrealistic expectations and demands, and will need to exercise restraint in administering silicone.

G. TREATMENT DURING PREGNANCY

To the best of our knowledge, there have been no adverse reports concerning the subcutaneous injection of injectable-grade silicone in pregnant women; however, definitive human studies have not been done.

H. ACTIVELY INFLAMED OR INFECTED SITES

Injection into depressed sites of active inflammation (i.e., bovine collagen reactions and allergic contact dermatitis) or active infection (i.e., acneiform lesions, ulcers, and herpes lesions) is best deferred until the underlying process has resolved.

I. SILICONE ALLERGY

Although never encountered in the authors' practice or review of the literature, should a patient develop a true allergic reaction (proven by appropriate serologic and intradermal skin testing) to injectable-grade silicone, he or she would not be a candidate for further silicone implantation.

XIII. ANIMAL TOXICITY AND LACK OF CARCINOGENICITY[12,128-142]

Polydimethylsiloxane of various viscosities were reportedly devoid of adverse reproductive, teratogenic, and mutagenic effects in the mice, rats, and rabbits studied. Injectable-grade fluid silicone has not been found to be carcinogenic in animal or humans.

The Dow Corning Corporation conducted a study which showed that one quarter of rats tested had tumors at the site of silicone gel implantation. The tumors were diagnosed as sarcomas, most of which were fibrosarcomas. All aspects of the response including tumor incidence, latency period, and histopathologic type were consistent with a phenomenon known as solid state tumorigenesis (SST), which is also called the "Oppenheimer effect." These and other investigators demonstrated in mice and rats that all relatively inert alloplastic materials such as cellophane, nylon, glass, metals, and silicone elastomer (rubber) induce sarcomas at the implantation site provided the size of the implant is sufficiently large. The effect is independent of chemical composition as supported by genetic toxicity testing of silicone gel showing no effects. They also concluded that this effect in rodents does not indicate a significant risk to human health.

An epidemiologic study of more than 3,100 women who had received silicone gel-bag breast implants showed no local soft-tissue sarcomas and no excess of ordinary breast cancers. Furthermore, prolonged living with solid and gel silicone materials imbedded internally has not been carcinogenic in over a million patients with synthetic devices, such as shunts for drainage of hydrocephalus; heart valves; coverings for pacemakers; joint, breast, and penile implants; arterial prostheses; and ocular bands installed for repair of detached retinas.

The methodology used to prove safety and efficacy in the above animal resports were state-of-the art when published. Clinical experience has supported their findings. Today, if a company were to seek FDA approval of injectable fluid silicone for soft-tissue augmentation, they would probably be required to utilize the latest methodology available to substantiate previous reports that demonstrated safety and efficacy.

XIV. METABOLISM AND EXCRETION

Fluid silicone is not known to be altered *in vivo*. Little dissipation of injectable-grade silicone from sites injected with the microdroplet serial puncture technique has been found. Minute quantities of the material may be phagocytized and transported through the reticuloendothelial system, but with no known harmful effects. Traces of the material may be found in urine and stool.

XV. DETECTION IN TISSUE SPECIMENS[13,18,23,24,31,34,36,41,43,73,89,94,113,131,143-146]

Fluid silicone is not stainable or retained during routine preparation of tissue for microscopic examination. It has been erroneously claimed, especially in examination of frozen preparations or thick sections stained with hematoxylin and eosin, that "silicone" may be discernible as thin refractile sheets or membranes lying in spaces surrounded by histiocytes. These are neither specific nor sensitive methods of identification. Electron microscopy cannot be used to positively identify fluid silicone in tissues. The location of silicone in tissue may be suspected from rounded extracellular spaces and vacuoles within cells; however, an identical picture may be produced by various nonsilicone oily substances.

Detection of silicone requires special tissue preparation and sophisticated equipment because of the inert character of the polymer *in vitro* (Section III).

Infrared spectroscopy is the only accurate physical method of detecting the silicon-carbon and silicon-oxygen bonds. Since the silicon-carbon bond is synthetically produced and does not occur spontaneously in nature, a positive test implies that one or more silicones are present. The test does not reveal the nature of the remainder of the silicone molecules; the source, quantity or purity of the material present; or the presence or absence of adulterants. Infrared spectroscopy is also able to detect linear hydrocarbons such as olive oil and paraffin (mineral oil) which were commonly added to injectable silicone.

X-ray spectroscopy or energy dispersive spectroscopy can only demonstrate the presence of elements, including silicon. Merely demonstrating the presence of silicon, the most abundant element on earth, does not prove that the silicon containing polydimethylsiloxane molecule is present. The element silicon may have been introduced during biopsy since medical-grade liquid silicone is used to coat may disposable instruments, needles, and scalpels. Furthermore, during processing, the tissue specimen comes into contact with fixatives, stains, and cutting and mounting equipment which may contaminate the specimen with silicon. A specimen of both normal and diseased tissue should be handled and analyzed in a similar fashion if meaningful conclusions are to be drawn.

XVI. COMPATIBILITY WITH OTHER SURGICAL/COSMETIC PROCEDURES[92,97,99,147,148]

Sites properly augmented by fluid silicone do not require special patient care. There have been no adverse interactions following exposure to the sun. Makeup may be applied in the usual manner.

Proper soft-tissue augmentation with injectable-grade silicone does not interfere with surgical procedures or wound healing. Dermabrasion, skin grafting, chemical peel, rhytidectomy, blepharoplasty and liposuction all have been performed without increased morbidity in patients previously treated with injectable-grade silicone. Dermabrasion has been successfully performed even in areas where excessive amounts of silicone have been deposited.

Additional cosmetic improvement may also be obtained with injectable-grade silicone augmentation in patients who have previously undergone the above surgical techniques.

REFERENCES

1. **Ashley, F. L., Braley, S., Rees, T. D., Goulian, D., and Ballantyne, D. L.,** The present status of silicone fluid in soft-tissue augmentation, *Plast. Reconstr. Surg.,* 39, 411, 1967.
2. **Braley, S.,** The silicones as tools in biological engineering, *Med. Electron. Biol. Eng.,* 3, 127, 1965.
3. **Scales, J. T.,** Discussion on metals and synthetic materials in relation to soft tissues; tissue reaction to synthetic materials, *Proc. R. Soc. Med.,* 46, 647, 1953.
4. **Kipping, F. S., Blackburn, J. C., and Short, J. F.,** Organic derivatives of silicon. XLIV, *J. Chem. Soc.,* 133, 1290, 1931.
5. **Braley, S.,** The chemistry and properties of the medical-grade silicones, *J. Macromol. Sci. Chem.,* A4 (3), 529, 1970.
6. **Noll, W.,** *Chemistry and Technology of Silicones,* Academic Press, New York, 1968.
7. **Dingman, R.,** Silicone injections, in *Skin Surgery,* 3rd ed., Epstein, E., Ed., Charles C Thomas, Springfield, IL, 1970, 578.
8. **Mullison, E. G.,** Silicones and their uses in plastic surgery, *Arch. Otolaryngol.,* 81, 264, 1965.
9. **Mullison, E. G.,** Current status of silicones in plastic surgery, *Arch. Otolaryngol.,* 83, 59, 1966.
10. **Mullison, E. G.,** Silicones in head and neck surgery, *Arch. Otolaryngol.,* 84, 91, 1966.
11. **Nedelman, C. I.,** Oral and cutaneous tissue reactions to injected fluid silicone, *J. Biomed. Mater Res.,* 2, 131, 1968.
12. **Blocksma, R. and Braley, S.,** Implantation materials, in *Plastic Surgery,* 2nd ed., Grabb, W. C. and Smith, J. W., Eds., Little, Brown, Boston, 1973, 131.
13. **McDowell, F.,** Complications with silicones—what grade of silicone? How do we know it was silicone?, *Plast. Reconstr. Surg.,* 61, 892, 1978.

14. **Ashley, F. L., Rees, T. D., Ballantyne, D. L., et al.,** An injection technique for the treatment of facial hemiatrophy, *Plast. Reconstr. Surg.,* 35, 640, 1965.

15. **Gonzalez Ulloa, M., Stevens, E., Loewe, P., Vargas de la Cruz, J., and Noble, G.,** Preliminary report on the subcutaneous perfusion of dimethyl-polysiloxane to increase volume and alter regional contour, *Br. J. Plast. Surg.,* 20, 424, 1967.

16. **Braley, S.,** The status of injectable silicone fluid for soft-tissue augmentation, *Plast. Reconstr. Surg.,* 47, 343, 1971.

17. **Klein, J. A., Cole, G., Barr, R. J., Bartlow, G., and Fulwinder, C.,** Paraffinomas of the scalp, *Arch. Dermatol.,* 121, 382, 1985.

18. **Chaplin, C. H.,** Loss of both breasts from injections of silicone (with additive), *Plast. Reconstr. Surg.,* 44, 447, 1969.

19. **Montgomery, H.,** *Dermatopathology,* Harper & Row, New York, 1967, 403.

20. **Edgerton, M. T. and Wells, J. H.,** Indications for and pitfalls of soft-tissue augmentation with liquid silicone, *Plast. Reconstr. Surg.,* 58, 157, 1976.

21. **Lever, W. F. and Schaumberg-Lever, G.,** *Histopathology of the Skin,* 6th ed., Lippincott, Philadelphia, 1983, 222.

22. **Rees, T. D.,** Silicone injection therapy, in *Cosmetic Facial Surgery,* Rees, T. D. and Wood-Smith, D., Eds., W. B. Saunders, Philadelphia, 1973, 232.

23. **Symmers, W. St. C.,** Silicone mastitis in "topless" waitresses and some other varieties of foreign-body mastitis, *Br. Med. J.,* 3, 19, 1968.

24. **Braley, S.,** Silicone fluids with added adulterants—letter to the Editor, *Plast. Reconstr. Surg.,* 45, 288, 1970.

25. **Aronsohn, R. B.,** Observations on the use of silicone in the face, *Arch. Otolaryngol.,* 82, 191, 1965.

26. **Aronsohn, R. B.,** A 22-year experience with the use of silicone injections, *Am. J. Cosmet. Surg.,* 1, 21, 1984.

27. **Berger, R. A.,** Dermatologic experience with liquid silicones, *N. Y. State J. Med.,* 66, 2523, 1966.

28. **Kagan, H. D.,** Sakurai injectable silicone formula. A preliminary report, *Arch. Otolaryngol.,* 78, 663, 1963.

29. **Ortiz-Monasterio, F. and Trigos, I.,** Management of patients with complications from injections of foreign materials into the breasts, *Plast. Reconstr. Surg.,* 50, 42, 1972.

30. **Berger, R. A.,** Use of silicone injections in facial defects, *Arch. Otolaryngol.,* 101, 525, 1975.

31. **Nosanchuk, J. S.,** Silicone granuloma in breast, *Arch. Surg.,* 97, 583, 1968.

32. **Arthaud, J. B.,** Silicone-induced penile sclerosing lipogranuloma, *J. Urol.,* 110, 210, 1973.

33. **Ellenbogen, R., Ellenbogen, R., and Rubin, L.,** Injectable fluid silicone therapy: human morbidity and mortality, *JAMA,* 234, 308, 1975.

34. **McCurdy, H. and Solomons, E. T.,** Forensic examination of toxicological specimens for dimethylpoly-siloxane (silicone oil), *J. Anal. Toxicol.,* 1, 221, 1977.

35. **Winer, L. H., Sternberg, T. H., Lehman, R., and Ashley, F. L.,** Tissue reactions to injected silicone liquids. A report of three cases, *Arch. Dermatol.,* 90, 588, 1964.

36. **Delage, C., Shane, J. J., and Johnson, F. B.,** Mammary silicone granuloma: migration of silicone fluid to abdominal wall and inguinal region, *Arch. Dermatol.,* 108, 104, 1973.

37. **Rae, V., Pardo, R. J., Falanga, V., and Blackwelder, P.,** Leg ulcers following subcutaneous injection of a liquid silicone preparation, *Arch. Dermatol.,* 125, 670, 1989.

38. **Orentreich, N. and Orentreich, D. S.,** Letter to the Editor: Leg ulcers following subcutaneous injection of a liquid silicone preparation, *Arch. Dermatol.,* 125, 1283, 1989.

39. **Blocksma, R.,** The voice of polite dissent: complications following silicone injections for augmentation of the contours of the face (By Pearl, R. M., Laub, D. R., Kaplan, E. N.), *Plast. Reconstr. Surg.,* 62, 109, 1978.

40. **Bulcao de Moraes, H.,** Liquid silicone in the dorsum of the hand, *Ann. Plast. Surg.,* 6, 500, 1981.

41. **Chastre, J., Basset, F., Viau, F., Dournovo, P., et al.,** Acute pneumonitis after subcutaneous injections of silicone in transsexual men, *N. Engl. J. Med.,* 308, 764, 1983.

42. **Karfik, V. and Smahel, J.,** Subcutaneous silicone granuloma, *Acta Chir. Plast.,* 10, 328, 1968.

43. **Kopf, E. H., Vinnik, C. A., Bongiovi, J. J., and Dombrowski, D. J.,** Complications of silicone injections, *Rocky Mount. Med. J.,* 73, 77, 1976.

44. **Kozeny, G. A., Barbato, A. L., Bansal, V. K., Vertuno, L. L., and Hano, J. E.,** Hypercalcemia associated with silicone-induced granulomas, *N. Engl. J. Med.,* 311, 1103, 1984.

45. **Milojevic, B.,** Complications after silicone injection therapy in aesthetic plastic surgery, *Aesth. Plast. Surg.,* 6, 203, 1982.

46. **Pearl, R. M., Laub, D. R., Kaplan, E. N.,** Complications following silicone injections for augmentation of the contours of the face, *Plast. Reconstr. Surg.,* 61, 888, 1978.

47. **Perry, R. P., Jaques, D. P., Lesar, M. S., et al.,** *Mycobacterium avium* infection in a silicone-injected breast. Case report, *Plast. Reconstr. Surg.,* 75, 104, 1985.

48. **Piechotta, F. U.,** Silicone fluid, attractive and dangerous: collective review and summary of experience, *Aesth. Plast. Surg.,* 3, 347, 1979.

49. **Travis, W. D., Balogh, K., and Abraham, J. L.,** Silicone granulomas: report of three cases and review of the literature, *Human Pathol.,* 16, 19, 1985.

50. **Zandi, I.,** Use of suction to treat soft tissue injected with liquid silicone, *Plast. Reconstr. Surg.,* 76, 307, 1985.

51. **Wilkie, T. F.,** Late development of granuloma after liquid silicone injections, *Plast. Reconstr. Surg.,* 60, 179, 1977.

52. **Achauer, B. M.,** A serious complications following medical-grade silicone injection of the face, *Plast. Reconstr. Surg.,* 71, 251, 1983.

53. **Wolff, K. and Tappeiner, G.,** Mycobacterial diseases: tuberculosis and atypical mycobacterial infections, in *Dermatology in General Medicine,* 3rd ed., Fitzpatrick, T. B., Eisen, A. Z., Wolff, K., Freedberg, I. M., and Austen, K. F., Eds., McGraw-Hill, New York, 1987, 2175.

54. **Rees, T. D., Ballantyne, D. L., and Seidman, I.,** Eyelid deformities caused by the injection of silicone fluid, *Br. J. Plast. Surg.,* 24, 125, 1971.

55. **Goin, J. M.,** Silicone for facial furrows, *JAMA,* 229, 1581, 1974.

56. **Klein, A. W. and Rish, D. C.,** Substances for soft-tissue augmentation: collagen and silicone, *J. Dermatol. Surg. Oncol.,* 11, 337, 1985.

57. **Vinnik, C. A.,** The hazards of silicone injections, *JAMA,* 236, 959, 1976.

58. **Sergott, T. J., Limoli, J. P., Baldwin, C. M., Jr., et al.,** Human adjuvant disease, possible autoimmune disease after silicone implantation: a review of the literature, case studies and speculation for the future, *Plast. Reconstr. Surg.,* 78, 104, 1986.

59. **Kumagai, Y., Shiokawa, Y., Medsger, T. A., Jr., et al.,** Clinical spectrum of connective tissue disease after cosmetic surgery, *Arthritis Rheum.,* 27, 1, 1984.

60. **Orentreich, N.,** Soft-tissue augmentation with medical-grade fluid silicone, in *Biomaterials in Reconstructive Surgery,* Rubin, L. R., Ed., C. V. Mosby, St. Louis, 1983, 859.

61. **Rees, T. D.,** Local and systemic response to injectable silicone fluid, in *Biomaterials in Reconstructive Surgery,* Rubin, L. R., Ed., C. V. Mosby, St. Louis, 1983, 529.

62. **Selmanowitz, V. J. and Orentreich, N.,** Medical-grade fluid silicone: a monographic review, *J. Dermatol. Surg. Oncol.,* 3, 597, 1977.

63. **Webster, R. C., Fuleihan, M. D., Gaunt, J. M., Hamdan, U. S., and Smith, R. C.,** Injectable silicone for small augmentations: twenty-year experience in humans, *Am. J. Cosmet. Surg.,* 1, 1, 1984.

64. **Webster, R. C., Fuleihan, N. S., Hamdan, U. S., Gaunt, J. M., and Smith, R. C.,** Injectable silicone for small augmentations: recommendations for controlled release to medical profession, *Am. J. Cosmet. Surg.,* 1, 11, 1984.

65. **Clauser, S. B., Fanta, C. M., Finkel, A. J., and Perlman, J. M., Eds.,** *Physicians' Current Procedural Terminology,* 4th ed., American Medical Association, Chicago, IL, 1985.

66. **Legal Opinion Letters to N.** Orentreich and on file at the Food and Drug Administration: March 8, 1983 from Dewey, Ballantine, Bushby, Palmer, and Wood, New York, N.Y.; and March 7, 1983 from Kleinfeld, Kaplan, and Becker, Washington, D.C.

67. **Ben-Hur, N., Ballantyne, D. L., Rees, T. D., and Seidman, I.,** Local and systemic effects of dimethylsiloxane fluid in mice, *Plast. Reconstr. Surg.,* 39, 423, 1967.

68. **Hueper, W. C.,** Cancer induction of polyurethan and polysilicone plastics, *J. Natl. Cancer Inst.,* 33, 1005, 1964.

69. **Andrews, J. M.,** Cellular behavior to injected silicone fluid: a preliminary report, *Plast. Reconstr. Surg.,* 38, 581, 1966.

70. **Hawthorne, G. A., Ballantyne, D. L., Rees, T. D., Seidman, I.,** Hematological effects of dimethylpolysiloxane fluid in rats, *J. Reticuloendothel. Soc.,* 7, 587, 1970.

71. **Kopf, E. H.,** Injectable silicones, *Rocky Mount. Med. J.,* 63, 34, 1966.

72. **Balkin, S. W.,** Plantar keratoses: treatment by injectable liquid silicone. Report of an eight-year experience, *Clin. Orthop.,* 87, 235, 1972.

73. **Nosanchuk, J. S.,** Injected dimethylpolysiloxane fluid. A study of the antibody and histologic response, *Plast. Reconstr. Surg.,* 42, 562, 1968.

74. **Ohmori, S. and Hirayma, T.,** Is it possible to produce adjuvant's disease in human beings by the injection of silicone?, *Jpn. J. Plast. Reconstr. Surg.,* 13, 132, 1966.

75. **Orentreich, D. S. and Orentreich, N.,** Acne scar revision update, *Dermatologic Clinics,* Vol. 5, No. 2, Balin, P. L., Ratz, J. L., and Wheeland, R. G., Eds., W. B. Saunders, Philadelphia, 1987, 359.

76. **Orentreich, N. and Durr, N. P.,** Rehabilitation of acne scarring, in *Dermatologic Clinics,* Vol. 1, No. 3, Symposium on Acne, Shalita, A. R., Ed., W. B. Saunders, Philadelphia, 1983, 405.

77. **Orentreich, N. and Selmanowitz, V. J.,** Cosmetic improvement of factitial defects, *Med. Trial Tech. Q.,* 17, 172, 1970.

78. **Selmanowitz, V. J. and Orentreich, N.,** Cosmetic treatment of factitial defects, *Cutis,* 6, 549, 1970.

79. **Wynn, S. K.,** Combining cosmetic rhinoplasty with nasolabial silicone injection, *Wisc. Med. J.,* 65, 179, 1966.

80. **Orentreich, N.,** Dermabrasion, *J. Amer. Med. Women's Assoc.,* 24, 331, 1969.

81. **Berman, W. E.,** Synthetic materials in facial contours, *Am. Acad. Ophthalmol. Otolaryngol.,* 68, 876, 1964.

82. **Ashley, F. L., Thompson, D. P., Henderson, T.,** Augmentation of surface contour by subcutaneous injections of silicone fluid. A current report, *Plast. Reconstr. Surg.,* 51, 8, 1973.

83. **Rees, T. D. and Ashley, F. L.,** Treatment of facial atrophy with liquid silicone, *Am. J. Surg.,* 111, 531, 1966.

84. **Rees, T. D. and Ashley, F. L.,** A new treatment for facial hemiatrophy in children by injections of dimethylpolysiloxane fluid, *J. Pediatr. Surg.,* 2, 347, 1967.

85. **Rees, T. D., Ashley, F. L., and Delgado, J. P.,** Silicone fluid injections for facial atrophy. A ten-year study, *Plast. Reconstr. Surg.,* 52, 118, 1973.

86. **Franz, F. P., Blocksma, R., Brundage, S. R., and Ringler, S. L.,** Massive injection of liquid silicone for hemifacial atrophy, *Ann. Plast. Surg.,* 20, 140, 1988.

87. **Blocksma, R.,** Experience with dimethylpolysiloxane fluid in soft-tissue augmentation, *Plast. Reconstr. Surg.,* 48, 564, 1971.

88. **Rees, T. D. and Coburn, R. J.,** Silicone treatment of partial lipodystrophy, *JAMA,* 230, 868, 1974.

89. **Ashley, F. L., Braley, S., and McNall, E. G.,** The current status of silicone injection therapy, *Surg. Clin. North Am.,* 51, 501, 1971.

90. **Balkin, S. W.,** Treatment of corns by injectable silicone, *Arch. Dermatol.,* 111, 1143, 1975.

91. **Balkin, S. W.,** Silicone injection for plantar keratoses. Preliminary report, *J. Am. Podiatry Assoc.,* 56, 1, 1966.

92. **Balkin, S. W.,** Silicone augmentation for plantar calluses, *J. Am. Podiatry Assoc.,* 66, 148, 1976.

93. **Stough, D. B.,** Silicone treatment of plantar keratoses, *Cutis,* 8, 575, 1971.

94. **Balkin, S. W.,** Treatment of painful scars on soles and digits with injections of fluid silicone, *J. Dermatol. Surg. Oncol.,* 3, 612, 1977.

95. **May, S. B. and Balkin, S. W.,** Plantar callus and diabetic ulceration treated by injectable liquid silicone, *Soc. Trans. Arch. Dermatol.,* 108, 287, 1973.

96. **Balkin, S. W.,** The fluid silicone prosthesis, *Clin. Podiatry,* 1, 145, 1984.

97. **Orentreich, N. and Durr, N. P.,** The four R's of skin rehabilitation, in *The Psychology of Cosmetic Treatments,* Graham, J. A. G., and Kligman, A. M., Eds., Praeger, New York, 1985, 227.

98. **Stough, D. B.,** Medical silicone in dermofacial defects, *Cutis,* 6, 1243, 1970.

99. **Sperber, P. A.,** Chemexfoliation and silicone infiltration in the treatment of aging skin and dermal defects, *J. Am. Geriatr. Soc.,* 12, 594, 1964.

100. **Le Van, P.,** The causes and prevention of poor cosmetic results from injection of fluid silicone, *J. Dermatol. Surg. Oncol.,* 4, 328, 1978.

101. **Selmanowitz, V. J. and Orentreich, N.,** Cutaneous corticosteroid injection and amaurosis, *Arch. Dermatol.,* 110, 729, 1974.

102. **Walsh, F. B. and Hoyt, W. F.,** *Clinical Neuro-Ophthalmology,* Vol. 3, 3rd ed., Williams & Wilkins, Baltimore, 1969, 2501.

103. **Durst, S., Johnson, B. S., and Amplatz, K.,** The effect of silicone coatings on thrombogenicity, *Am. J. Roentgenol. Rad. Ther. Nucl. Med.,* 20, 904, 1974.

104. **Jaques, L. B., Fidlar, E., Feldsted, E. T., and MacDonald, A. G.,** Silicones and blood coagulation, *Can. Med. Assoc. J.,* 55, 26, 1946.

105. Zyderm Collagen Implant Safety Notice, Collagen Corporation, Palo Alto, CA, 1983.

106. **Rich, J. D., Shesol, B. F., and Gottlieb, V. G.,** Supraclavicular migration of breast-injected silicone: case report, *Military Med.,* 147, 404, 1982.

107. **Capozzi, A., Du Bou, R., and Pennisi, V. R.,** Distant migration of silicone gel from a ruptured breast implant. Case report, *Plast. Reconstr. Surg.,* 62, 302, 1978.

108. **Huang, T. T., Blackwell, S. J., and Lewis, R. S.,** Migration of silicone gel after the "squeeze technique" to rupture a contracted breast capsule. Case report, *Plast. Reconstr. Surg.,* 61, 277, 1978.

109. **Mason, J. and Apisarnthanarax, P.,** Migratory silicone granuloma, *Arch. Dermatol.,* 117, 366, 1981.

110. **Van Nunen, S. A., Galenby, P. A., and Basten, A.,** Post-mammoplasty connective tissue disease, *Arthritis Rheum.,* 25, 694, 1982.

111. **Speira, H.,** Scleroderma after silicone augmentation mammoplasty, *JAMA,* 260, 236, 1988.

112. **Medsger, T. A. and Masi, A. T.,** Epidemiology of systemic sclerosis (scleroderma), *Ann. Intern. Med.,* 74, 714, 1971.

113. **Solomons, E. T. and Jones, J. K.,** The determination of polydimethylsiloxane (silicone oil) in biological materials: a case report, *J. Forensic Sci.,* 20, 191, 1975.

114. **Kuiper, D.,** Silicone granulomatous disease of the breast simulating cancer, *Mich. Med.,* 72, 215, 1973.

115. **Lewis, M. C.,** Inflammatory carcinoma of the breast following silicone injections. Case report, *Plast. Reconstr. Surg.,* 66, 136, 1980.

116. **Parsons, R. W. and Thering, H. R.,** Management of the silicone-injected breast, *Plast. Reconstr. Surg.,* 60, 534, 1977.
117. **De Cholnoky, T.,** Augmentation mammoplasty: survey of complications in 10,941 patients by 265 surgeons, *Plast. Reconstr. Surg.,* 45, 573, 1970.
118. **Wustrack, K. O. and Zarem, H. A.,** Surgical management of silicone mastitis, *Plast. Reconstr. Surg.,* 63, 224, 1979.
119. **Datta, N. S. and Kern, F. B.,** "Silicone" granuloma of the penis, *J. Urol.,* 109, 840, 1973.
120. **Zalar, J. A., Jr., Knode, R. E., and Mir, J. A.,** Lipogranuloma of the penis, *J. Urol.,* 102, 75, 1969.
121. **May, J. A. and Pickering, P. P.,** Paraffinoma of the penis, *Calif. Med.,* 85, 42, 1956.
122. **Christ, J. E. and Askew, J. B., Jr.,** Silicone granuloma of the penis, *Plast. Reconstr. Surg.,* 69, 337, 1982.
123. **Lighterman, I.,** Silicone granuloma of the penis. Case reports, *Plast. Reconstr. Surg.,* 57, 517, 1976.
124. **Arduino, L. J.,** Sclerosing lipogranuloma of male genitalia, *J. Urol.,* 82, 155, 1959.
125. **Newcomer, V. D., Graham, J. H., Schaffert, R. R., and Kaplan, L.,** Sclerosing lipogranuloma resulting from exogenous lipids, *AMA Arch. Dermatol.,* 73, 361, 1956.
126. **Smetana, H. F. and Bernhard, W.,** Sclerosing lipogranuloma, *Arch. Pathol.,* 50, 296, 1950.
127. **Brown, A. F. and Joergenson, E. J.,** Geritomammary paraffin oil granulomas in the male, *Ann. Western Med. Surg.,* 1, 301, 1947.
128. **Kennedy, G. L., Jr., Keplinger, M. L., and Calandra, J. C.,** Reproductive, teratologic, and mutagenic studies with some polydimethylsiloxanes, *J. Toxicol. Environ. Health,* 1, 909, 1976.
129. **Grasso, P., Goldberg, L., and Fairweather, F. A.,** Injections of silicones in mice. Letters to the Editor, *Lancet,* 2, 96, 1964.
130. **Rees, T. D., Platt, J., and Ballantyne, D. L.,** An investigation of cutaneous response to dimethylpolysiloxane (silicone liquid) in animals and humans: a preliminary report, *Plast. Reconstr. Surg.,* 35, 131, 1965.
131. **Rees, T. D., Ballantyne, D. L., Seidman, I., and Hawthorne, G. A.,** Visceral response to subcutaneous and intraperitoneal injections of silicone in mice, *Plast. Reconstr. Surg.,* 39, 402, 1967.
132. **Rees, T. D., Ballantyne, D. L., and Coburn, R. J.,** Liquid silicone therapy—a decade's experience, in *Drug Induced Clinical Toxicity,* McMahon, F. G., Ed., Future Publishing, Mt. Kisco, NY, 1974, 169.
133. **Ballantyne, D. L., Rees, T. D., and Seidman, I.,** Silicone fluid: response to massive subcutaneous injections of dimethylpolysiloxane fluid in animals, *Plast. Reconstr. Surg.,* 36, 330, 1965.
134. **Rees, T. D., Ballantyne, D. L., and Hawthorne, G. A.,** Silicone fluid research. A follow-up summary, *Plast Reconstr. Surg.,* 46, 50, 1970.
135. **Harris, H. I.,** Survey of breast implants from the point of view of carcinogenesis, *Plast. Reconstr. Surg.,* 28, 81, 1961.
136. **Ben-Hur, N. and Neuman, Z.,** Malignant tumor formation following subcutaneous injections of silicone fluid in white mice, *Israel Med. J.,* 22, 15, 1963.
137. **Ben-Hur, N. and Neuman, Z.,** Siliconoma—Another cutaneous response to dimethylpolysiloxane. Experimental study in mice, *Plast. Reconstr. Surg.,* 36, 629, 1965.
138. **Freeman, B. S., Bigelow, E. L., and Braley, S. A.,** Experiments witn injectable plastic. Use of silicone and silastic rubber in animals and its clinical use in deformities of the head and neck, *Am. J. Surg.,* 112, 534, 1966.
139. **Frisch, E. E.,** Technology of silicones in biomedical applications, in *Biomaterials in Reconstructive Surgery,* Rubin, L. R., Ed., C. V. Mosby, St. Louis, 1983, 73.
140. **Rylee, R. T. and Dillon, C. F.,** Letter from Dow Corning Corporation: Information summary concerning experimental animal tumors associated with silicone gel. Dow Corning Corporation, P.O. Box 994, Midland, MI, 1988.
141. **Brand, K. G.,** Foam covered mammary implants, *Plast. Reconstr. Breast Surg.,* 15, 533, 1988.
142. **Deapen, D. M., Pike, M. C., Casagrande, J. T., and Brody, G. S.,** The relationship between breast cancer and augmentation mamoplasty: an epidemiologic study, *Plast. Reconstr. Surg.,* 77, 361, 1986.
143. **Vinnik, C. A.,** Silicone mastopathy, presented at the 8th Ann. Meet. of The American Society for Aesthetic Plastic Surgery, Vancouver, BC, May 5, 1975.
144. **Urbach, F., Wine, S. S., Johnson, W. C., and Davies, R. E.,** Generalized paraffinoma (sclerosing lipogranuloma), *Arch. Dermatol.,* 103, 277, 1971.
145. **Abraham, J. L. and Etz, E. S.,** Molecular microanalysis of pathological specimens in situ with a Laser-Raman microprobe, *Science,* 206, 716, 1979.
146. **Pucevich, M. V., Rosenberg, E. W., Bale, G. F., and Terzakis, J. A.,** Widespread foreign-body granulomas and elevated serum angiotensin-converting enzyme, *Arch. Dermatol.,* 119, 229, 1983.
147. **Rees, T. D., Ballantyne, D. L., Jr., Hawthorne, G. A., and Seidman, I.,** The effects of dimethylpolysiloxane fluid on rat skin autografts, *Plast. Reconstr. Surg.,* 41, 153, 1968.
148. **Orentreich, N.,** Preventive and therapeutic measures for aging skin, *Proc. Sci. Sec. Toilet Goods Assoc.,* 41, 37, 1964.

Chapter 15

INJECTABLE COLLAGEN: A TEN-YEAR EXPERIENCE

Michael M. Churukian, Alfred Cohen, Frank M. Kamer, Lawrence Lefkoff, Francis R. Palmer, III, and Carol A. Ross

TABLE OF CONTENTS

I. INTRODUCTION

Injectable collagen was introduced to a wary audience by Knapp et al. in 1977,[1] with a report of 28 patients receiving human and/or bovine collagen implants. Formal clinical trials followed in September 1979, and were thoroughly monitored by the manufacturer until final FDA approval was granted in July 1981. During these two years, over 700 physicans entered 5,109 patients into the investigational treatment protocol.

Subsequent clinical reports established techniques, relative safety, and efficacy of injectable collagen.[2-4] The original collagen implant (Zyderm I, 35 mg/ml collagen) was joined in 1983 by a more concentrated form (Zyderm II, 65 mg/ml collagen). More recently in 1987, a glutaraldehyde cross-linked implantable collagen (Zyplast) became commercially available.

From the start, both patient and physician interest has been keen. Within only 2 to 3 years of FDA approval over 100,000 patients had been treated with collagen in the United States and that number has exceeded 400,000 to date. This unprecedented success of injectable collagen was aided by steadily increasing patient demand, as well as skillful management and promotion by the parent organization. The experience gained by the authors during the last 10 years includes over 10,000 treatments in over 1,000 patients. The following discussion will focus on practical aspects of collagen use in a clinical setting.

II. INDICATIONS AND SITE SELECTION

At this time, the relative safety and efficacy of injectable collagen has been well established and the overriding consideration has become cost-effectiveness. The patient must be able and willing to commit the financial resources to initiate and maintain collagen treatments. Likewise, the physician or a specifically trained registered nurse must make adequate time available to carefully treat each patient and obtain acceptable results. Without these obvious prerequisites, injectable collagen cannot survive in a practice, much less flourish.

All three forms of collagen constitute intradermal implants and as such are most effective for defects of dermal depth. Highly superficial fine lines as in the lower eyelids are difficult to correct as are deep folds and creases with overhanging ptotic cheeks or jowls.

Appropriate lesions generally fall into the categories of age, gravity and actinic rhytids or dermal defects due to acne, viral pox, and trauma. The horizontal lines of the forehead are generally less aesthetically disturbing than the vertical glabellar lines and furrows which are also more consistently correctable. The lateral peri-orbital Crow's feet may be treated if the skin is thick enough to accept the implant without immediate overcorrection and lumping. Any tendency toward lumping is greatest over a bony prominence such as the orbital rim or the margin of the mandible. The nasolabial lines and creases generally respond well to collagen as do the vertical peri-oral rhytids. The upper vermilion border and Cupid's Bow are frequently augmented with pleasing results. The oblique folds at the oral commissures are particularly annoying to patients and are routinely treated although they tend to quickly recur. More lateral mimetic lines of the cheeks respond well if the skin is not overly thin. Defects due to dermal atrophy respond according to their shape rather than their origin. Soft, sloping saucer-shaped depressions respond well to correction, whereas sharply defined, vertically edged crater-like depressions are difficult to correct and generally have little residual dermis in which to implant collagen. Dilated "ice-pick" pilosebaceous pores resist any improvement with collagen. These observations correlate with previously reported clinical experiences.[5-6] Postrhinoplasty irregularities are generally best treated by more permanent means.

Flexibility and a graded approach of trial and observation will yield the proper combination of site selection and mix of specific collagens for each particular patient. At this

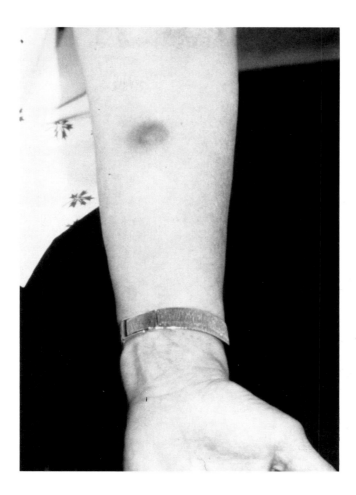

FIGURE 1. A single skin test is mandatory and a double test is prudent to decrease the incidence of hypersensitivity reactions on the face.

time, it remains preferable to avoid bovine collagen treatment and any possible antigenic stimulus for individuals with a personal history of autoimmune disorders.

III. TECHNIQUE

All new patients undergo two skin tests one month apart prior to treatment. A dermal wheel is raised with 0.05 cc to 0.1 cc in a uniform location on the left volar forearm to facilitate subsequent identification. Instructions and pamphlets are reinforced by phone contact at 48 to 72 h. If the test site shows any response at this time the patient returns for palpation and a visual check (Figure 1).

At 4 weeks a second skin test is placed in the glabellar frown lines or more conservatively on the opposite forearm. If the original skin test is in any way ambiguous, the opposite forearm is used. Patients actively observe their test sites and report any erythema, pruritus, edema, color change or induration. The reduced probability of hypersensitivity is nonetheless reiterated at the time of the second test. A consistent 3% of patients show a positive response to the initial skin test. Just over 1% still have a hypersensitivity reaction at the site of the second test despite a negative initial skin test.

The amount of collagen and the specific type of collagen used are governed by the severity and location of the patient's soft tissue defects and the response to the initial two collagen implantations. If the test sites show an obvious residual implant which is firm to palpation, much less collagen is used and the thin skin of the peri-orbital region and any other marginal areas are initially avoided. Zyderm I has been most useful in patients with a strong tendency to form visible or palpable lumps. Conversely, if there is no residual at the test sites, overcorrection is desirable and more sites can be treated with the inclusion of Zyplast for deeper defects in thicker skin. Thereafter, the areas treated, the amounts used, the treatment intervals, and the specific types of collagen implanted are adjusted to suit the individual patient's needs and the physician's preferences.

The single most important element of technique is the depth of implantation. Zyderm is most effective in the superficial dermis whereas Zyplast may be implanted slightly deeper in the mid-dermis in thicker skin. Individual blanching wheals are raised and overlapped with the skin firmly stabilized and the needle close to parallel with the skin. The orientation of the bevel is a matter of personal preference. In deep nasolabial creases overcorrection with Zyderm and/or Zyplast may be maximal to the limits of the dermis. Conversely, in fine lateral peri-orbital lines, the minimum amount of Zyderm possible is injected at each needle site without raising a visible wheal. Even the slightest overcorrection is accentuated directly over the lateral orbital rim. The glabella is treated exclusively with Zyderm since overlying skin necrosis may occur following Zyplast in this area. Collagen Corporation has advised against the use of Zyplast for the glabella.

Immediately preceding and following collagen implantation, the skin is thoroughly scrubbed with alcohol. All treatment areas are marked with the patient sitting and with overhead lighting. The patient confirms the treatment objectives with a hand mirror just prior to starting. After implantation, a steroid cream and massage are applied to the treatment areas. Most patients apply ice for 20 to 30 min following treatment.

Occasionally patients with low pain thresholds will take an oral analgesic such as acetaminophen 1 h prior to treatment. Topical anesthetics have been minimally useful with the recent exception of a combination anesthetic from England termed EMLA.[7] This cream is applied over the treatment areas several times and occluded starting 1 h prior to implantation. A standard infra-orbital block is offered to patients undergoing upper lip, vermilion, or Cupid's Bow augmentation with a majority preferring the block. This is performed using a 30-gauge needle through the superior buccal sulcus and infiltrating 0.5 cc to 1.5 cc of 1% plain lidocaine (buffered to avoid pain) on each side. A mental block for the lower lip is minimally effective and infrequently performed. A supra-orbital block has not been necessary.

IV. RESULTS

Well over a thousand patients and more than ten thousand treatments have been performed between 1979 and 1989. The nasolabial creases were treated most frequently followed by the glabella, lips, cheeks, peri-orbital rhytids, forehead, acne, and other depressions. The first full treatment occurs 2 months after the initial skin test. By combining the second skin test with a partial treatment in the glabellar region, most patients sense an improvement and anticipate further treatments while appreciating the caution of a double test.

The first full treatment averages 1 cc of collagen, primarily Zyderm. If the patient obtains a good correction without visible or palpable lumping after 2 weeks, another full treatment follows including the lateral peri-orbital skin or other marginal locations and including Zyplast for thicker skin regions. A combination of Zyderm and Zyplast in different locations, or together in the same location, at different depths is used for maximal effectiveness.

A. ZYDERM I VS. ZYDERM II

Zyderm II was introduced to improve both the degree and longevity of correction attainable per treatment. Ten patients were treated for their nasolabial creases with Zyderm I randomly assigned to one side and Zyderm II to the other side. As expected the doubly concentrated Zyderm II afforded roughly twice the correction of Zyderm I at 2 weeks (Figure 2A, B, and C). Most patients tolerated both but noted more lumpiness with Zyderm II. In 3 patients, the Zyderm II coalesced into an unacceptably obvious and persistent white lumpy line. This visible lumpiness was particularly aggravating because it was not due to over-correction of the defect (as can occur with Zyderm I) and it persisted from several weeks to two months. Zyplast is now available for the same indications and has virtually replaced Zyderm II.

B. ZYDERM VS. ZYPLAST

Glutaraldehyde cross-linked collagen (GAX) was formulated to reduce antigenicity and prolong correction. The initial clinical studies included subdermal implantations but final results confirmed its usefulness as an intradermal implant (Zyplast). Being partially cross-linked, Zyplast is inherently less pliable in consistency.

Our initial experiences as investigators for the subdermal study were inconclusive. Following clinical release of Zyplast, ten patients who had positive skin tests to Zyderm were retested with Zyplast. Three were weakly but persistently positive. A fourth was tested twice with Zyplast but not treated. Of the remaining six, five had either one or two treatments with a maximum of 0.5 cc. Despite adequate results, in the face of uncertain risks it was elected not to attempt Zyplast in anyone with a positive skin test to Zyderm.

Personal preference plays the strongest role in selection of Zyderm or Zyplast. Although good results are attainable with either product, thin skin has a minimal margin between adequate correction and annoyingly lumpy overcorrection. Some patients readily become visibly or palpably lumpy while others never experience any induration. Zyplast may also leave a persistent brawny pigmentation (Figure 3). In this series, the authors vary widely in their preferences for Zyderm vs. Zyplast.

C. FIBREL®

Fibrel® is composed of absorbable gelatin powder and aminocaproic acid. Before use, it is reconstituted with plasma from the patient and injected intradermally to elevate the dermal defect. It is hypothesized that when this gelatin matrix is implanted intradermally, the injury leads to entrapment of clotting factors essential for wound healing. It has also been suggested that the gelatin powder acts as a chemotactic agent for monocytes and fibroblasts,[8] while aminocaproic acid helps to stabilize the fibrinogen and other clotting factors.[9]

A history of keloid formation, autoimmune disease, hypersensitivity to components of Fibrel®, and bleeding disorders are contraindications to Fibrel® injections. Patients on anticoagulant therapy should not receive Fibrel®. Each candidate should be given an intradermal skin test and be evaluated for 4 weeks. Of the patients who had a clinical trail with Fibrel®, only 1.8% had a positive skin test.[10]

Lidocaine is injected along the periphery of scars or wrinkles. For injection of scars, a #21-gauge needle has been utilized to make a small pocket under the scarred area followed by a 50 to 100% correction. For treatment of wrinkles, the technique varies from the standard multiple puncture technique recommended for injecting collagen. Most of the wrinkles can be treated via a linear or zig zag method of injection in the mid to deep dermis utilizing a #27-gauge needle.

Most patients require two consecutive treatments approximately 2 weeks apart to achieve the desired effect. Studies indicate that 50% of scars are at least 65% improved, and the correction lasts approximately one year. With wrinkles, the Fibrel appears to be less effective and may have a shorter duration of correction.

Fibrel® is a suitable alternative to collagen as a dermal filler material. Adverse reactions reported with Fibrel® are approximately 5%, and the most common reactions are erythema,

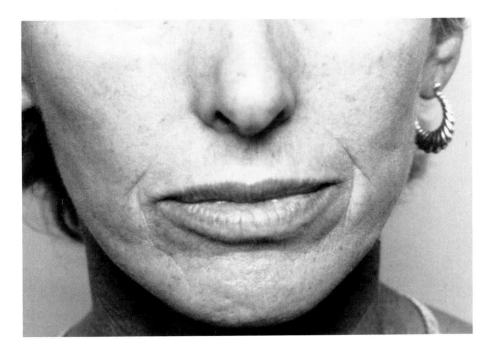

FIGURE 2A.   Nasolabial lines prior to collagen injection.

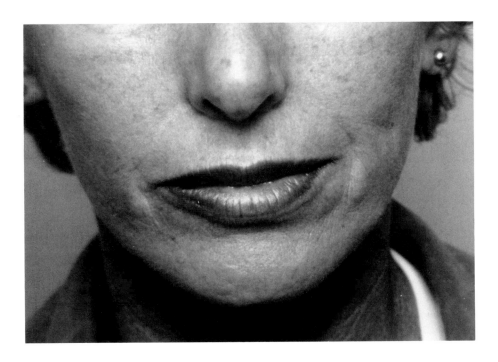

FIGURE 2B.   Following one treatment of 0.3 cc Zyderm I on the patient's left and 0.3 cc of Zyderm II on her right. Zyderm II in equal amounts affords an obviously greater correction than Zyderm I.

swelling, and nodules at the treatment site. The nodules might be related to injecting Fibrel too superficially. The disadvantages of Fibrel® include its preparation time, the need to perform a venipuncture, the need for local anesthesia before injection, and a somewhat more complicated technique of injection. At the present time, we are using Fibrel® as an alternative

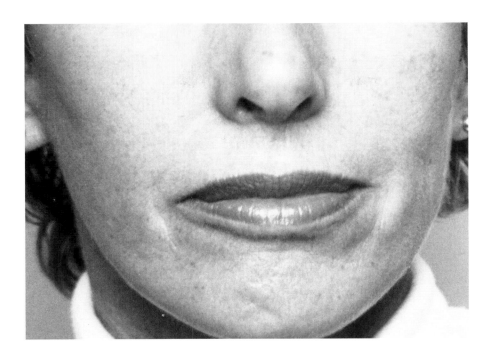

FIGURE 2C. Following the second treatment of 0.3 cc Zyderm I on the patient's left and no further treatment on her right. As expected, double the volume of Zyderm I (in two sessions) is roughly equivalent in correction to the doubly concentrated Zyderm II.

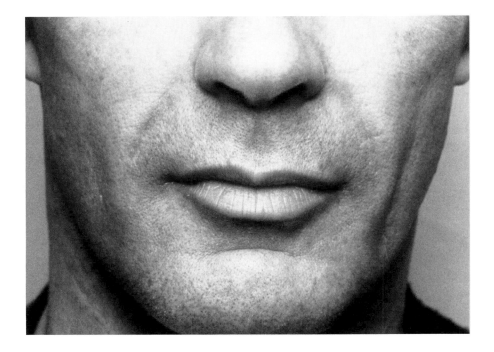

FIGURE 3. A diffuse brawny discoloration resulting from Zyplast in the nasolabials.

for patients with hypersensitivity to Zyderm. For depressed scars, Fibrel® has been as effective or better than Zyderm or Zyplast with a longer lasting correction. Additional clinical experience is necessary to document the relative efficacy of Fibrel® for facial rhytides and expressive lines. Fibrel® is difficult to use for fine lines in thin skin. (Fibrel/Serono Laboratories, Randolph, MA)

D. KOKEN ATELOCOLLAGEN

Available in Japan and Europe but not FDA approved is still another form of bovine injectable collagen (KOKEN Atelocollagen). This is not a dispersion such as Zyderm and Zyplast but a solution. The difference is that a solution is monomolecular, containing only molecules of collagen and appearing as a nearly transparent liquid. Zyderm and Zyplast are dispersions of collagen containing variable proportions of molecules, fibrils, and fibers. This gives the familiar opaque white product.

Two clinicians in Belgium compared Zyderm and Atelocollagen in a single blind series of 60 patients with 3 months and 6 months follow-up.[11] Paradoxically, when the codes were broken, the 2% solution of collagen (Atelocollagen) yielded a subjective correction of 71% whereas the 3.5% dispersion of collagen (Zyderm) yielded 51% correction. Ultrastructural analysis showed that the solution, once implanted, formed a more finely structured matrix than the dispersion, trapping more water and glycosaminoglycans. In a French series of 705 patients treated with Atelocollagen, 3.8% had a positive skin test and 2.3% of the remaining patients developed a subsequent adverse reaction.[12]

E. CLINICAL EXPERIENCE

Our treatment population consists of most age groups, primarily females and most often for age-related rhytids. The initial full treatment generally follows a forearm skin test and a subsequent glabellar test. Two full treatments using a total of 3 cc is usually adequate to initiate collagen therapy. The majority of patients return at routine 4 to 6 month intervals or when they reach approximately 50% of their original correction. Patients requiring intervals of less than 3 months are discouraged from continuing and nearly 10% fall into this category. Another 5% require intervals of 12 months or even longer. The longest lasting corrections are those for scar depressions and occasionally for glabellar lines. A single "booster" treatment is used unless most of the correction has been lost in which case two treatments separated by 2 weeks are used.

More recently, lip enhancement has become popular and some patients have their upper and lower vermilion borders, Cupid's Bows, and lips themselves injected with 1 to 2 cc of collagen. Zyderm has been used to augment the upper vermilion border and lip since 1981, and Zyplast following its introduction. An infraorbital nerve block is almost essential. The collagen implant is introduced into the very superficial subcutaneous space parallel to the vermilion border with the vermillion isolated firmly between thumb and index finger. This creates a pleasing pout and youthful upper lip and can be extended to augment the bulk of the lips themselves although the duration of this effect is only from 2 to 4 months (Figure 4). Many other unique applications of injectable collagen exist. The learning curve for a physician using injectable collagen seems to reach a natural plateau within 2 years. By this time treatment patterns allow the maximum longevity of results with the least amount of collagen and fewest adverse reactions.

V. ADVERSE REACTIONS AND COMPLICATIONS

The most accurate data concerning localized hypersensitivity reactions to collagen skin testing were collected during the initial clinical trials in which 3% of 9427 subjects tested positive. Of the 5109 patients subsequently treated just over 1% experienced a hypersensitivity reaction despite a negative skin test. Since a hypersensitivity reaction represents both

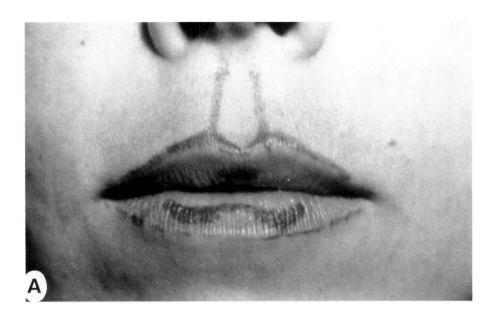

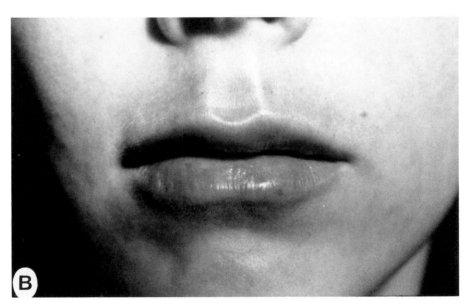

FIGURE 4. (A) The upper lip vermilion and Cupid's bow as well as the lower lip marked for injection. (B) Immediately following injection with Zyderm I and Zyplast.

a treatment failure and a persistently annoying complication of collagen implants, the problem bears further examination (Figure 5).

A single skin test eliminates 3% of positive responders, leaving another 1% to react at a subsequent provocation. In a prospective series Elson compared a single test to a double test.[13] He single tested 200 consecutive patients followed by double testing the next 200 patients. In both groups there were 5 positive tests (2.5%). In the first group the remaining 195 patients were treated following the single negative skin test. Fully 6 patients (3.1%) developed subsequent hypersensitivity reactions. In the second group, 7 patients (3.5%) were positive to a second skin test. Of the 171 remaining patients, none became hypersensitive during the course of this study. The rate of reaction following a negative single test was

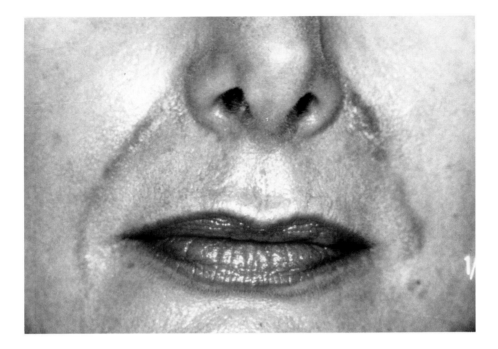

FIGURE 5.   A mild to moderate collagen hypersensitivity reaction following the initial treatment. This patient was not double skin tested.

unusually high in this series. Of note, the second skin test was performed only 14 days following the initial test and negative responders to both tests commenced facial treatment at 4 weeks.

Four weeks may not be an adequate interval following skin testing. A report of two patients who became positive 6 weeks after single testing confirms similar experiences in our series.[14] A routine second test allows a total of 8 weeks to elapse after the initial skin test prior to a full facial treatment.

Despite double testing, some patients react even years after starting multiple collagen treatments. The incidence in this series has been relatively consistent at 3 to 4 per thousand to Zyderm. The most frequent preceding event has been an infection, usually viral. This presumably triggers the body's general immune response. Collagen Corporation reviewed the characteristics of voluntary reports of hypersensitivity reactions during the 4 years following FDA approval. Although these reports represent only a fraction of the total, the following proportions should be representative: of the hypersensitivity reactions reported following one negative skin test, 56% occurred after the first treatment, 28% after the second, 10% after the third and 6% after subsequent treatments.[15] The lesson is clear that more than one half of the hypersensitivity reactions to Zyderm can be avoided by initially double testing (instead of single testing) all patients. Hypersensitivity to Zyplast treatment has not yet been identified in this series. Elson has reported a similar disparity.[16]

Attempts to ameliorate hypersensitivity reactions with systemic steroids, anti-inflammatory or antihistamines have proven disappointing. Effective and safe when properly performed is direct subdermal injection of a dilute steroid at 1 to 2 month intervals. For a typical glabellar reaction triamcinolone 10 mg/ml is diluted to 1 or 2 mg/ml (5- to 10-fold dilution) and a maximum of 0.5 mg injected subdermally for a severe hypersensitivity. Atrophy has been avoided by injecting only a dilute solution, subdermally, and titrating not more than once a month until resolution.

Fortunately, few adverse reactions have been more serious than localized hypersensitivity. At least one patient has been reported with unilateral loss of vision following implantation in the glabella. Zyplast has been followed by skin slough, again in the glabella. In this series one patient came close to a glabellar skin loss following Zyplast. Glabellar treatment is currently limited to Zyderm.

Possible long-term autoimmune sequelae of bovine collagen implantation have been addressed from the earliest clinical trials by the Collagen Corporation. Temporary anticollagen antibodies are frequently demonstrated in patients during localized hypersensitivity reactions but these are specific to bovine collagen and do not cross-react with human collagen. Sera from 126 patients having antibovine collagen antibodies were tested and found negative to human types I or III collagen. Antihuman dermal collagen antibodies can exist due to trauma or disease but are not associated with any known autoimmune disease. The greatest reassurance of long term safety is derived from epidemiological data. Injectable collagen and multiple other bovine collagen containing products and devices have been used for decades in literally millions of patients without a demonstrable increase in the incidence of autoimmune disease.

VI. DISCUSSION

Injectable collagen has achieved unprecedented success in a relatively short time despite its costs, limited longevity, and occasional hypersensitivity. An early survey of patients having collagen treatments, between 1979 and 1982, revealed disappointment due to adverse reactions and shorter than expected longevity of results. Fortunately, hypersensitivity can now either be avoided or adequately treated. Longevity remains a major drawback. Compared to autologous fat, collagen has the advantage of being easier and less traumatic to use although the indications for these two modalities have limited overlap. Compared to silicone, collagen has the advantage of causing exceedingly rare permanent complications and is FDA approved.

The ideal soft-tissue implant would replace the deficiency with a readily available like substance, at a reasonable cost, with great ease and accuracy and without adverse reactions. Should the resulting correction last permanently? Oddly enough, in the case of a dermal filler the answer is an emphatic NO. Since there is an unavoidable learning curve for each practitioner and since each patient's esthetic desires and skin responses vary widely, the margin for error can become uncomfortably narrow. Permanent lumps, or bumps, or irregularities due to overcorrection or misplacement would prove far more distressing than the original natural defects and could not easily be removed or corrected. In addition, for mimetic folds and furrows, by the time collagen has been gradually displaced from its original implantation site by the same muscle action which formed the furrow, it has been degraded. Otherwise, as can happen with a permanent substance (silicone), as the furrow reforms, any adjacent undesirable fullness may be accentuated.

Currently, both Zyderm and Zyplast achieve their results in two stages. First the defect is filled by the bovine collagen, then a host response gradually degrades the implant and replaces this with host collagen. By 4 months the original Zyderm bovine collagen is no longer detectable in the human dermis.[17] Zyplast remains identifiable up to 6 months.[18] Clinical correction beyond these intervals is due to host collagen first replacing the bovine implant then gradually remodeling itself. Zyplast achieves its greater longevity with a sacrifice in pliability.

A form of collagen with the characteristics of Zyderm but with reduced antigenicity and therefore increased longevity should prove very close to the imagined ideal. Collagen Corporation may finally achieve this elusive goal with human placenta-derived collagen in the future.

VII. SUMMARY

Ten years of actively using injectable collagen in a diverse clinical setting has yielded an appreciation of the indications and techniques of treatment as well as a respect for the limitations and possible adverse reactions. The rapid pace of acceptance and usage of injectable collagen speaks loudly for its current status as the foremost superficial soft-tissue implant. Eventually the antigenicity will be further reduced, thereby increasing its longevity and bringing it very close to the elusive ideal of a soft-tissue implant.

REFERENCES

1. **Knapp, T. R., Kaplan, E. N., and Daniels, J. R.,** Injectable collagen for soft tissue augmentation, *Plast. Reconstr. Surg.,* 60, 398, 1977.
2. **Stegman, S. J. and Tromovitch, T. A.,** Implantation of collagen for depressed scars, *J. Dermatol. Surg. Oncol.,* 6, 450, 1980.
3. **Klein, A. W.,** Implantation techniques for injectable collagen: Two-and-one-half years of personal clinical experience, *J. Am. Acad. Dermatol.,* 9, 224, 1983.
4. **Kamer, F. M. and Churukian, M. M.,** The clinical use of injectable collagen: A three-year retrospective study, *Arch. Otolaryngol.,* 110, 93, 1984.
5. **Klein, A. W. and Rish, D. C.,** Injectable collagen update, *J. Dermatol. Surg. Oncol.,* 10, 519, 1984.
6. **Robinson, J. K. and Hanke, C. W.,** Injectable collagen implant: histopathologic identification and longevity of correction, *J. Dermatol. Surg. Oncol.,* 11, 124, 1985.
7. **Hanks, G. W. and White, I.,** New uses suggested for EMLA anaesthetic cream, *Pharmaceutical,* 242, 1989.
8. **Postlethwaite, A. E., Seyer, J. M., and Kangah,** Chemotactic reaction of human fibroblast to type I, II and III collagens and collagen-derived peptides, *Proc. Natl. Acad. Sci. U.S.A.,* 75, 871, 1978.
9. **Nilsson, I. M., Sjoerdsma, A., and Waldenstron, J.,** Antifibrinolytic activity and metabolism of E-aminocaproic acid in man, *Lancet,* 1, 1233, 1960.
10. **Millikan, L., Rosen, T., Manheit, G., et al.,** Treatment of depressed cutaneous scars with gelatin matrix implant, *J. Am. Acad. Dermatol.,* 16, 1155, 1987.
11. **Dierickx, P. and Derumeaux, L.,** Comparative study of the clinical efficiency of a 2% collagen solution and a 3.5% collagen dispersion on 60 patients, presented at the 5th Int. Congr. of Dermatol. Surg., Jerusalem, Israel, October, 1984.
12. **Charriere, G., Bejot, M., Schnitzler, L., Ville, G., and Hartmann, D.,** Reactions to a bovine collagen implant, *J. Am. Acad. Dermatol.,* 21, 1203, 1989.
13. **Elson, M. L.,** The role of skin testing in the use of collagen injectable materials, *J. Dermatol. Surg. Oncol.,* 15, 301, 1989.
14. **Labow, T. A. and Silvers, D. N.,** Late reactions at Zyderm® skin test sites, *Cutis,* 35, 154, 1985.
15. **DeLustro, F., et al,** Reaction to injectable collagen: Results in animal models and clinical use, *Plast. Reconst. Surg.,* 79, 581, 1987.
16. **Elson, L. M.,** Clinical assessment of Zyplast implant: a year of experience for soft tissue contour correction, *J. Am. Acad. Dermatol.,* 18, 707, 1988.
17. **Burke, K. E., Naughton, G., and Cassai, N.,** A histological, immunological, and electron microscopic study of bovine collagen implants in the human, *Ann. Plast. Surg.,* 14, 515, 1985.
18. **Kligman, A. M. and Armstrong, R. C.,** Histologic response to intradermal Zyderm and Zyplast collagen in humans, *J. Dermatol. Surg. Oncol.,* 12, 351, 1986.

Chapter 16

AUTOLOGOUS FAT TRANSPLANTATION

Michael M. Churukian

TABLE OF CONTENTS

I. INTRODUCTION

Few topics in aesthetic surgery currently evoke more controversy and divergent opinion than free-fat autografts. Clinical reports vary widely in techniques and results. This is despite a hundred years of usage, multiple clinical and basic research studies, and a strong resurgence of interest in the wake of blunt suction lipectomy.

Free-fat grafts and dermal-fat grafts enjoyed widespread popularity for a half century until eclipsed by the availability of liquid silicone. The recent advent of liposuction conveniently provided an enormous supply of potential donor material and created an abundance of new recipient sites.

The early pioneers in fat transplantation established the important general relationship of atraumatic technique to long-term graft retention. Now in the context of blunt suction extraction, the question of optimal techniques of harvest and reinjection, as well as donor and recipient site selection are again addressed.

II. HISTORY

A. FROM NEUBER TO PEER

Free-fat grafting was introduced by Neuber[1] in 1893, at the 23rd Congress of the German Surgical Society. He reported the original transplant of pearl-sized grafts from the proximal upper extremity to a peri-orbital defect resulting from tuberculous osteitis. He was satisfied with the results and continued this work[2] emphasizing the use of small grafts as his attempts at large grafts all failed. Neuber's work was confirmed in 1896 by Silex.[3]

Also at this time, Czerny[4] gained renown by transplanting a large lipoma to replace a breast removed for chronic cystic mastitis. He was satisfied with the results despite noting that the breast was smaller and darker. Venderame[5] in 1909 reviewed the progress to date and claimed a 10 year personal experience with autologous fat in the peri-orbital region. He advocated overcorrection to compensate for graft shrinkage. By 1910, Lexer[6] helped popularize fat grafts by reporting extensively on their use for a wide variety of indications.[7,8] The first reported fat injection is credited to Brunings[9] in 1911, who tried this for nasal defects following rhinoplasty. Other early research found that, under some circumstances, transplanted fat was replaced by fibrous tissue,[10] while under different circumstances it retained its original qualities and even grew with patient weight gain.[11]

Early basic research included a well-conceived study reported by Gurney[12] in 1938. He utilized fat from either the groin or the abdominal cavity of 185 white rats and placed it into a subcutaneous pocket in the thorax. The groin fat required greater dissection and manipulation and averaged 23% survival at one year. A strand or intraabdominal (testicular) fat was obtained with minimal trauma and averaged 51% survival at one year. Some grafts were first crushed or sharply cut into smaller pieces and showed poor survival. All seven cases of infection and complete graft loss occurred in the cut or crushed grafts. Fibrous tissue initially replaced lost graft material but failed to persist long-term.

The best known and often cited work of Peer[13,14,15] capped this period. In 1950, he reported his results in 13 human subjects. He removed abdominal subcutaneous fat and first divided it into two identical grafts by weight. He then implanted one graft intact and sharply cut the other into 20 segments. The recipient site was the rectus sheath. The longest follow-up was at 12 to 14 months when the original grafts were retrieved from five subjects. The single unit grafts retained an average of 55% by weight while the 20 unit grafts retained 21%. One graft increased in size as the patient had gained considerable weight. The histology of these grafts shortly after transplantation showed greatest cell damage at the cut periphery and possible early direct host to graft vascular anastomoses. The histology at one year demonstrated normal fat appearance. Peer later preferred dermal-fat grafts and made the interesting observation that lean individuals had the greatest graft retention.

To summarize, there were several pertinent observations of this early animal and human work. First, using careful sharp dissection with atraumatic handling approximately 50% of the original graft was found to survive at one year or longer. Second, either manipulating the graft or sharply slicing it into smaller segments reduced long term survival to approximately 20%. Finally, the residual graft was histologically normal lobular fat at one year without fibrous scar tissue.

B. CURRENT ERA

The record now jumps from Peer in the lat 1950s to Yves-Gérard Illouz, credited by many as the "father of blunt suction lipectomy." Illouz first wrote of recycling the suctioned fat in 1984, in French.[13] He reached a wide American audience with a letter published in July 1986, describing the fat obtained by strong vacuum as a "fat cell culture."[14] His initial experience with 37 patients resulted in 9 (or 25%) with partial resorption. Fine dermal defects as well as deeper subcutaneous defects were treated. The letter immediately following was written by Bahman Teimourian describing his good results with a "semiliquid fat graft" in 6 patients.[15] Chajchir and Benzaquen from Buenos Aires reported enthusiastically on their initial 38 patients, noting resorption of 30% to 60% at 10 to 12 months.[16] Also in 1986, a report of sharp surgical fat excision and implantation reminiscent of a prior era was published.[17]

In the next year, Bircoll initiated the controversy over fat injection to the breast with two case reports.[18,19] By 1989, multiple anecdotal reports of fat injection for lipodystrophy and hemifacial atrophy demonstrated apparent good results with various periods of follow-up using widely different techniques.[20-22] Chajchir and Benzaquen compiled a more detailed review of their first 253 patients from 1984 to 1988 with continuing enthusiasm for their results.

The widespread clinical use of free fat obtained from liposuction has outpaced supporting basic research. Fournier observed in 1983, that lipocytes were not damaged by extraction with 6-, 8-, or 10-mm cannulas under high vacuum. Recent studies have focused on both the immediate metabolic and histomorphological fate of harvested and reinjected fat.

Biochemical analysis of adipocyte metabolism was undertaken by Campbell et al. as a sensitive indicator of cell function following extraction and reinjection.[15] Human fat harvested by blunt wall suction was washed with warm saline containing bovine serum albumin. The effects of injecting this fat through different sized needles was measured as a function of adipocyte glucose oxidation and lipid synthesis. Both of these basic activities are centered within the mitochondria providing a sensitive measure of cell injury.

The results of glucose oxidation measurements showed that relative to a 16-gauge needle, adipocyte activity after passage through an 18-gauge needle was reduced to approximately 87%. The effect of a 20-gauge needle dropped the relative activity to 25%.

Assays of lipid synthesis after passing the fat through these three needle sizes echoed the results of glucose oxidation. The 18-gauge needle showed a reduced activity of 61% compared to the 16-gauge needle and the 20-gauge needle was down to 34%. Taken together, these show a clear trend of increasing cell damage with decreasing needle size, although the figures are relative and confidence limits are not stated.

The histology of subcutaneous fat is straightforward and the effects of trauma and damage are readily studied. Adipose tissue exists as an arboreal network of individual lobules in a connective tissue matrix. Each lobule contains from hundreds to thousands of cells and is an independent unit both morphologically and functionally. A terminal circulation supplies the lobule through a pedicle of one or two axial arteries and geminate veins. This arrangement provides the fragile adipocytes with adequate connective tissue protection and a rich capillary network for metabolic activity.

Cutting the vascular pedicle is stated to cause ischemic necrosis of the lobule within 24 h. If invariably so, then little if any fat obtained by blunt suction could be expected to

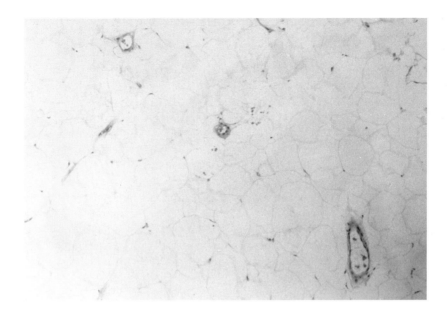

FIGURE 1.   Histological appearance of a well-preserved sample of fat.

survive transplantation. Conversely, if the lobule is disrupted and intact adipocytes released to form a free cell culture, then some fraction of cells could survive initially by imbibition. Historically a 50% volume retention is the maximum attainable at 1 year with atraumatic sharp dissection technique. Current blunt suction extraction subjects the fragile adipocytes and the lobular architecture to new and sometimes extreme trauma. A recent histomorphological study set out to delineate the effects of suction harvesting and reinjecting fat.[17]

A total of 90 samples of fat were examined over a 6-month period by two independent pathologists blinded to the protocol. The technique related variables studied were the size of the cannula for extraction, the degree of vacuum, donor sites, the time delay before reinjection, needle diameter for reinjection and centrifugation. Both the lobular architecture and individual cell morphology were assessed (Figure 1).

A trend favoring the larger sized cannulas became apparent but lost importance beyond the 6-mm size. Vacuum at 600 mmHg was found to preserve cells far better than full vacuum of nearly 760 mmHg. The combination of a blunt 6-mm standard Illouz cannula with 600 mgHg vacuum yielded near perfect results. The only specimens better preserved had no vacuum during collection.

Collection of fat as an office procedure was tested with a variety of luer-lock needles and cannulas and a 10-cc disposable syringe. All sharp or blunt needles from 14-gauge to 18-gauge caused considerable damage whereas the 14-gauge blunt cannulas yielded useable graft material. The vacuum induced by syringe harvest does not approach 760 mmHg except at the very start of the procedure when the barrel of the syringe is empty.

There was no significant histological difference in donor sites. Of note, peri-orbital fat was highly fibrous and after chopping for injection, the cells were badly damaged. Also, fat obtained by a flat spatula cannula from the neck at full vacuum contained fragments of platysma muscle and very poorly preserved adipocytes.

Time delay at room temperature showed no ill effects until 4 h after harvest. By 8 h, there was obvious histological distortion of individual cell morphology.

Reinjection of fat through a 22-gauge needle caused considerable trauma. A single passage through the 18-gauge needle showed no difference but repeated injections of the same specimen five times did result in damage. Using a 16-gauge needle did not result in histological damage either once or after five passages.

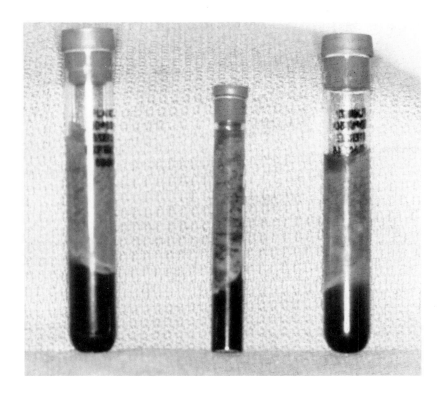

FIGURE 2. Centrifuged samples of harvested fat demonstrating a fatty supernatant, a layer of fat, and a blood clot.

Centrifugation at 500 or 1000 rpm for one to ten minutes caused no histological disruption. Ten minutes at 1500 rpm did result in visible trauma. The proportions of fatty supernatant and blood clot following centrifugation provided an independent index supporting the conclusions of the histological studies (Figure 2).

Another histological study focused on the effects of injecting different volumes of fat in a single site. The grafts were obtained from the left abdomen of two patients by blunt suction and injected with a dye marker into recipient sites in the right abdomen in boluses of 1, 3, 5, 10, and 15 cc. Three months later during abdominoplasty, the grafts were removed and examined histologically. All showed a minimal host reaction and little fibrosis. The 1-cc and 2-cc grafts contained microcysts of lipid. The 5-cc grafts had larger and more numerous microcysts. The 10-cc and 15-cc grafts contained macrocysts and preserved but nonviable fat. A total of 28 specimens were examined.

III. FAT INJECTION IN A CLINICAL SETTING

A. PATIENT POPULATION

Over 400 patients underwent over 1000 fat injections from 1985 through 1989. Ages ranged from eighteen to seventy-six. The majority of patients were females between thirty-five and sixty-five. Donor sites included the knees, medial or lateral thighs, abdomen, hips, flanks, submentum, or occasionally another site. Recipient sites included the glabella, nasolabial folds, lips, malar complex, angle of the mandible, paramental depressions, degrees of hemifacial atrophy or asymmetry, and various trunk or limb defects.

B. TECHNIQUE

Most fat injections have been done as an independent office procedure using local anesthesia with or without oral sedation. Patients choose the donor site based upon areas

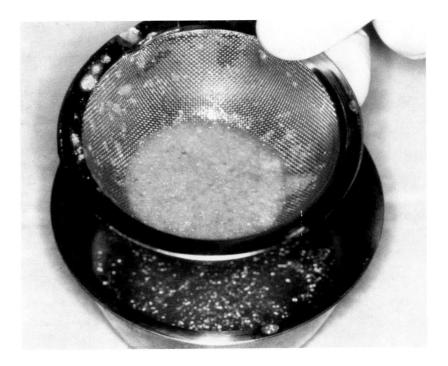

FIGURE 3.   Fat is thoroughly washed with lactated Ringer's solution prior to injection.

most recalcitrant to volume loss regardless of weight and exercise. If the patient has no preference then the fat is taken from the lower abdomen or hips. Cold packs are applied for 20 min followed by local infiltration, using plain lidocaine with sodium bicarbonate added to greatly reduce the pain of injection. Further infiltration with lidocaine and epinephrine (again with bicarbonate) provides vasoconstriction. Large volumes of local anesthetic with a long 30-gauge or 27-gauge needle have been used.

A 12-gauge blunt multiple port luer-lock cannula is introduced through a stab incision made with a 16-gauge needle or a #11 blade. The 10-cc syringe plunger is withdrawn to the 5-cc mark and the fat harvested from the middle layer of subcutaneous fat with one hand as the skin is stretched flat and taut with the other hand. The fat is washed with lactated Ringer's solution through a fine mesh stainless steel tea strainer (Figure 3), and placed initially into a 10-cc or 20-cc syringe. The residual fat for injection is usually one half the original volume. The syringe is allowed to stand vertically and layer into fat and supernatant, while the recipient site is marked and infiltrated with plain lidocaine (Figure 4). Overcorrection of up to 100% is the end point of an even subcutaneous injection using an 18-gauge needle and 3-cc syringe for the face (Figure 5). For larger volumes in the trunk or extremities, a 10-cc syringe and 16-gauge needle allow less trauma to the fat (Figure 6).

C. RESULTS

A carefully conceived and controlled clinical study has yet to be attempted. Nonetheless, using the described technique, an empirical average of three injections at 3- to 12-month intervals gives a satisfactory lasting result in nonmimetic areas. The leaner the patient the less resorption: a small minority of thin young patients require only one or two injections. The average long-term retention ranges from 10% to 20% for each injection. The best results are obtained in the malar-submalar complex, the angle of the mandible (squaring the jawline), degrees of hemifacial atrophy or asymmetry, and traumatic or iatrogenic soft tissue defects. Results are highly subjective and variable for constantly mobile areas such as glabellar

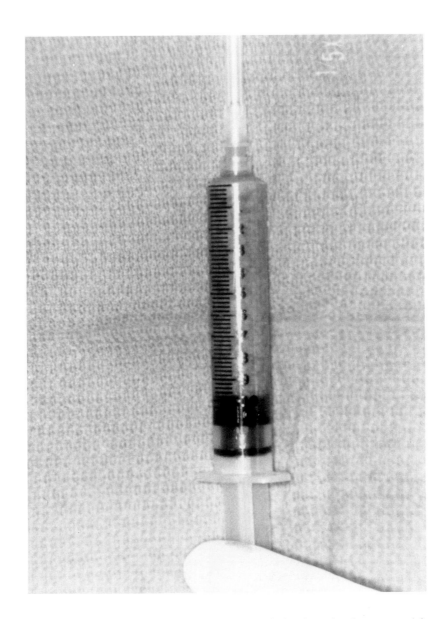

FIGURE 4. After 10 min in a vertical position, the fat has layered and concentrated for injection.

furrows and nasolabial folds (Figure 7). Some patients prefer the fat injection to collagen for these mimetic folds but Zyplast remains easier and has the theoretical advantage of not being permanent. Any residual permanent substance such as fat or silicone will eventually be displaced from mimetic folds to adjacent areas by the constant muscle action. Fat is a subcutaneous filler and not appropriate for dermal defects such as fine lines or wrinkles.

D. COMPLICATIONS

Three patients were placed on antibiotics for localized infection and one was drained. One patient requested removal of the graft at 6 months and this was done with 14-gauge cannula and syringe. There have been reports of visual loss following collagen or fat injection to the glabella. One patient noted a subtle but persistent pigmentary change in a previously radiated cheek after a single fat injection.

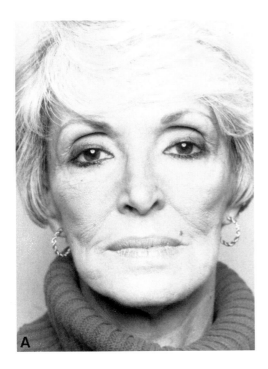
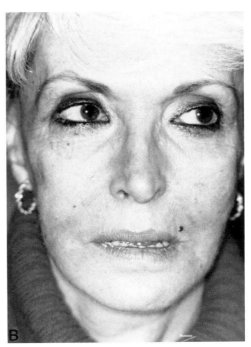

FIGURE 5.   (A) Preinjection, submalar and para-oral soft tissue atrophy. (B) Immediately following the initial fat injection with a mild (approximately 50%) overcorrection.

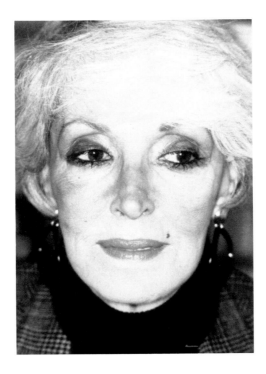

FIGURE 5C.   First follow-up visit at one month.

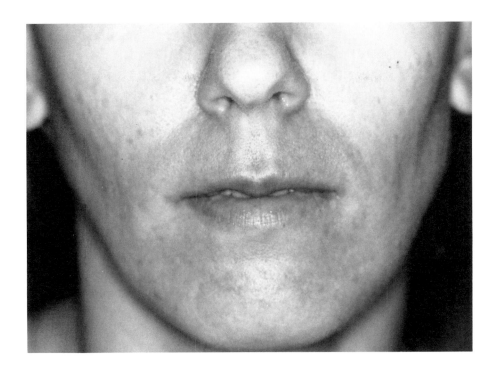

FIGURE 6A. Pre-injection of fat to thin upper lip.

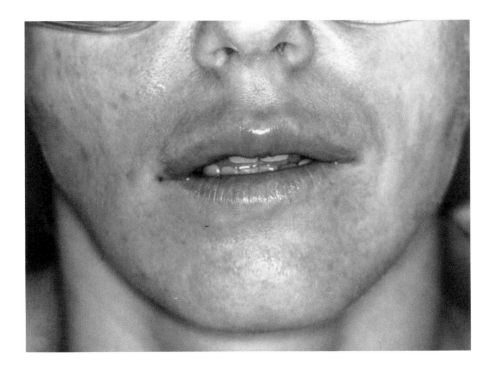

FIGURE 6B. Immediately following injection of 2 cc to the upper lip from the oral commissures.

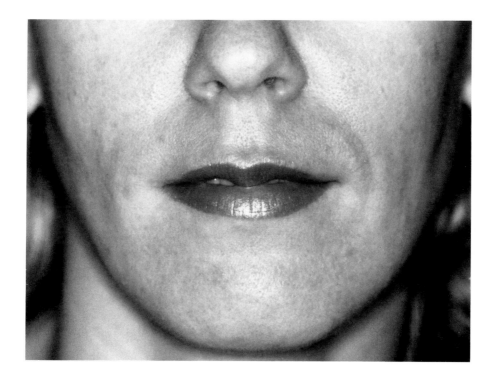

FIGURE 6C.   Results at 3 month follow-up visit.

IV. SUMMARY

As with all aesthetic procedures, patient and physician satisfaction depends primarily on realistic expectations. With consistent careful technique, appropriate patient and recipient site selection, and the understanding that an average of three treatments are necessary at intervals of up to 12 months, autologous fat transplantation should attain a reliable and important permanent status in aesthetic surgery (Figure 8).

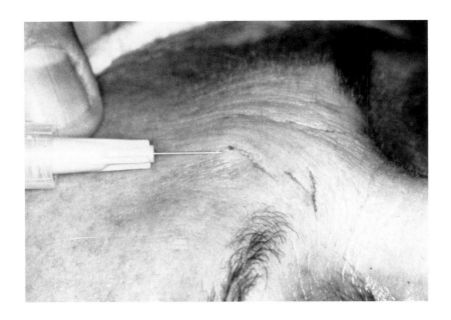

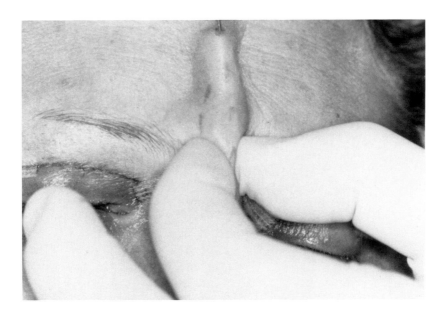

FIGURE 7. Technique of superficial dermal wheal using collagen in glabella with a 30-gauge needle.

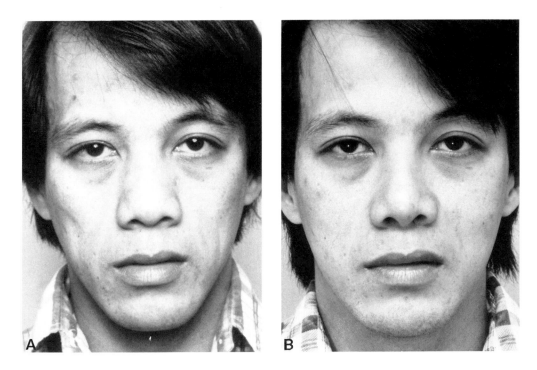

FIGURE 8.   (A) Pre-op young, thin male patient with long face and submalar hollows. (B) Six months following one cc fat injection to each submalar region with a 16-gauge needle. Fat was obtained with difficulty from a thin abdominal SQ.

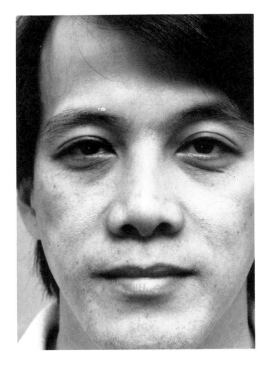

FIGURE 8C.   Twelve-month follow-up with good persistence of fat. A second fat injection was planned at this time for a pleasing permanent result.

REFERENCES

1. **Neuber, F.,** Fat grafting, *Chir. Kongr. Verh. Dtsch. Ges. Chir.,* 22, 66, 1893 (in German).
2. **Neuber, F.,** Fat grafting, *Chir. Kongr. Verh. Dtsch. Ges. Chir.,* 39, 188, 1910 (in German).
3. **Silex, P.,** Ueber Lidbildung mit stiellosen Hautlappen (Fettgewebe zur Unterfutterung), *Klin. Monatshefte f. Augenh.,* 626, 1896 (in German).
4. **Czerny, M.,** Reconstruction of the breast with a lipoma, *Chir. Kongr. Verhandl.,* 2, 216, 1895 (in German).
5. **Verderame, F.,** Ueber Fett transplantation bei adharenten Knochennarben am Orbitalrand, *Klin. Monatshefte f. Augenh.,* 47, 433, 1909.
6. **Lexer, E.,** Free fat grafting, *Dtsch. Med. Wochenschr.,* 36, 640, 1910 (in German).
7. **Lexer, E.,** Free fat grafting, *Ann. Surg.,* 60, 166, 1914.
8. **Lexer, E.,** Fatty tissue transplantation, in *Transplantation, Part I,* Lexer, E., Ed., Ferdinand Enke, Stuttgart, 1919, 265 (in German).
9. **Brunings,** As cited by Newman, J. and Ftaiha, Z., The biographical history of fat transplant surgery, *Am. J. Cosmet. Surg.,* 4, 85, 1987.
10. **Tuffier,** Treatment of pulmonary gangrene and abscesses, 3 ème Congrès Société Internationale Chirurgie, Brussels, 1911, 780 (in French).
11. **Strandberg, J.,** A case of skin transplantation with unique results, *Hygiea Stockholm,* 77, 372, 1915; as quoted in **Newman, J. and Ftaiha, Z.,** The biographical history of fat transplant surgery, *Am. J. Cosmet. Surg.,* 4, 85, 1987.
12. **Gurney, C. E.,** Experimental study of the behavior of free fat transplants, *Surgery,* 3, 679, 1938.
13. **Illouz, Y.-G.,** L'avenir de la réutilisation de la graisse après liposuccion, *Rev. Chir. Esthet. Franc.,* Vol. 9, 1984.
14. **Fournier, F. P. and Otteni, F. M.,** Lipodissection in body sculpturing: the dry procedure, *P.R.S.,* 72, 598, 1982.
15. **Campbell, G. L., Laudenslager, N., and Newman, J.,** The effect of mechanical stress on adipocyte morphology and metabolism, *Am. J. Cosmet. Surg.,* 4, 89, 1987.
16. **Smahel, J.,** Adipose tissue in plastic surgery, *Ann. Plast. Surg.,* 16(5), 444, 1986.
17. **Churukian, M., Zemplenyi, J., Martin, C., and Thomas, P.,** Autologous fat injection for soft tissue augmentation: a prospective, blind comparative histological study, unpublished.

Chapter 17

FACIAL AUGMENTATION WITH SOLID ALLOPLASTIC IMPLANTS: A RATIONAL APPROACH TO MATERIAL SELECTION

Jeanne S. Adams

TABLE OF CONTENTS

I. INTRODUCTION

Throughout the history of medicine, physicians have sought to restore anatomically deficient areas of the human body. Grafts of autologous, homologous, and heterologous bone, cartilage, fat, and dermis have been used for years and are still used in some form today. But autologous grafts require a second surgical procedure to obtain the material. Homologous grafts carry the risk of disease transmission—especially important now with the AIDS pandemic, and heterologous grafts are little used with the exception of injectable bovine collagen (Zyderm).

Because of the disadvantages of implants derived from living animals, the search for a well-tolerated implant material has been underway for generations. Among the earliest substances used at the beginning of the century were vaseline (injected), celluloid, various metals, gutta percha, and even stones from the Black Sea.[1-3] Earlier in the century, surgeons were occupied for years with removing the granulomatous "paraffinomas" which resulted from paraffin injections. Most of the other materials were extruded or required surgical removal because of low tissue tolerance. Ivory was the one exception, for there have been reports of a number of ivory implants which have persisted for years.[1]

In 1953, Scales[4] outlined the properties of an ideal implant.

1.   Not physically modified by tissue fluids
2.   Clinically inert
3.   No inflammatory or foreign body reaction
4.   Noncarcinogenic
5.   Produces no state of allergy or foreign body reaction
6.   Capable of resisting mechanical strain

7. Capable of fabrication in the form desired
8. Capable of being sterilized

In addition to these, the ideal soft tissue substitute should remain in good position and maintain a consistency similar to surrounding tissues without apparent joint or seam. While the implant's pores may be invaded by the host's tissue, the implant's structure should not be replaced, removed, or deformed by the host.[1] Since it may be rejected, it should also be relatively inexpensive, available in a variety of forms, and easily removable, if it is rejected.

After the dawn of polymer chemistry, many materials were tested as possible alloplastic implants. Plasticizers and additives were used to soften the polymer or to ensure chemical and thermal stability. Many were initially discarded because of exuberant tissue reactivity leading to a high rate of rejection. With time it became clear that polymers needed to be pure or "medical grade"; i.e., that they contain no plasticizers or additives which could leach out, causing adverse local or systemic reactions.

Four other factors were then noted to influence implant rejection.

1. Soft tissue coverage—Firm nonreactive alloplastic materials can survive indefinitely when buried deep in the soft tissues. Scant soft-tissue coverage or coverage by poor quality, poorly vascularized skin often leads to extrusion.
2. Mobility—Implants placed in highly mobile areas such as the nose are subject to dislodgement from frequent trauma. In addition, it is very important that any porous implant have a period of initial stability with regard to adjacent tissue if the desired tissue ingrowth response is to occur; fibroblasts have difficulty catching a moving target.
3. Infection—A third factor leading to extrusion is infection. Some infections occur immediately after surgery, resulting in a draining, open wound that is frequently unresponsive to antibiotic therapy. This usually necessitates removal of the implant. Implant materials can also become infected months to years after surgery, presumably from bacteremia or a local infection such as a dental or skin abcess.
4. Closure under Tension—A fourth factor is closure under tension. Frequently an area that needs augmentation is deficient in soft tissues and/or scarred from previous surgery or trauma. The surgeon is then faced with the problem of a tight closure to accommodate an appropriately sized prosthesis. This unfortunately leads to extrusion.

As surgeons have come to understand the limitations and advantages of solid alloplastic implants, they have found increasing numbers of uses for them. This chapter looks at two widely used materials—Silastic and Proplast—and two less well known solid implants—polyethylene and acrylic.

II. SILICONE RUBBER (SILASTIC)

A. PHYSICAL AND CHEMICAL PROPERTIES

Silastic, in use since the 1950s, is one of the most widely used alloplastic implant materials. It can fill a variety of rolls from cheek augmentation to buttock and calf augmentation. It is available as soft gel-filled implants, such as are used for chin and breast augmentation, and solid implants which may be either very firm or soft and rubbery (Table 1). Clearly this physical variability had expanded Silastic's popularity among soft tissue surgeons.

A second property which has lead to the popularity and ever increasing variety of uses is its low tissue reactivity and low rejection rate. Third, Silastic is easily inserted. Its surface is smooth and slippery, and it can be folded upon itself for insertion through small incisions.

TABLE 1
Summary of Augmentation Materials and Uses

	Silastic	Proplast	Polyethylene	Acrylic
Chin	+ + + +	+ + + +	+ + + ?[g]	+ + + +
Geniomandibular groove	+ + + +	NA	NA	NA
Malar	+ + + +	+ + +[c]	+ + + ?[g]	+ + +[i]
Submalar	+ + + +	NA[d]	NA[d]	NA
Temple & forehead	+ + +	+ + +	?[h]	+ + + +
Premaxilla	+ + + + ?[a]	+ + +[e]	NA[h]	NA[j]
Nose	?[b]	+ + +[f]	O	O

Note: + = poor-fair results; + + + + = excellent results; O = material not used;
NA = preformed implant not available.

[a] Only one clinical series (Dr. Guinta).
[b] Possible use in non-Caucasian nasal augmentation.
[c] Successful, but limited number of preformed shapes available.
[d] Would probably be successful; must custom carve implants.
[e] Successful in reports by Silver and Sheen.
[f] Good results in non-Caucasian rhinoplasty.
[g] Preformed shapes available; no reported clinical series.
[h] No reported cases; should theoretically be successful.
[i] Not implant of choice for this area (see text).
[j] No reported cases; probably too cumbersome for this use.

1. Chemistry

Silastic is an organosilicone polymer with the formula

$$\left[\begin{array}{c} CH_3 \\ | \\ -O-Si-O- \\ | \\ CH_3 \end{array} \right]_n$$

These subunits are linked together producing polydioxsone. Very fine silica particles (0.02 μm) are added to silicone fluid. This mixture is then vulcanized by using dichlorobenzoyl peroxide, producing a true rubber. Chain length determines the firmness of the implant: short chains produce silicone fluid while longer chains produce a rubber.

The resulting rubber is nonwettable. It repels blood, tissue fluids, and plasma proteins. Additionally Silastic is inert in host tissues. Its chemical composition and its shape are not altered by tissue fluids after implantation. Because the chemical composition is not altered and because it is a pure "medical grade" polymer, Silastic is not toxic to the host. It is heat stable and easily autoclaved or dry heat sterilized.

2. Tissue Response

Since Silastic is nonwettable and has low toxicity, the tissue response is very mild. A thin but tough fibrous tissue capsule is laid down around the implant. Typically this collagen containing capsule demonstrates only a few chronic inflammatory cells. Host tissues outside the capsule are unaffected.[5]

B. GENERAL PRINCIPLES FOR IMPLANTATION

All alloplastic implant materials act as foreign bodies in host tissues and therefore, require special handling. The "no touch" technique is used. Implants are handled only with instruments to avoid contamination with glove powder and any other substances which may have accumulated on the gloves of the operating team. Each implant is opened onto the Mayo stand and then carefully placed into antibiotic solution. Gentamicin or Cleocin are the choice of most surgeons. After the implant is thoroughly wetted, it is ready for placement into the waiting soft-tissue pocket.

It is common practice for all patients to receive i.v. antibiotics at least 30 min prior to insertion of the implant. A broad spectrum antibiotic such as Ancef is adequate. This antibiotic is continued i.v. while the patient is still in the hospital or outpatient surgical facility. After discharge an oral Cephalosporin is then continued for a total of at least 72 h to seven d postoperatively.

While both early and late extrusion can occur regardless of technique, adherence to the above procedure will reduce this complication.

C. USE IN FACIAL AUGMENTATION

Silastic implants work best in areas of good soft-tissue coverage. Its success in mentoplasty has been well documented, and a variety of silicone implant types are available.[6,8,10-13] Other areas which are successfully augmented with Silastic are the zygoma for both post-traumatic defects and cosmetic recontouring,[7,9,14-16] the submalar area,[17] the geniomandibular groove, the temple,[18] and forehead.[19]

However, in nasal augmentation, its use is limited. Thin soft-tissue coverage, constant movement of the nose, and frequent midface trauma lead to an unacceptably high incidence of dislodgement and extrusion.[20-22]

For the most part, Silastic is well anchored in the tissues by the tough, fibrous capsule which develops around it. Traumatic disruption or tearing of this capsule probably accounts for the high extrusion rate in the nose. To gain additional anchoring, many implants have preformed holes to allow for tissue ingrowth or holes can be easily placed where none exist. Tissue ingrowth through the holes has been demonstrated histologically[5] and probably occurs in most instances. However, Tobin[15] reports removing malar implants which showed no fibrous tissue ingrowth but had developed a well-defined fibrous capsule. Additionally, the author has removed chin implants—patients who decided after several months that they did not like their appearance—which showed no tissue ingrowth. It may be then, that fibrous tissue growth through perforations cannot always be relied upon for fixation.

1. Chin

Chin augmentation is a popular and generally very successful procedure—the primary reasons being that soft-tissue coverage is good, and that motion and stresses are small and mostly absorbed by the mandible itself. The chin is also a forgiving site. Because of the good soft tissue coverage, minor changes in the contour or position of the implant are not nearly as aesthetically significant as in areas with thinner soft-tissue coverage. Silastic is the implant of choice for most plastic surgeons.

a. Advantages of Silastic™ Implants

The advantages of Silastic chin implants are several: (1) ease of insertion secondary to the smooth surface and ability to be deformed; (2) good fit over the curve of the mandible insuring no dead space and possible late implant malposition from scar contracture; (3) availability in a wide variety of sizes and shapes; (4) easy carvability should a customized implant be desired.

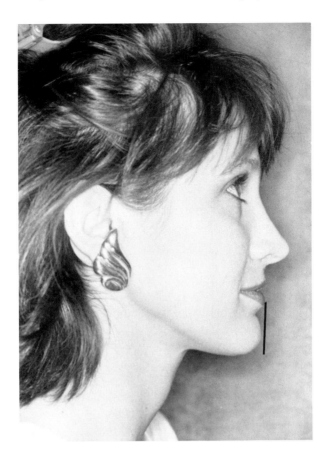

FIGURE 1.   Vertical line drawn from lip analyzing the appropriate
length of projection of chin in a female.

b. Preoperative Analysis

The simplest method of preoperative analysis to determine the need for augmentation mentoplasty is to drop a vertical line from the lower lip. In women, the mentum should approach or ideally touch this line (Figures 1 and 2). Males, however, require a stronger chin, and the mentum should approximate a vertical line dropped from the upper lip.

c. Surgical Technique

Both intraoral and extraoral insertion are accepted and are commonly used. There is at least one advantage to the intraoral route: it leaves no external scars. This approach has been widely used, probably because the intraoral route was used initially for introducing autogenous bone grafts.[23] Later, when alloplastic materials came along this incision seemed the logical choice. Synthetic implants can be placed via the intraoral approach with a surprisingly low complication rate. However, certain factors militate against optimal results from the intraoral approach. A short mandibular body and shallow labial sulcus may cause the implant to be placed in too high a position. Even without this anatomic variation, the incidence of superior migration of the implant is higher with the intraoral approach.

The extraoral approach, an alternative to the intraoral, has gained in popularity because it allows access to the submental area, upper platysma, and neck through the same incision. Submental lipectomy, platysma tightening, and neck liposuction can be easily performed at the same time. This approach also reduces the chances of superior migration of the implant because the superior attachments of the mentalis and depressor labii inferioris muscles remain intact.[24]

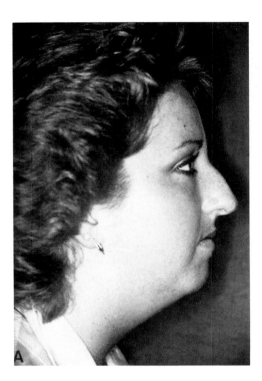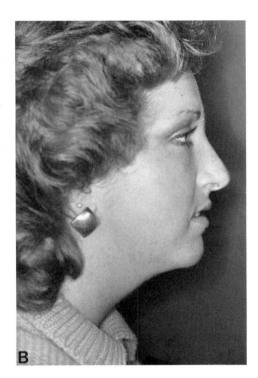

FIGURE 2. Pre- and postoperative views of a patient who underwent mentoplasty. (A) Preoperative lateral view indicating a mild degree of micrognathia; (B) postoperative view following insertion of a small Silastic™ chin implant and rhinoplasty.

The extraoral insertion of the Silastic implant is performed through a 1 to 2 cm incision placed in the submental crease. The muscles which insert on the inferior margin of the mandible are then divided sharply down to the periostium. The soft tissue is elevated above the periostium. The horizontal pocket is created low along the border of the mandible so that the implant will not extend into or above the labiomental sulcus. The pocket need be only large enough to accept the Silastic implant. Since the submental nerves exit approximately 2 to 2.5 cm on either side of the symphysis menti at the level of the mental crease,[24] care must be taken to keep the dissection low on the mandibular border (Figure 3). The implant is then inserted, handling it with Allis clamps or forceps, again the "no touch" technique.

The muscle layer is closed securely and then the skin is closed with a layered closure. There is no need to drain the wound.

d. Current Concepts in the Choice of Chin Implants

Until recently, Silastic chin implants were all generally sized and shaped in a standard fashion. The variation in size depended on the amount of projection desired, usually from about 4 mm to about 14 mm. The lateral extension of most implants was confined to the distance between the oral commissures (Figure 4). The choice exists between solid, silicone rubber or gel-filled implants as well as contoured backs to fit the curve of the chin. They are also available with coated backings to prevent slippage.

For most mentoplasties, these standard shapes were adequate. However, the chin-jaw shape and relationship does vary somewhat. In the individual with a wide jaw and/or narrow chin, the jowl may become prominent or a groove may develop between the chin and the jowl. The standard implants tend to exaggerate this problem. The new anatomic shaped

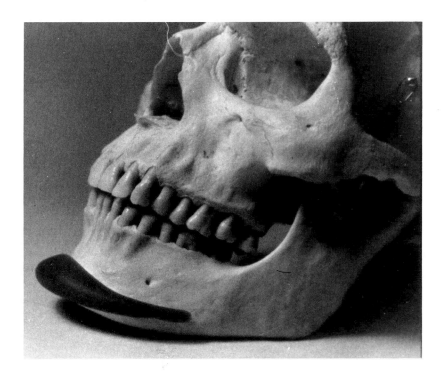

FIGURE 3.   Placement of extended chin implant on skeleton indicating relationship to mental foramen. (Photograph courtesy of McGhan Medical.)

implants, which extend laterally to the jowl region, reduce the problem and produce a better contour (Figure 5). They are also available in a variety of sizes. The Mittleman implant advances this concept another step and augments the lateral extension of the anatomical implant to fill in the geniomandibular groove. These implants are useful in reducing the prominence of the jowl as well as augmenting the chin (Figure 6). They may be used as part of a facelift procedure where indicated. They are available in three sizes from McGhan.

e. Complications

While complications of augmentation mentoplasty are rare, extrusion, malposition, bone erosion, infection, bleeding, and hypoesthesia of the lip sometimes occur. Infection and extrusion may occur in the immediate postoperative period but usually occur later, frequently after dental manipulation or infection.[25] Patients usually present with tenderness, swelling, and erythema around the implant. In most cases the findings are not dramatic. If an abcess is present (it rarely is), it is evacuated, cultured, and drained. Treatment consists of high dose, broad spectrum, oral antibiotics for 3 weeks. In most cases this will improve the situation, but infection will often recur. Additional courses of antibiotics may be given. However, if the infection fails to clear completely after two to three courses, the implant must be removed. Unlike Silastic malar implants which seem to have an amazing ability to survive infection without extrusion,[14,15] most infected chin implants require removal.

A number of articles have documented bone resorption beneath firm alloplastic implants in the chin, skull, orbit, and experimentally in rabbit skulls.[26-29] In reviewing these articles, it appears that bone resorption occurred largely in implants placed subperiosteally and also in a few implants placed over the periosteum. This does not appear to be a commonly reported problem now (Figure 7).

Bleeding and hematoma should be treated by early evacuation, drainage, and application of compressive dressings. Rarely does this complication necessitate removal of the implant.

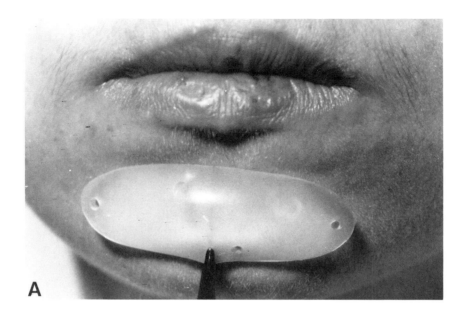

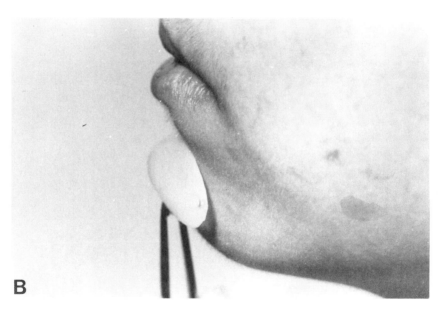

FIGURE 4. Placement of a standard Silastic™ implant on the chin. (A) Anterior view — note lateral extent of implant; (B) lateral view of implant.

Malposition, seen more commonly in the intraoral insertion technique, is often caused by creation of a pocket which is significantly larger than the implant and/or creation of a pocket which does not hug the lower border of the mandible.

Transient hypoesthesia of the lower lip is often seen secondary to postoperative swelling. This usually lasts from only a few days to a week or two. Hypoesthesia secondary to submental nerve injury can last up to 6 months. Severe crush injury and transection of the nerve can result in permanent anesthesia.[34]

2. Malar Augmentation

High cheekbones have always been recognized as a sign of beauty and youth in Western

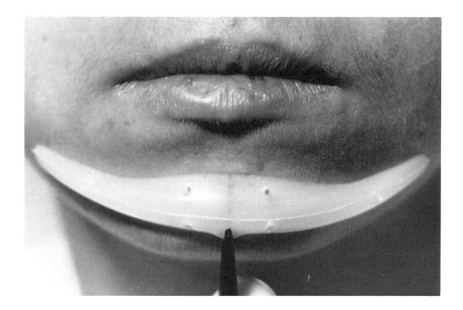

FIGURE 5.   Anterior view of position and lateral extent of an "anatomical" shaped chin implant.

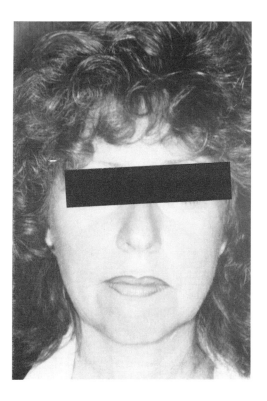 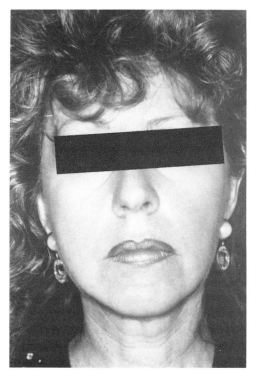

FIGURE 6.   (A) Preoperative view of a patient with evident jowls and prominent geniomandibular groove; (B) postoperative view of the same patient following insertion of a Mittleman implant to reduce the effect of jowling and eliminate the geniomandibular groove. (Photographs courtesy of Dr. Alvin I. Glasgold.)

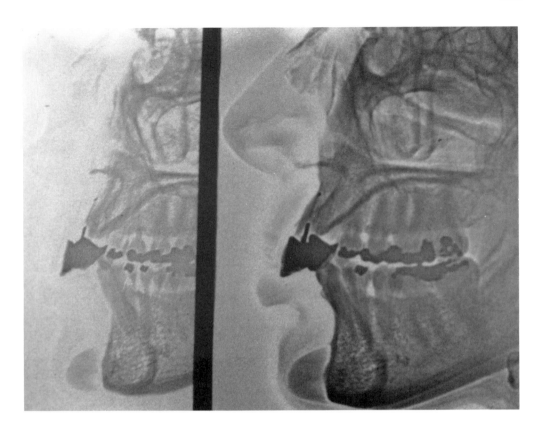

FIGURE 7. Radiographs of Silastic™ implant at 6 months and 30 months postoperatively indicating the absence of any significant bone erosion. (Photograph courtesy of Dr. Sidney Feuerstein.)

culture. Men and women with high cheek bones retain their youthful appearance longer. In addition, malar augmentation gives a long narrow face a more oval shape—the ideal facial configuration.

Unilateral malar onlay grafting has been performed for years for traumatic malar depressions using bone grafts,[30] Silastic,[3,9,14-16] Proplast™,[31-34] polyethylene,[35] and acrylic.[19] Aesthetic bilateral malar augmentation is relatively new. It was first performed by Hinderer in 1971 who used Kiel-Braun bone grafts.[30] Spadafora used polyethylene implants, and in 1973 Gonzalez-Ulloa employed silicone rubber implants of three basic shapes—the "Half Moon", the "Submarine", and the "Collar Button."[9]

In the ensuing 18 years malar augmentation has very gradually been accepted and employed by cosmetic surgeons. As at least one author points out,[15] the public knows relatively little about this procedure. At the present time malar augmentation must usually be suggested to patients.

a. Implant Types

Malar implants of bone, polyethylene, Silastic, acrylic, and Proplast have been used. At this writing Silastic implants are the most popular. (Proplast and polyethylene implants are discussed below.)

The first preformed implants were developed by Hinderer in 1974.[30] These were oval, perforated, curved discs of Silastic and came in three sizes—small, medium, and large. Perforations were made to allow ingrowth of fibrous tissue to anchor the implant.[9]

Anatomically the malar area is a tripod. The oval shape of the early implants can give a pointy unnatural appearance in some patients or resulted in demarcation of the implant's

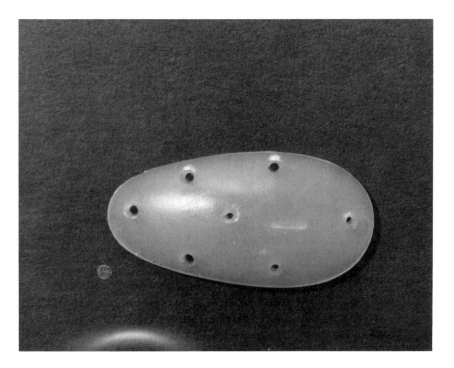

FIGURE 8.   Photograph of an extended malar implant. (Courtesy of McGhan Medical.)

edge in thin skinned individuals. To overcome these problems Wilkinson in 1976 designed extended perforated Silastic implants available through McGhan (Figure 8).

The extended implants have a narrow posterior extension over the zygoma and a superior extension over the lateral orbital rim. These extensions give an aesthetic, sculptured appearance and allow for greater variability in size and shape. The anatomical shaped malar implants have been designed to better conform to the contour of the orbital rim and zygomatic arch (Figure 9).

Silastic has worked very well in the malar area. Published series of malar implants do not report a high extrusion rate.[7,9,14,16,36] In this respect, Silastic malar implants function very much like chin implants. Presumably soft tissue coverage is adequate and mobility is low—two factors important to the success of Silastic implants.

b. Preoperative Analysis

As with all cosmetic procedures, preoperative analysis is important to the success of the procedure and to patient satisfaction. Two points must be evaluated: (1) is the patient an appropriate candidate for augmentation malarplasty? and (2) what size and shape does the augmentation need to take? Photographs—frontal, oblique (34° from the saggital plane), basal, and lateral views—are essential. O'Quin and Thomas[37] recommend roentgenograms of the face combined with cephalometry. They further suggest that three-dimensional computerized tomography can be helpful. Prendergast and Schoenrock[38] have recently published a detailed article describing their technique for preoperative computer analysis.

c. Surgical Technique

While Hinderer[30] described six approaches for insertion of malar prostheses—an adjacent incision, a preauricular incision, a rhytidectomy incision, a lower blephroplasty incision, a lower nasal osteotomy incision, and an intraoral incision—the lower lid blephroplasty (or

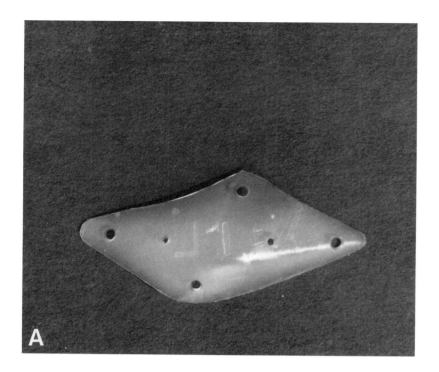

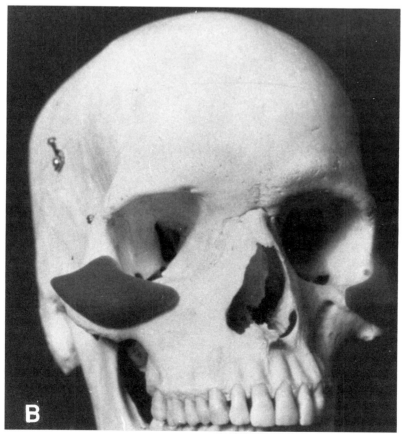

FIGURE 9. (A) Example of an anatomical shaped implant; (B) position of an anatomical shaped malar implant on the facial skeleton. (Photograph courtesy of McGhan Medical.)

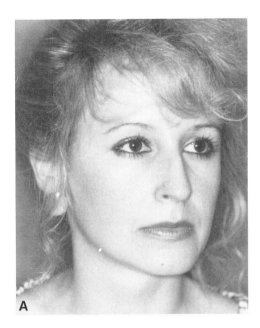
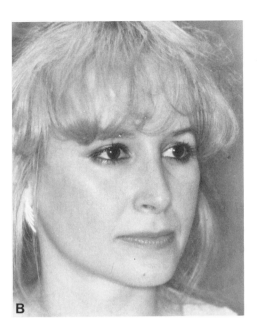

FIGURE 10.   (A) Pre- and (B) postoperative photographs of patients with extended malar implants to accentuate malar eminence. (Photographs courtesy of Dr. Alvin I. Glasgold.)

transconjunctival) approach and the intraoral approach were most commonly used in the early 1980s.[9] The lower eyelid subciliary incision seems to be fraught with numerous possible complications—such as ectropion and implant extrusion.[14,39] Consequently the majority of surgeons rely upon the intraoral approach, for it requires a minimum of dissection, provides excellent exposure, facilitates medial dissection, and circumvents the problems of external scarring and damage to the facial nerve.

A sublabial incision is made and a subperiosteal pocket is developed. The infraorbital nerve and zygomatic arch are identified. This deeper plane of dissection is used to avoid damage to branches of the facial nerve and has the advantage of being almost bloodless. The dissection is continued in the laterosuperior direction over the zygomatic arch, where the pocket is made just large enough to accommodate the implant. At times the dissection over a portion of the zygomatic arch is not truly subperiosteal because the periosteum becomes thinned out and blends into the insertion of the masseter and temporalis muscles. Here the dissection is carried over the fascia of the masseter and the temporalis muscles. The dissection at this point is guided by external palpation of the inferior orbital rim to prevent inadvertent entrance into the orbit. Precaution must be taken to place the implant at least 6 mm away from the inferior orbital rim. Closer placement of the prosthesis to the orbital rim may result in patient discomfort and extrusion.

After the implant is pulled into proper position, it is stabilized by 0 silk stay sutures which had been previously placed in the implant. These sutures are brought out through the temporal scalp within the hairline and tied over a Silastic button, or may be brought out directly over the cheek and tied over a dental roll over a Silastic button. The reader is referred to the articles by Newman[14] and Tobin[15] for more details. Postoperatively patients are placed on a Cephalosporin antibiotic for one week. They are instructed to use ice packs to both cheeks for 24 h. A soft diet is prescribed and instructions are given to rinse the mouth after eating with a mixture of 1/2 Peroxide and 1/2 Cepacol mouthwash (Figure 10).

d. Complications

Complications are few and relatively minor. The most common complication is infection.

Most of these occur in the immediate postoperative period, but may be delayed indefinitely. Interestingly, most of these infections were cleared by antibiotics and drainage and did not require removal of the implant.

There has been much written about bone erosion beneath firm alloplastic implants. Most of this has been with regard to chin implants. For malar implants, this issue was addressed by Brennan[7] who examined ten patients xeroradiographically 2 to 4 years postoperatively. These ten patients showed no bone erosion beneath implants placed subperiosteally.

Many patients show some asymmetry postoperatively. This is so common as to not be a true complication. It is fortunately slight. It is therefore necessary that patients be informed of this common occurrence preoperatively.

In nearly every series, as with most cosmetic procedures, there has been some patient dissatisfaction. This has been rare and usually consists of complaints that the implants are not big enough or are too big.[14,15]

3. Submalar Augmentation

Submalar augmentation is a relatively new technique. Binder[6] recently published a paper in which he reviews his 6-year experience with submalar augmentation in 78 patients. As he points out, the aging process results in atrophy of subcutaneous fat in addition to accumulation of fat in unwanted areas such as the jowls and submentum. This fat atrophy leads to hollows and depressions in the cheeks and nasolobial folds giving a cadaver-like appearance. According to Binder this appearance is often seen in patients in the 38 to 50 year age group. These patients often present to cosmetic surgeons seeking face-lift surgery. While they may have some laxity of the cheek and neck tissues, in many cases, the primary problem is fat atrophy in the cheek and nasolobial fold areas. Patients such as these then benefit from submalar augmentation as an alternative to rhytidectomy (Figure 11).

a. Implant Types

As with the cheek and chin, the submalar region has sufficient soft tissue coverage and lack of motion to successfully accept Silastic implants. Preformed Binder submalar facial implants are manufactured by Implant Tech and distributed by Byron Medical. Four sizes are available (Figure 12).

b. Surgical Technique

The technique is similar to the canine fossa approach used for malar augmentation. The area of deficiency is marked with the patient in the sitting position. The patient is asked to smile broadly to determine the medial extent of the implant.

The incision is made in the sublabial sulcus and carried down through the periosteum. The periosteum is elevated superiorly off the face of the maxilla exposing the infraorbital nerve, the lateral malar-zygomatic area, and medial maxilla. The implant is then inserted into the pocket and its position adjusted. A stay suture of 0 silk is double threaded through the holes in the implant around the undersurface and then threaded onto two Keith needles. The needles are threaded through the pocket and out through the cheek tissues. The implant is pulled gently into the pocket and positioned. The sutures are tied on the cheek over dental rolls to stabilize the implant (Figure 13). After the implant is in good position the incision is closed in two layers. An external pressure dressing is used to immobilize the implants further. On postop day one, the dressing is removed and the dental rolls are covered with bandages. The bolsters are removed on the third or fourth postoperative day. Perioperative antibiotics are given.

c. Complications

Binder[6] reports a 12.8% complication rate. As with the other Silastic implants that we have seen, infection occurred in two patients. Both were treated successfully with drainage

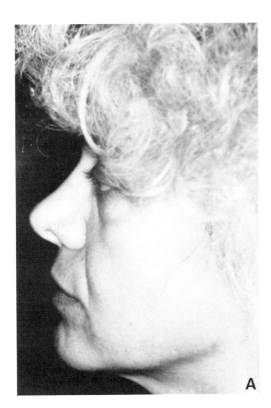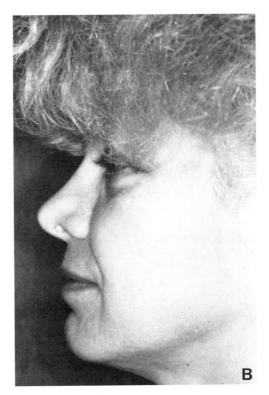

FIGURE 11.   (A) Preoperative photo of patient exhibiting fat atrophy in the submalar region; (B) postoperative photo correcting the submalar deficiency utilizing binder submalar implant. (Photographs courtesy of Dr. Alvin I. Glasgold.)

and antibiotics. Neither required removal of the prosthesis. Three experienced unilateral slightly reduced lip mobility which resolved in 4 weeks. Five complained of lip numbness. All resolved within 3 months. Five cases had sufficient asymmetry to require adjustment of the implant. This was accomplished without difficulty.

4. Temple and Forehead Augmentation
a. Temple

Temple augmentation has probably been performed for years, but there is very little in the Western literature about this procedure—probably because there are few series large enough to publish. Watanabe,[18] a Japanese plastic surgeon, published a series of 21 cases in 1984. He points out that this procedure is popular in Japan because Japanese people are mesocephalic and tend to have relatively broad faces secondary to protrusion of the zygoma: this may give a "coarse" impression. He goes on to say that the concavity in the temporal area also gives the face a "seedy" look and causes the person to look older than he or she really is. Temple augmentation gives definition to the forehead laterally.

In cases of extreme zygomatic protrusion, Onizuka et al.[40] recommend zygoma reduction. In most cases, however, simple temporal augmentation will suffice.

The temporal area has been augmented with "injectable materials" according to Watanabe, but these would often migrate giving a lumpy supraorbital protuberance. Some patients also developed "induration". This "injectable material" was probably the Japanese Sakurai injectable silicone long associated with a high incidence of siliconomas.[41-44] Autologous fat was used, but it was difficult to obtain symmetry both in volume and position.

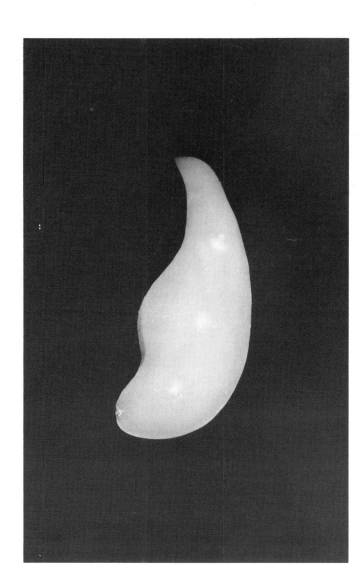

FIGURE 12.   Binder Silastic® submalar implant. (Photograph courtesy of Dr. William Binder.)

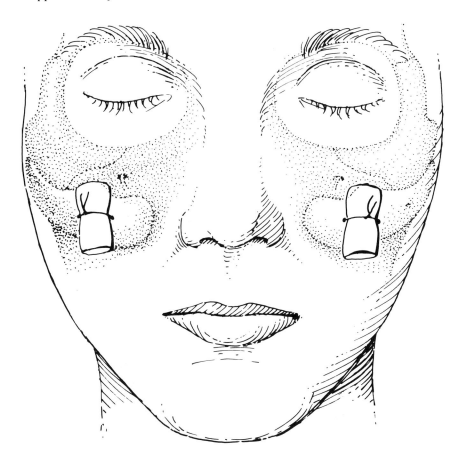

FIGURE 13.   Placement of implant and bolsters for submalar augmentation. (Courtesy of Dr. William Binder.)

Also, the fat was placed subcutaneously, a technique which endangers the temporal branch of the facial nerve. Watanbe's technique uses custom designed Silastic implants which he makes at the time of surgery. The implants are shaped either like a quarter-circle or like the tip of an airplane propeller that is slightly curved. The edges are feathered and holes are dotted throughout.

The plane of insertion in Watanabe's technique is beneath the temporalis fascia. Prior methods for insertion have included submuscular insertion which carries an increased risk of hemorrhage and is technically more difficult and subcutaneous insertion which carries the risk of injury to the temporal brach of the facial nerve. Another problem with subcutaneous insertion is that the margin of the prosthesis often becomes conspicuous postoperatively.

Watanabe does not list complications. One expects that they would be the same as for Silastic® implants in other areas—infection, extrusion, hematoma, etc.

b. Forehead

Augmentation of forehead defects has probably been performed for years but again, as with temporal augmentation, little has been written. Silver[32] describes the use of Proplast for this (see below), and in 1981 Schultz[19] published a paper in which he discussed the use of Silastic and acrylic (methylmethacrylate) for reconstruction of facial bone deformities.

For supraorbital and glabellar defects, Schultz uses implants carved from silicone rubber blocks or molded from a room temperature-vulcanizing silicone rubber. The silicone blocks are carved with a scalpel and then finely contoured and smoothed with a rotating burr. These are then heat autoclaved.

Silastic implants can also be molded instead of carved, using room temperature-vulcanizing silicone rubber. These are modeled from a moulage of the facial defect or from the defect itself before surgery. The room temperature-vulcanizing rubber can be molded in sites where heat cannot be tolerated as opposed to acrylic which produces much heat (see Section V). After molding, the implants can be heat autoclaved without losing their shape.

Molding an implant over the skin surface or over a moulage taken from the skin surface never produces a piece that will fit the defect precisely. However, to achieve the best possible fit, the implant can be carved after the defect is exposed surgically.

For most frontal and supraorbital defects the implant is placed subcutaneously, for the soft-tissue coverage there is adequate to cover the implant well without fear of erosion or visibility. The incision is ideally placed in a preexisting scar, forehead wrinkle, or at the junction of the brow and forehead skin. Baring these possibilities, a gull-wing incision can be used, although in some situations a coronal incision would be a good choice.

5. Premaxilla Augmentation

Augmentation of the premaxilla is frequently necessary as an adjunct to rhinoplasty for increasing the nasolabial angle, correction of bimaxillary protrusion, rotating the tip upward, and increasing projection. The need may be minimal and a small amount of autologous septal cartilage will suffice. But some noses require large amounts of augmentation—too large to be adequately augmented with autologous cartilage without the need for a second operative site such as the ear or rib.

In 1981, Dr. Stephen Guinta[45] developed a Silastic premaxillary implant which he implanted into 108 individuals over a 6-year period. Only one rejection occurred early on—probably because the implant was too large. Dr. Guinta attributes this surprising success rate to his implantation technique.

The surgical technique has two important aspects: (1) a sublabial approach and (2) preservation of the depressor septi-nasi muscle when possible. The technique is as follows: after infiltrating the sublabial area with Xylocaine and with epinephrine, a midline, transfrenular incision is carried down to the periosteum. Using a small periosteal elevator, a small pocket is created under the depressor septi-nasi muscle. Small relaxing incisions in the muscle are sometimes necessary to permit introduction of the implant. The dissection is continued across the base of the pyriform aperture and into the naso-alar groove on each side. The implant is inserted "feet first". Suture fixation is generally not required. The incision is closed with 3 to 0 chromic, and external tape fixation is used. As with all alloplastic implants, perioperative antibiotics are given for 7 d.

The implant is available through Byron Medical and comes in two sizes—male and female (Figure 14). It can be easily carved to make any necessary size and contour alterations.

6. Nose

The nose presents several particular problems not encountered elsewhere on the face. It occupies a unique position of prominence on the face, and as such, receives frequent microtrauma and often major blows. The lower two fifths of the nose is highly mobile, and nasal soft-tissue coverage is thin. Any implant placed here is subject to frequent stress, because the soft, thin, mobile tissues are unable to absorb much of the force. The forces of trauma can often result in dislodgement of an implant from within its fibrous capsule and subsequent extrusion. For this reason Silastic has been generally abandoned for nasal augmentation.[20,21,46]

The above has been well demonstrated. Silastic can survive indefinitely when buried deep in the soft tissues. However, when used in the nose, especially in the nasal dorsum, the extrusion rate is increased. Beekhuis reports a 34% extrusion rate[46] with Silastic nasal implants, Davis and Jones report 18%,[22] and Milward 30%.[21]

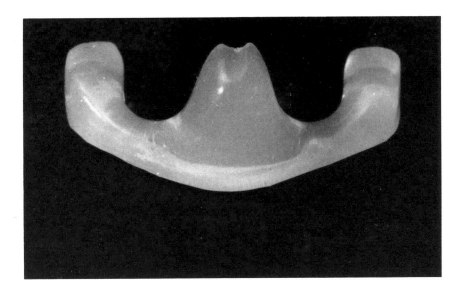

FIGURE 14A.   Photograph of Guinta premaxillary implant.

The above point has been demonstrated experimentally. Brown et al.[29] found a higher rate of extrusion and flap necrosis with rigid, nonporous Plasti-Pore and Silastic implanted into rabbit ears as compared to Proplast and Supramid.

In contrast to other reports, McCurdy[47] reported in 1989 his experience with Silastic nasal augmentation in 743 Oriental noses. He reported a 1.7% incidence of infection and removal and a 1.5% incidence of late extrusion. McCurdy speculates that his success is probably a result of the greater thickness of skin and subcutaneous tissues in the Oriental nose. He also emphasizes that the implant should not fit too snugly in the dorsum and that one should avoid excessive tension in the lobular region—two factors that appear linked to delayed extrusion.

III. PROPLAST™

A. PHYSICAL AND CHEMICAL PROPERTIES

While polytetrafluoroethylene polymer was synthesized in the 1940s, the product known as Proplast was developed by Homsey[31] in 1970, and first used as a coating material over metal orthopedic and temporomandibular joint implants. Proplast was initially manufactured in sheets and blocks and used primarily for implant stabilization, then gradually evolved into use in soft-tissue augmentation, and preformed implants became available.

1. Chemistry

Proplast is made of Teflon fluorocarbon polymer (polytetrafluoroethylene) combined with either black vitreous carbon fibers (Proplast I) or white aluminum oxide fiber (Proplast II). In both animal and human experiments, Proplast II is physiologically similar to the earlier product Proplast I.[48] Its white color improves its value for use in superficial subcutaneous locations.

Teflon alone has a low surface energy and is minimally wetted by body fluids. The addition of carbon fibers or aluminum oxide renders Proplast extremely wettable, thus permitting adsorption of plasma proteins and subsequent tissue ingrowth, creating a solid unit with the surrounding tissues and minimizing implant migration. When experimentally exposed to pseudoextracellular fluid, Proplast has the least reactivity of any known material.[49]

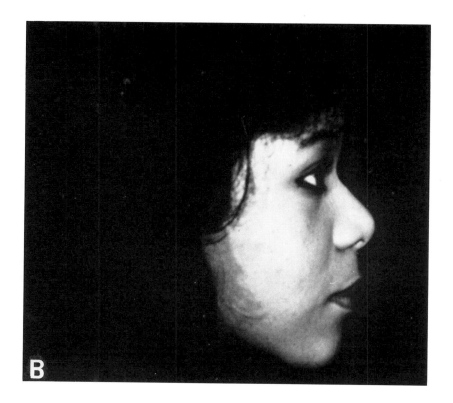

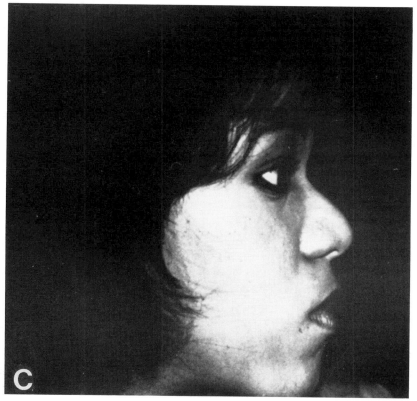

FIGURE 14B and C. Preoperative view of patient (B); postoperative view of patient (C) following insertion of premaxillary implant. (Photographs courtesy of Dr. Stephen Guinta.)

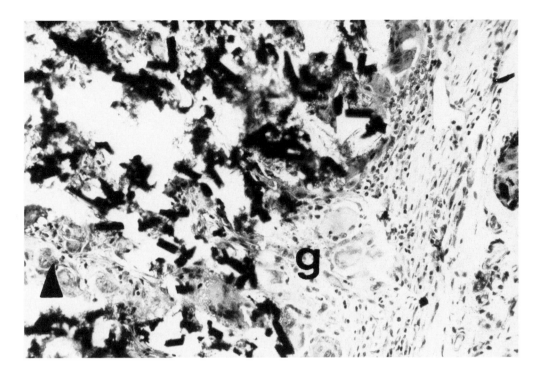

FIGURE 15.   Thick, continuous granulomas (g) cover the cut surface and infiltrate the pores of the Proplast. Adjacent foreign body giant cells (arrowhead) are apparent primarily within the Proplast.

Proplast is manufactured as a firm but compressible sponge. The pores occupy approximately 70% of its volume. There is some controversy regarding pore size but it is in the 70—100 μm to 400—500 μm range with dendritic pore interconnections greater than 80 μm. It is easily shaped with a knife, scissors, or even a high-speed grinder. This gives Proplast a significant advantage over other solid implants, allowing easy sculpting of custom designed implants and subtle contouring.[34] Silver[32] points out that the black Proplast I is easier to carve and that its edges can be carved and feathered more precisely than Proplast II, which is harder and can be very difficult to carve with precision. Westfall et al.[48] also report that Proplast II deforms and compresses more than Proplast I when equal stresses are applied.

2. Tissue Response

In the tissues Proplast elicits, initially, an exuberant response.[5] At 7 weeks the implant is surrounded by contiguous granulomas which infiltrate into the pores of the material. The granulomas are composed primarily of mature macrophages and within the Proplast numerous foreign body giant cells are also present. In the center of the implant is loose granulation tissue with a moderate chronic inflammatory response containing primarily mononuclear cells and some plasma cells (Figure 15). Organizing fibrous tissue is seen in the granulation tissue surrounding the implant and strands of fibrous tissue are present throughout. After several months, this reaction subsides and the implant is completely surrounded and infiltrated by fibrous tissue.[50]

B. GENERAL PRINCIPLES FOR IMPLANTATION

Proplast like all alloplastic implant materials acts as a foreign body. The ''no touch'' technique is again used. Implants are handled only with instruments to avoid contamination with glove powder and any other substances which may have accumulated on the gloves of the operating team. Alternatively, fresh, sterile, rinsed gloves can be used to handle the implant.

Silver[32] recommends that Proplast be sculpted sometime prior to the surgical procedure. Care must be taken not to compress the implant. This not only alters the implant's shape but reduces pore size inhibiting local tissue ingrowth. It is then sterilized with a slow steam autoclave at 250°C for 30 min. Fine shape alterations if necessary can then be made at the time of surgery.

NovaMed, the sole manufacturer and distributor of Proplast, recommends vacuum antibiotic impregnation of Proplast implants. The implant is placed in a large (60 cc or larger) irrigation syringe with an adequate amount of sterile antibiotic solution (e.g., 1 g of a Cephalosporin in normal saline) to cover the implant. The syringe is held in a vertical position with the open end pointed up. The implant along with an air bubble will be at the open end of the syringe. All of the air is expelled from the syringe. The open end of the syringe is closed with the finger and the plunger retracted several times creating a vacuum. The air is again expelled from the syringe and the above process repeated several times until no further air bubbles are elicited from the implant. The implant will sink in the solution when fully impregnated. After the implant is thoroughly wetted, it is ready for placement into the waiting soft-tissue pocket.

All patients receive i.v. antibiotics at least 30 min prior to insertion of the implant. A broad spectrum antibiotic such as Ancef is adequate. This antibiotic is continued i.v. while the patient is still in the hospital or outpatient surgical facility. After discharge, an oral Cephalosporin is then continued for a total of 7 d postoperatively.

While both early and late extrusion can occur regardless of technique, adherence to the above procedures will reduce this complication.

C. USE IN FACIAL AUGMENTATION

Proplast has been in use for almost two decades. Initially utilized in orthopedic surgery as a stabilizing interface between the femoral head and a total hip prosthesis,[49,51] it subsequently found application in facial plastic surgery for augmentation of the nasal dorsum,[52] maxilla (nasolabial angle),[52-54] mentoplasty,[52,55] orbital floor reconstruction,[52] malar augmentation,[52] and as a mandibular onlay graft.[52] In middle ear surgery it has been incorporated into "TORPS"[56] and has been used for posterior canal wall reconstruction.[57] Oral surgeons have used it for alveolar ridge augmentation[58] and as part of TMJ replacement prostheses.[58,59]

Proplast has worked well in facial augmentation surgery including nasal augmentation. Unlike Silastic, extrusion has not been a major problem in the nose. Homsey[60] reports the results of a 1977 retrospective evaluation of Proplast by the USDA. In 117 patients followed for 24 to 63 months only four complications were reported.

1. Chin Augmentation

Chin augmentation using Proplast is not as prevalent as is augmentation with Silastic. Several reasons are probably responsible. Silastic is easily inserted because its surface is smooth and slippery. Additionally, it can be folded and easily inserted through a small incision. Proplast is porous and tends to stick to tissues as it is inserted. It can be bent only slightly. In addition, harsh handling causes pore compression. A larger incision is often necessary for insertion. A final reason for Proplast's reduced usage is that preformed Proplast chin implants are available in only two shapes—standard (four sizes) and dimpled (three sizes) (Figure 16). While Proplast can be custom carved from blocks and the preformed implants can be easily altered, many plastic surgeons prefer Silastic because it is available in a very large number of shapes and sizes. This offers the time-saving convenience of not having to custom carve or make significant alterations.

Preoperative analysis and implantation technique are the same as for Silastic (see above section).

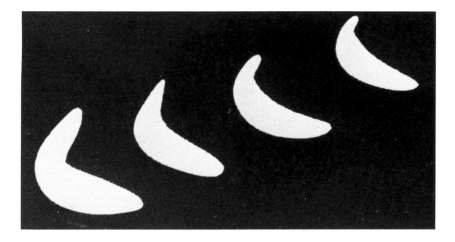

A

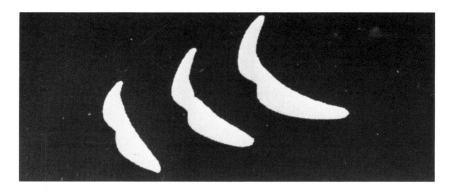

B

FIGURE 16.   Photograph of standard (A) and dimpled (B) Proplast® chin implants. (Courtesy of NovaMed.)

Complications

A number of articles have documented bone resorption beneath firm alloplastic implants in the chin, skull, orbit, and experimentally in rabbit skulls.[26-29] The vast majority of this work was done with Silastic implants. However, in 1981, Kent et al.[34] published a paper in which Proplast was used for chin augmentation in 33 patients who were followed radiographically for up to 6 years. Patients were divided into five groups—one group had Proplast chin augmentation only. The other four had chin augmentation combined with maxillary and/or mandibular surgery. Some loss of augmentation was noted in all groups of patients. Most loss occurred within 1 year of augmentation and was complete by 2 years. The overall loss of augmentation in patients with Proplast chin implant only was 30%. In the remaining groups the loss of augmentation was greater. The implants themselves showed 98% stability. The Proplast implant did not shrink, deform, or change in any way. The authors state that "the major contribution to loss of augmentation in each group is redistribution of soft tissue rather than posterior migration of the implant into bone".[34]

Bone erosion was seen in the groups which combined augmentation with maxillary and/or mandibular surgery. The authors felt that this was consistent with the theory that posterior migration of the implant into bone was secondary to increased mentalis muscle strain to accomplish lip closure. By extension, one can postulate thinning of the soft tissues as well, due to this increased pressure.

In reviewing previously published articles concerning bone erosion with Silastic implants,[26-28] it appears that bone resorption occurs mainly in implants placed subperiosteally and in a few implants placed over periosteum as well. Bone erosion is not a commonly reported phenomenon these days. I suspect that it is largely due to the fact that in recent years most implants are being placed over the periosteum. Kent et al.[34] have shown that bone resorption and soft-tissue flattening appear to be linked to the tightness of closure and of the surrounding soft tissues, which may be related to implant size.

Complications of Proplast augmentation mentoplasty are the same of those with Silastic (see Section II.C.1.e). One major difference exists: because of the tissue ingrowth into Proplast, removal is more difficult should rejection occur.

2. Malar Augmentation

Implants of bone,[30] polyethylene,[35] Silastic,[9,14-16,30] Proplast,[31-34] and acrylic[19] have been used for malar augmentation. At this writing Silastic implants are the most popular. However, Proplast has been used for years for augmentation of posttraumatic malar defects.[33] Silver[32] uses custom-made Proplast implants for cosmetic malar augmentation, and four different types of preformed malar/zygomatic implants are available—notched zygomatic (two sizes), plain malar (three sizes), high/low profile zygomatic (two sizes), and laterally extended zygomatic (two sizes) (Figure 17).

Proplast works well in the malar area. Published series of malar implants for posttraumatic defects do not report a high extrusion rate.[33] Since these defects are often scarred, tense, and poorly vascularized, Proplast should be successful in normal tissues for cosmetic malar augmentation. In this respect, Proplast malar implants behave very much like chin implants. Presumably there is adequate soft-tissue coverage and obvious low mobility—two factors important to the success of Proplast implants.

Complications

Complications are few and relatively minor. Since there are few articles on Proplast malar augmentation and no large reported series of complications, the reader is directed to the section on Silastic malar implants for further information. In general the clinical behavior of Proplast and Silastic is quite similar with the exception of the nose.

3. Temple and Forehead Augmentation

Correction of frontal bony defects with Proplast is included in Silver's article (see Reference 32). He uses custom-designed Proplast implants placed in a subcutaneous pocket. The implants are fashioned using a moulage of the patient's face. For more details of the implantation technique, see Section II.4 above.

4. Premaxilla

One type of premaxillary implant is available in Proplast II. This was designed by Sheen and comes in four sizes (Figure 18). For those interested in a custom designed implant, Sheen describes his technique for fashioning the implant and also for its insertion in his book *Aesthetic Rhinoplasty.*[54]

This premaxillary implant is similar to the Guinta Silastic premaxillary implant in that the highest point is at the anterior nasal spine. Like its Silastic counterpart, the Sheen implant also extends laterally along the base of the pyriform aperture, but then tapers off so it does not afford the increased projection of the ala and flattening of the nasolabial fold that the Guinta implant provides. In Sheen's description of the custom designed implants,[54] the

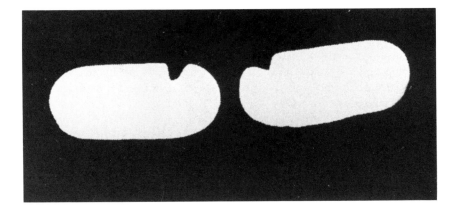

A

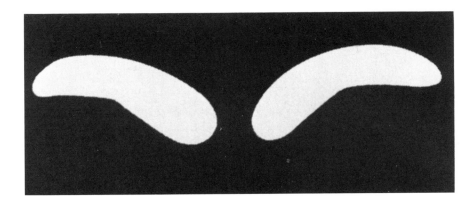

B

FIGURE 17.   Photograph of Proplast™ malar implants. (A) Notched zygomatic implant; (B) extended malar implants. (Photographs courtesy of NovaMed.)

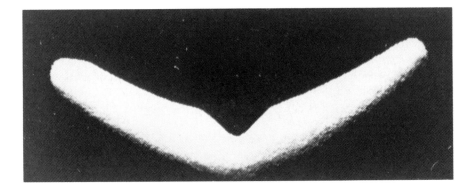

FIGURE 18.   Sheen premaxillary Proplast™ implant. (Photograph courtesy of NovaMed.)

central strut is at least 1 cm in height and is placed between the feet of the medial crura. In the preformed implants this central strut is not so prominent and ranges from 3 to 6 mm in height. This indicates to me that, as most rhinoplastic surgeons have observed, the degree of augmentation needed for the nasolabial/premaxilla area is highly variable.

The implantation technique, as described by Sheen, is relatively simple. A stab incision is made in the middle third of the nasal sill. A periosteal elevator is inserted to the anterior nasal spine and a pocket created which extends from the spine across the base of the pyriform aperture and then postero-laterally past the nasolabial fold on each side. The implant is inserted, first one side and then when the central part of the implant is just past the midline, the skin edge on the opposite side is retracted and the remaining arm of the implant is placed against the maxilla. Care is taken to not crush or squeeze the implant. Sheen says that the implant should be "intimate with the bone" but does not say whether or not the dissection is sub- or supraperiosteal. The incision is closed with interrupted 5—0 chromic.

5. Nasal Augmentation

Proplast has worked well in nasal augmentation for years[32] despite the fact that it, like Silastic, is a firm alloplast. This is presumably because Proplast's porosity allows it to become integrated with the surrounding tissues through tissue ingrowth and less subject to dislodgement by trauma. It has been used primarily in non-Caucasian rhinoplasty and the thicker skin and subcutaneous tissues also may account for its success. A great concern would be the difficulty in removal of an infected implant.

IV. POLYETHYLENE

In 1947, Rubin[35,62] began using polyethylene as a synthetic replacement for deformed or deficient facial bones and cartilage. Rubin made his own implants from granular polyethylene manufactured by the Bakelite Company. In 1968, he reported his 21-year experience with 281 patients.[62] The results showed that polyethylene survived the test of time and was a good synthetic replacement for bone in the face. Cartilage replacement did not fare so well (see below). Despite this success, polyethylene is used in only a limited fashion in facial reconstruction.

Rubin's implants were solid and smooth. He describes them as being cartilage-like in consistency. Today this type of polyethylene implant is not commercially available. Today's polyethylene is linear, high-density, high molecular weight polyethylene. This substance differs from Rubin's polyethylene in that the linear type of material has the molecules arranged in a straight line making the product much harder and nonwettable.[62] In addition the polyethylene manufactured today is porous.

Porous, high-density polyethylene (PHDPE) is used in facial augmentation, as an ossicular chain prosthesis[64] and in orthopedic surgery. It has tremendous tensile strength and is resistant to tissue stresses and fatigue. The porosity allows for fibrous and/or bony ingrowth which firmly fixes the material in the host tissues. The porosity of the surface tends to grab at tissues but does provide good initial fixation before tissue ingrowth occurs. This is important since a period of immobility is necessary for tissue ingrowth to begin.[65]

A. PHYSICAL AND CHEMICAL PROPERTIES
1. Chemistry

Polyethylene is a straight chain aliphatic hydrocarbon synthesized by the polymerization of ethylene at high temperature and pressure. The formula is

$$\begin{bmatrix} & H & H \\ & | & | \\ -C & -C- \\ & | & | \\ & H & H \end{bmatrix}_n$$

The molecular weight can vary from 1000 to 38,000—low molecular weight polyethylene is a grease, whereas very high molecular weights are firm, hard materials. The pore size ranges from 100 to 250 (av 100), and pore volume is about 50%.

Polyethylene is chemically inert. It reacts neither with concentrated hydrochloric and sulfuric acids nor with concentrated NaOH. It does not conduct heat or electricity. It is not changed or degraded by tissue fluids. Its size, shape, and consistency remain constant since it does not contain a plasticizer or hardener.

2. Tissue Response

The tissue response to polyethylene is very mild. Brown et al.[29] implanted porous polyethylene (20 to 30 μm pore size) into rabbit ears—beneath the perichondrium and into subcutaneous forehead pockets above the perichondrium. Animals were sacrificed and the implants studied histologically at 6 weeks, 6 months, and 1 year. A small amount of fibrous tissue was seen in and around the implants at all data points. A few histiocytes and foreign body giant cells were also seen. Interestingly, these cells appeared to increase with time.

Since porous polyethylene is primarily used today in orthopedic surgery, another key aspect of the tissue response is that of bony ingrowth. This clearly has significance for stabilization of orthopedic prostheses. Spector et al.[66] implanted porous polyethylene plugs (pore size = 400 μm) into the lateral diaphyseal cortex of the femurs of eight dogs. At 2 weeks new bone spicules were found in the surface pores and fibrous tissue was found in the deep pores of the polyethylene. By 8 to 10 weeks, bone spicules and marrow were seen throughout the pores of the implant. In the discussion, the authors state that previous studies demonstrated that interconnecting pore sizes of about 100 μm was required to accommodate bone ingrowth. Brown et al.[29] also cite work which shows that bone will infiltrate polyethylene if the pore size is 100 to 130 μm. Recall that in their study the pore size was 20 to 30 μm.

A second factor significantly affecting bony ingrowth is location of the implant. Brown et al.[29] did observe a "moderate" amount of bone and cartilage growing into 5 of the 17 polyethylene implants places subperichondrially in rabbit ears. Implants which were placed in subcutaneous pockets in the forehead showed no bone ingrowth. A small amount of fibrous tissue was seen around and in the implants in both locations. Sauer,[67] using MEDPOR porous high density polyethylene implants (pore size = 100 to 250 μm), demonstrated ingrowth of bone and fibrous tissue in implants placed subperiosteally in the supraorbital and malar areas of dogs. Bony ingrowth was limited to the surface pores at the bone-implant interface. The implants were firmly attached to the underlying bone. Deep in the body of the implants fibrous tissue was observed. Interestingly he reported no fibrous capsule formation.

Sauer also placed some implants in a large subcutaneous pocket in the mental area. These were loosely attached to the bone by a fibrous tissue layer, but no capsule formation was observed nor was bone ingrowth seen except in one out of six implants in the mental area. This study spanned a 2-year period, but is not specific about the intervals at which the animals were sacrificed and the implants examined.

It appears, then, that to achieve bony ingrowth and stabilization, porous polyethylene implants with a pore size of at least 100 μm be placed beneath the periosteum in direct contact with bone. Fibrous tissue ingrowth occurs where the implant is placed subcutaneously. This is probably sufficient for soft tissue augmentation.

B. GENERAL PRINCIPLES FOR IMPLANTATION

As with all alloplasts polyethylene requires careful handling with the no-touch technique. Patients should be given i.v. Ancef or other broad spectrum antibiotic one-half hour prior to implantation. The implant must be impregnated in antibiotic (Gentamicin) solution by

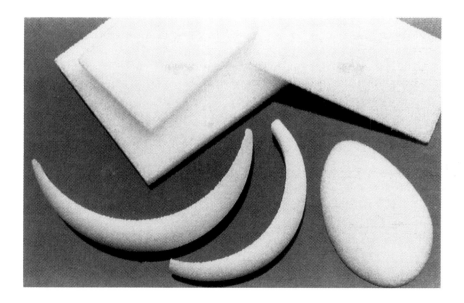

FIGURE 19. Photograph of porous polyethylene in the form of blocks, cheek implants, and chin implants. (Photograph courtesy of POREX.)

submersion and gentle agitation in the solution. The surgical pocket should be large enough to accommodate the implant. Unlike Silastic which slips easily across tissue, porous polyethylene grabs at the tissues. While this allows for early stabilization of the implant, it also makes positioning more difficult. Since only firm implants are available now, the inability to fold and bend the implant and its tendency to grab tissue could require creation of a larger pocket or a change in surgical technique for accurate positioning.

Polyethylene implants survive well in areas of adequate soft-tissue coverage with low mobility. Rubin[35] abandoned the use of polyethylene in the septum, nasal tip, and ears because of the high extrusion rate. His series reports an 18.2% extrusion rate in the nose and a 53.8% extrusion rate in the ear. Brown et al.[29] reported increased flap necrosis and extrusion with polyethylene implants implanted beneath the thin skin of the mobile rabbit ear.

Porous polyethylene is available from POREX Medical in blocks, sheets, as preformed chin "shapes" (four sizes) and as malar "shapes" (standard and extended) (Figure 19). It can be carved with a grinding wheel or with a special carving set available from POREX Medical. Carving and grinding do not alter pore size.

Implants are supplied in sterile packaging. Unsterile implants can be gas sterilized, but it is necessary to wait at least 3 days before use. POREX does not recommend resterilization because of the difficulty with adequately outgasing the ethylene oxide.

C. USE IN FACIAL AUGMENTATION

Rubin[35,62] reports using solid polyethylene successfully as malar and skull onlay grafts, in the orbital floor and to augment the chin. His writings do not give details of his operative technique—supra- vs. subperiosteal implantation. Most extrusions occurred within one month postoperatively. Eleven implants extruded between 18 and 30 months after implantation; in all cases these extrusions took place after trauma. Most of these involved the nose or ear. One ear implant broke through the skin after a period of 10 years. No inciting event is stated. As stated previously, Rubin has abandoned the use of polyethylene in these areas.

Berghaus[68] reported the use of polyethylene for correction of frontal and orbital rim defects in four patients. The author does not state whether the insertion plane is supra- or subperiosteal. Follow-up was 3 months to $2^1/_2$ years. The only complication was a small seroma tapped once shortly after the operation. The cosmetic results were reported as good. He has also reconstructed the external ear in four patients with 6 months to $2^1/_2$ years follow-up. One patient had a small suture dehiscence just following the operation. No extrusions are reported except in a fifth patient who manipulated the wound himself immediately after surgery.

V. ACRYLIC (METHYL METHACRYLATE)

A. CHEMICAL AND PHYSICAL PROPERTIES
1. Chemistry

Acrylic is the polymerized ester of acrylic acid, $CH_2=CHCOOH$, or an ester of methacrylic acid, $CH_2=C(CH_3)COOH$. Acrylic implants can be formed prior to surgical implantation and then heat sterilized just prior to the procedure, or the acrylic can be mixed just prior to use and molded *in situ* since the newly prepared material is sterile.

Powdered polymer granules are mixed with a liquid monomer at room temperature. Because the speed of setting leaves insufficient time for complete polymerization, polymer granules do not become completely fused into a homogeneous mass. This makes the material slightly porous. Monomer is for the most part lost by evaporation during the mixing process, but at least 4% residual monomer always remains.

Since it is the free monomer which is responsible for adverse reactions to methyl methacrylate, the mixing technique is critical. Mixing time should take about $2^1/_2$ to 3 min. Monomer loss has been shown to be related more to frequency than to duration of stirring. Therefore the material should be beaten as rapidly as possible during the mixing period before being molded. The mixing and fitting time together can last up to 7 min; hardening takes another 7 min. The material should be worked until it is tacky and then molded *in situ* or formed into a preformed implant.

When molded *in situ* the now tacky material is worked from the center out directly over the defect. If the material becomes inadvertently mixed with blood it may become laminated. This can be minimized by manual pressure on the methyl methacrylate mass as it hardens.

As the compound polymerizes, the exothermic reaction generates temperatures up to 100°C. Since proteins coagulate at 56°C, it is necessary to cool the surrounding tissues by irrigation as the cement sets. The highest temperature generated experimentally by methyl methacrylate in the tissues was 68°C, reached in 4 to 5 min after implantation.

Several hazards have been reported with the use of methyl methacrylate, fortunately none in facial or skull augmentation. Orthopedic surgeons have reported deformation of the implant when subjected to heavy loads. The monomer (see details of preparation above) has been responsible for allergic reactions, hypotension, and cardiac arrest. These have occurred in orthopedic surgical procedures where large volumes of methyl methacrylate have come into contact with large raw surfaces of bone and soft tissue.

Acrylic implants have several advantages. The fact that they can be formed in the operating room and actually molded into the defect makes them highly desirable for irregular posttraumatic or congenital defects, allowing for more precise contouring. Since acrylic is hard, like bone, it is useful for augmentation of bony defects. Small changes in the contour can be made *in situ* with a rotating burr. This also allows precise feathering of the implant's edges to avoid palpable and visible step-offs. The rejection rate is extremely low. Acrylic is strong, does not conduct electricity, and is noncarcinogenic.

2. Tissue Response

The tissue response to methyl methacrylate is minimal though not quite as mild as with

Silastic. Initially a few foreign-body giant cells are seen on the spheres of polymer. Later this subsides and the implant becomes surrounded with a thin layer of fibrous tissue. Later a small amount of new bone formation can be seen around this fibrous capsule. It is well tolerated by soft tissue, bone, and dura.[63]

B. GENERAL PRINCIPLES FOR IMPLANTATION

As with every solid implant two factors significantly influence the success of augmentation with acrylic implants: (1) the amount and quality of the covering tissue and (2) the frequency and intensity of external trauma. Consequently, acrylic implants do better in the chin, forehead, and skull than over the basal bones.

Preoperative antibiotics are necessary—usually 1 g of Ancef given $1/2$ h prior to insertion. I.v. Ancef is continued throughout the hospital stay and then oral Keflex or Ceftin is given for a total of 7 days postoperatively. Drains are not used. They are rarely necessary but more importantly can be a route for bacterial contamination of the implant.

C. USE IN FACIAL AUGMENTATION

1. Chin Augmentation

In the early 1960s Dr. Benito Rish[63] first described his experience with acrylic chin implants. These prostheses are still available but are rarely used today by most cosmetic surgeons who prefer Silastic implants.

There are four major objections to the Rish acrylic chin implant. Three of the complaints appear to be unfounded, a fourth—unsubstantiated in the literature—could potentially indeed be a problem.

The first major objection to acrylic implants is their extreme difficulty of insertion through a small incision. In contrast, the Silastic implants can be easily compressed and bent for insertion through a small incision. Newman et al.[69] described their technique for insertion of the Rish acrylic chin implant and report very satisfactory results in 640 patients. In their hands, the procedure takes only 10 min.

Another major concern with the Rish implant is that of bone resorption. Rish does not address this issue specifically nor does he mention any apparent loss of correction. Newman et al.[69] state that they did not see bone resorption, but this is unsubstantiated by X-ray or xeroradiography. (For a complete discussion of bone resorption beneath alloplastic implants see Section II.C.1 and Section III.C.1 above.)

The third major complaint of the Rish acrylic implant is that its firmness gives an unnatural feel.[70] This complaint seems unfounded. Firm implants such as acrylic and Silastic actually give a more natural feel since they are augmenting a deficiency of hard tissue—bone. A last objection to the Rish acrylic implant is that it may, in thin skinned individuals, leave a palpable and/or visible step-off at the lateral edge.[70] This can be avoided by thinning the edges with a small burr attached to a small hand engine.

Serson[70] mention ''slipping and dislocation'' of acrylic chin implants as a fourth detractor. He does not site personal experience or references for this. However, one could speculate that the migration could be the result of rocking of the implant over a mandible with a curvature smaller than that of the implant. Additionally, the potential for dead space between the implant and a differently shaped mandible could lead to pulling by scar tissue and implant displacement.

The Rish acrylic implant is available in nine sizes, #1 through #5. Newman et al.[69] state that half-size gradations are available, but information obtained from Dr. Rish[71] does not mention these. The amount of projection ranges from 1.0 to 1.4 cm, the height from 0.6 to 1.0 cm, and the width from 3.9 to 4.6 cm. The posterior contour of the implants is standard. The anterior aspect of the implant is fairly standard but can be altered using a rotating burr. These preformed implants incorporate a lip to avoid obliteration of the normal sulcus between the lower lip and the chin. A center notch allows for easy placement and accurate identification of implant location.

2. Malar Augmentation

Methyl methacrylate acrylic has been used for augmentation of posttraumatic malar defects. Schultz[19] discusses in some detail his technique for augmenting these defects with acrylic. While it is technically possible to use acrylic for malar augmentation, it seems to offer little advantage over custom carved Silastic or Proplast. Schultz himself states that his choice of materials for malar augmentation are, in order of preference, autologous iliac crest; Silastic; solid heat cured acrylic formed from a moulage prior to surgery; and lastly, acrylic molded to the defect at the time of surgery. Since the surgical approaches to the malar area involve incisions distant to the zygomatic arch, it would appear to be technically very difficult to quickly mold acrylic deep inside the pocket. Add to this the need to irrigate to cool the tissues, and the task seems formidable.

3. Forehead

This area differs from the malar/zygomatic arch area in that exposure is much better and acrylic can be easily molded *in situ*. The previous scar, a gull wing incision or a coronal flap are frequently used. Also it is easier to judge the final contour and size based on the well-visualized surrounding bony and soft tissue structure (Figure 20).

Since acrylic molds well to irregular bony contours, it could offer a real advantage over Silastic or Proplast in that there is almost no potential for dead space beneath the implant.

VI. SUMMARY

Clearly, facial augmentation can be accomplished with many different materials. The choice is dictated by many factors—acceptance by host tissues, ease with which the material can be removed should rejection occur, ease of insertion, availability of preformed shapes, the surgeon's own personal experience and expertise, and many others.

The chin and malar area lend themselves well to augmentation with any of the four materials discussed—Silastic, Proplast, polyethylene and acrylic. These areas are blessed with good soft-tissue coverage and low mobility, factors important for solid alloplast acceptance.

The submalar area and geniomandibular groove have both been successfully augmented with Silastic. Since these are relatively new procedures, no reports exist regarding the use of Proplast, polyethylene or acrylic. Based on the anatomic location alone, these materials should also be successful. It will be interesting to see what future clinical trials will show.

The temple and forehead both do well with Silastic, Proplast, and acrylic. While there are no reports of polyethylene, the author has had success with polyethylene forehead augmentation.

The nose remains a difficult area to augment with alloplastic materials. Guinta (Silastic) and Sheen (Proplast) have had success with premaxillary augmentation and McCurdy has used Silastic successfully in a large series of non-Caucasian rhinoplasties. While their results are impressive, most studies have demonstrated high rates of rejection and extrusion. Perhaps only by limiting the use of solid implants to the premaxilla with good soft-tissue coverage, or the non-Caucasian nose with thicker skin, will solid implants be successful in augmentation rhinoplasty. It will be interesting to follow the use and development of solid alloplasts in this area.

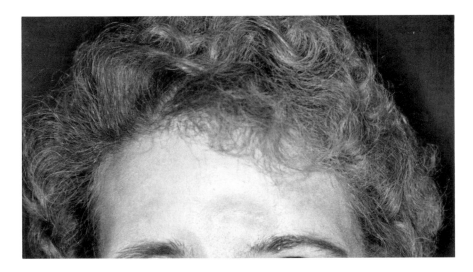

A

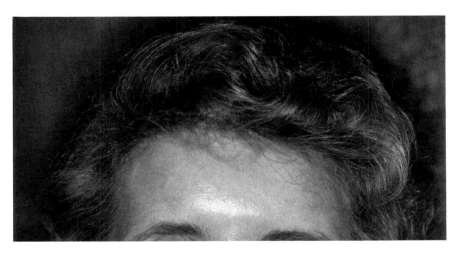

B

FIGURE 20.   (A) Preoperative view of a patient with substantial forehead defect; (B) postoperative view of the same patient following acrylic augmentation. The defect was a result of removal of frontal sinus osteoma.

REFERENCES

1. **Beekhuis, G. J.,** Saddle nose deformity: etiology, prevention, and treatment; augmentation rhinoplasty with polyamide, *Laryngoscope,* 84, 2, 1974.
2. **Landman, M. D., Strahan, R. W., and Ward, P. H.,** Chin augmentation with polytef paste injection, *Arch. Otolaryngol.,* 95, 72, 1972.
3. **Regnault, P. C. L.,** Reconstructive rhinoplasty with nasal implants, *Aesthetic Plast. Surg.,* 4, 79, 1980.
4. **Scales, J. T.,** Tissue reactions to synthetic materials, *Proc. R. Soc. Med.,* 46, 647, 1953.
5. **Adams, B. J. S., and Feuerstein, S. S.,** Looking under the epidermis: a histologic study of implants, in *Plastic and Reconstructive Surgery of the Head and Neck,* Proc. 4th Int. Symp., Vol. I, Ward, P. and Berman, W. E., Eds., C. V. Mosby, St. Louis, 1984, 148.

6. **Binder, W. J., Kamer, F. M., and Parkes, M. L.,** Mentoplasty—a clinical analysis of alloplastic implants, *Laryngoscope,* 91, 383, 1981.
7. **Brenna, H. G.,** Augmentation malarplasty, *Arch. Otolaryngol.,* 108, 441, 1982.
8. **Dmytryshyn, J. R.,** Mentoplasty, *J. Otolaryngol.,* 10, 181, 1981.
9. **Greenwald, A. E.,** Malar augmentation—high cheek bones, *Am. J. Cosm. Surg.,* 1, 29, 1984.
10. **Mahler, D.,** Chin augmentation—a retrospective study, *Ann. Plast. Surg.,* 8, 468, 1982.
11. **Parkes, M. L., Kamer, F. M., and Bassilios, M.,** Experience with gel-filled implants in augmentation mentoplasty, *Arch. Otolaryngol.,* 103, 292, 1977.
12. **Snyder, G. B. et al.,** A new chin implant for microgenia, *Plast. Reconstr. Surg.,* 61, 854, 1978.
13. **Toranto, I. R.,** Mentoplasty: a new approach, *Plast. Reconstr. Surg.,* 69, 875, 1982.
14. **Newman, J., Nguyen, A., and Anderson, R.,** Retrograde suspension malarplasty, *Am. J. Cosm. Surg.,* 3, 7, 1986.
15. **Tobin, H.,** Malar augmentation as an adjunct to facial cosmetic surgery, *Am. J. Cosm. Surg.,* 3, 13, 1986.
16. **Jabaley, M. E., Hoopes, J. E., and Cochran, T. C.,** Transoral Silastic augmentation of the malar region, *Br. J. Plast. Surg.,* 27, 98, 1974.
17. **Binder, W. E.,** Submalar augmentation. An alternative to face-lift surgery, *Arch. Otolaryngol.,* 115, 797, 1989.
18. **Watanabe, K., Miyagi, H., and Tsurukiri, K.,** Augmentation of temporal area by insertion of silicone plate under the temporal fascia, *Ann. Plast. Surg.,* 13, 309, 1984.
19. **Schultz, R. C.,** Reconstruction of facial deformities with alloplastic material, *Ann. Plast. Surg.,* 7, 434, 1981.
20. **Mackay, I. S. and Bull, T. R.,** The fate of Silastic in the management of saddle deformity in the nose, *J. Laryngol. Otol.,* 97, 43, 1983.
21. **Milward, T. M.,** The fate of Silastic and vitrathene nasal implants, *Br. J. Plast. Surg.,* 25, 276, 1972.
22. **Davis, P. B. K. and Jones, S. M.,** The complications of Silastic implants. Experience with 137 consecutive cases, *Br. J. Plast. Surg.,* 24, 405, 1971.
23. **Converse, J. M.,** Restoration of facial contour with bone grafts introduced through the oral cavity, *Plast. Reconst. Surg.,* 6, 295, 1950.
24. **Seltzer, H. M. and Feuerstein, S. S.,** Anatomic considerations in augmentation mentoplasty, in *Plastic and Reconstructive Surgery of the Head and Neck, Proc. 4th Int. Symp.,* Vol. 1, Ward, P. H. and Berman, W. E., Eds., C. V. Mosby, St. Louis, 1984, 442.
25. **Hoffman, S.,** Loss of a Silastic chin implant following dental infection, *Ann. Plast. Surg.,* 7, 484, 1981.
26. **Jobe, R., Iverson, R. and Vistnes, L.,** Bone deformation beneath alloplastic implants, *Plast. Reconstr. Surg.,* 51, 169, 1973.
27. **Peled, I. J. et al.,** Mandibular resorption from Silicone chin implants in children, *J. Oral Maxillofac. Surg.,* 44, 346, 1986.
28. **Robinson, M.,** Bone resorption under plastic chin implants, *Arch. Otolaryngol.,* 95, 30, 1972.
29. **Brown, B. L., Neel, H. B., and Kern, E. B.,** Implants of Supramid, Proplast, Plasti-Pore, and Silastic, *Arch. Otolaryngol.,* 105, 605, 1979.
30. **Hinderer, U. T.,** Malar implants for improvement of the facial appearance, *Plast. Reconstr. Surg.,* 56, 157, 1975.
31. **Freeman, B. S. and Wiemer, D. R.,** Clinical uses of Proplast: Experience and results, in *Biomaterials in Reconstructive Surgery,* Rubin, L., Ed., C. V. Mosby, St. Louis, 1983, 494.
32. **Silver, W. E.,** The use of alloplast material in contouring the face, *Facial Plast. Surg.,* 3, 81, 1986.
33. **Block, M. S., Zide, M. F., and Kent, J. N.,** Proplast augmentation for posttraumatic zygomatic deficiency, *Oral Surg., Oral Med., Oral Pathol.,* 57, 123, 1984.
34. **Kent, J., Westfall, R., and Carlton, D.,** Chin and zygomaticomaxillary augmentation with Proplast, *J. Oral Surg.,* 39, 912, 1981.
35. **Rubin, L. R.,** Polyethylene as a bone and cartilage substitute: a 32 year retrospective, in *Biomaterials in Reconstructive Surgery,* Rubin, L., Ed., C. V. Mosby, St. Louis, 1983, 474.
36. **Wilkinson, T.,** Complications in aesthetic malar augmentation, *Plast. Reconstr. Surg.,* 71, 643, 1983.
37. **O'Quin, B. and Thomas, J. R.,** The role of Silastic in malar augmentation, *Facial Plast. Surg.,* 3, 99, 1986.
38. **Prendergast, M. and Schoenrock, L. D.,** Malar augmentation, *Arch. Otolaryngol. Head Neck Surg.,* 115, 964, 1989.
39. **Agban, G.,** Augmentation and corrective malarplasty, *Bull. Int. Acad. Cosmet. Surg.,* 6, 3, 1981.
40. **Onizuka, T. et al.,** Reduction malarplasty, *Aesthetic Plast. Surg.,* 7, 121, 1983.
41. **Kagan, H. D.,** Sakurai injectable silicone formula, *Arch. Otolaryngol.,* 78, 663, 1963.
42. **Ben-Hur, N. and Neuman, Z.,** Siliconoma—another cutaneous response to dimethylpolysiloxane. Experimental study in mice, *Plast. Reconstr. Surg.,* 36, 629, 1965.
43. **Pearl, R. M., Laub, D. R., and Kaplan, E. N.,** Complications following silicone injections for augmentation of the contours of the face, *Plast. Reconstr. Surg.,* 61, 888, 1978.

44. **Wilkie, T. F.,** Late development of granuloma after liquid silicone injection, *Plast. Reconstr. Surg.,* 60, 179, 1977.

45. **Guinta, S. X.,** Pre-maxillary augmentation. Uses of a new implant in rhinoplasty, Presented at the 3rd Annual Scientific Meeting of the AACS, February 1987 and at the Annual Meeting of the AAFPRS, May 1988.

46. **Beekhuis, G. J.,** Use of silicone-rubber in nasal reconstructive surgery, *Arch. Otolaryngol.,* 86, 88, 1967.

47. **McCurdy, J. A.,** Augmentation rhinoplasty in the oriental nose: Autogenous or alloplastic implants, *Am. J. Cosmet. Surg.,* 6, 33, 1989.

48. **Westfall, R. L., Homsey, C. A., and Kent, J. N.,** A comparison of porous composite PTFE/graphite and PTFE/aluminum oxide facial implants in primates, *J. Oral Maxillofac. Surg.,* 40, 771, 1982.

49. **Homsey, C. A., Cain, T. E., Kessler, F. B., et al.,** Porous implant systems for prosthesis stabilization, *Clin. Orthop.,* 89, 220, 1972.

50. **Arem, A. J., Rasmussen, D., and Madden, J. W.,** Soft tissue response to Proplast: quantitation of scar ingrowth, *Plast. Reconstr. Surg.,* 61, 214, 1978.

51. **Homsey, C. A.,** Implant stabilization. Chemical and biomechanical considerations, *Orthop. Clin. N.A.,* 4, 295, 1973.

52. **Epstein, L. I.,** Clinical experiences with Proplast as an implant, *Plast. Reconstr. Surg.,* 63, 219, 1977.

53. **Whitaker, L. A.,** Facial Proportions in aesthetic surgery, in *Anthroprometric Facial Proportions in Medicine,* Farkas, L. G. and Munro, I. R., Eds., Charles C Thomas, Springfield, 1987, 103.

54. **Sheen, J. H.,** Maxillary augmentation, in *Aesthetic Rhinoplasty,* 2nd ed., Sheen, J. H., Ed., C. V. Mosby, St. Louis, 1987, 283.

55. **Parkes, M. L., Kamer, F. M., and Merrin, M. L.,** Proplast chin augmentation, *Laryngoscope,* 86, 1829, 1976.

56. **Janeke, J. B. and Shea, J. J.,** Self stabilizing Proplast total ossicular replacement prosthesis in tympanoplasty, *Laryngoscope,* 85, 1550, 1975.

57. **Shea, J. J. and Homsey, C. A.,** The use of Proplast in otologic surgery, *Laryngoscope,* 84, 1835, 1974.

58. **Kent, J. N., Homsey, C. A., Gross, B. D., et al.,** Pilot studies of a porous implant in dentistry and oral surgery, *J. Oral Surg.,* 30, 608, 1972.

59. **Hinds, E. C., Homsey, C. A., and Kent, J. K.,** Use of a biocompatible interface for binding tissues and prostheses in temporomandibular joint surgery, *Oral Surg.,* 38, 512, 1974.

60. **Homsey, C. A.,** Biocompatibility of perfluorinated polymers and composites of these polymers, in *Biocompatibility of Clinical Implant Materials,* Vol. 2, Williams, D. F., Ed., CRC Press, Boca Raton, FL, 1980, 59.

61. **Silver, W. E.,** Personal communication.

62. **Rubin, L. R., Bromberg, B. E. and Walden, R. H.,** Long term human reaction to synthetic plastics, *Surg. Gynecol. Obstet.,* 132, 603, 1981.

63. **Rish, B. B.,** Profile-plasty. Report on plastic chin implants, *EENT Monthly,* 41, 274, 1962.

64. **Shea, J. J.,** Biocompatible ossicular implants, *Arch. Otolaryngol.,* 104, 191, 1978.

65. **Homsey, C. A.,** Letters to the editor, *J. Biomed. Mater. Res. Applied Biomaterials,* 22, 351, 1988.

66. **Spector, M., Harmon, S. L., and Kreutner, A.,** Bone growth into porous high-density polyethylene, *J. Biomed. Mater. Res.,* 10, 595, 1976.

67. **Sauer, B. W.,** The use of Medpor surgical implants for craniofacial surgery: a two-year animal study, *Porex Clin. Rep.,* 2, 1985.

68. **Berghaus, A.,** Porous polyethylene in reconstructive head and neck surgery, *Arch. Otolaryngol.,* 111, 154, 1985.

69. **Newman, J., Dolsky, R. L., and Imber, P.,** The Rish acrylic mentoplasty: a re-introduction, *Am. J. Cosmet. Surg.,* 1, 43, 1984.

70. **Serson, D.,** A new technique for chin augmentation, *Plast. Reconstr. Surg.,* 46, 406, 1970.

71. **Rish, B. B.,** Personal communication.

Chapter 18

MESH MATERIALS FOR FACIAL AUGMENTATION

G. Jan Beekhuis and Jeffrey J. Colton

TABLE OF CONTENTS

I. INTRODUCTION

Alloplastic mesh products can successfully be used in facial augmentation. In this chapter, we examine three products—Vicryl mesh, Supramid mesh, and Mersilene mesh. We examine their reaction when implanted in the body, their longevity, and their practical applications and uses. We also discuss our personal experience with Mersilene mesh as it relates to nasal augmentation and reconstruction. We believe strongly that alloplastic mesh products have a definite place in nasal and facial augmentation.

II. MESH PRODUCTS

A. VICRYL™ MESH

Vicryl is polyglactin 910. It is manufactured by Ethicon, Inc. and has been used as an absorbable suture for sometime. In the early 1980s this material was woven into a mesh product and became available for use.

It is well known that Vicryl suture and mesh have a finite life expectancy. Histological analysis has shown that Vicryl is absorbed by 60 d.[1] Studies in the mid-1980s using Vicryl as a dural substitute showed that, although the graft material was resorbed, there was a substantial neomembrane which formed over the zone of the mesh graft.[2] It was also demonstrated that there was little reaction to adjacent cortical zones. If during the absorption period some kind of fibrotic layer (such as this neomembrane) formed, it might be a useful product in certain situations in facial augmentation.

Both Glasgold[3] and Gilmore[4] have utilized Vicryl mesh in rhinoplasty. In cases where the skin is extremely thin and there are slight dorsal irregularities they have placed Vicryl mesh over these irregularities (Figure 1). Both have experienced satisfactory healing. The irregularities have been nicely smoothed and virtually unnoticeable. It is speculated that the deposition of a fibrous layer accounts for this.

Because of its lack of persistence, Vicryl mesh would not be a satisfactory product for significant nasal or facial augmentation. However, as a covering for irregular areas it may be useful.

B. SUPRAMID™ MESH

Supramid is polyamide, a form of nylon. It is available in a variety of products (S. Jackson, Inc.), including suture material and mesh products. The mesh can be obtained in sheet form or prerolled for use in mentoplasty (Figure 2). Supramid mesh has been used in nasal and facial augmentation since the mid-1970s.

Once implanted, Supramid elicits a moderate foreign body response in the host tissues. The response consists of loose granulation tissue and dense granulomas containing mature macrophages and foreign body giant cells[5] (Figure 3). This reaction gradually subsides and may cease at the end of one to two years. Any nylon will give rise to some tissue reaction. Nylon products also undergo hydrolytic degradation. This will cause a reversal of the polymerization reaction which was initially used to form the polymer. This phenomenon results at a gradual loss of tensile strength which may occur at a rate of up to 20% per year. If nylon has been improperly sterilized, this *in vivo* degradation may proceed significantly faster.[6,7] Brown et al. have shown that Supramid strands appear to disintegrate at 6 to 12 months in rabbit face and ear.[8]

Our initial experience with mesh products involved Supramid. We found it useful and easy to use.[9] Clinically, we noticed that over several years there was a loss of correction. This indeed may be related to the phenomenon mentioned in the previous paragraph.

C. MERSILENE™ MESH

Mersilene is a polyester fiber constructed from polyethylene terephthalate. This material

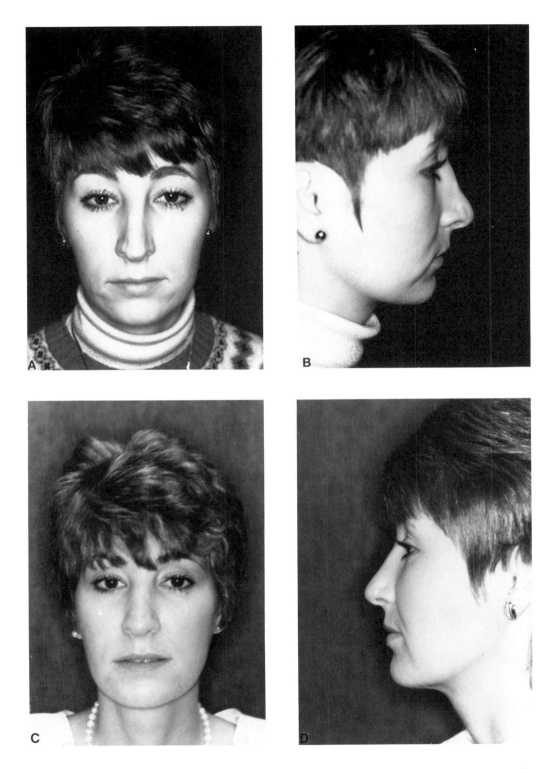

FIGURE 1A—D. Preoperative views of a woman who had previous rhinoplasty surgery (A and B). Postoperative views after revision surgery (C and D). Vicryl mesh was used along the dorsum of the nose as an onlay to smooth irregularities. These postoperative views show a nice smoothing and regular appearance of the nasal dorsum.

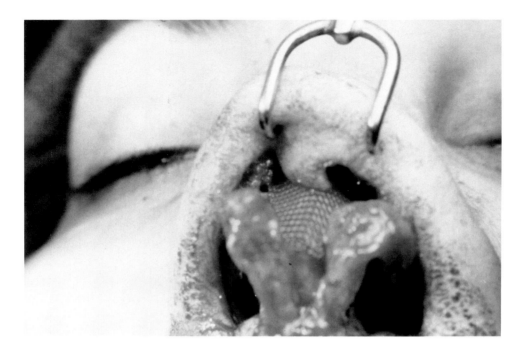

FIGURE 1E.   Vicryl mesh in place along the dorsum of the nose as an onlay to smooth irregularities. This is done through an open technique. (Photographs courtesy of Alvin I. Glasgold, M.D.)

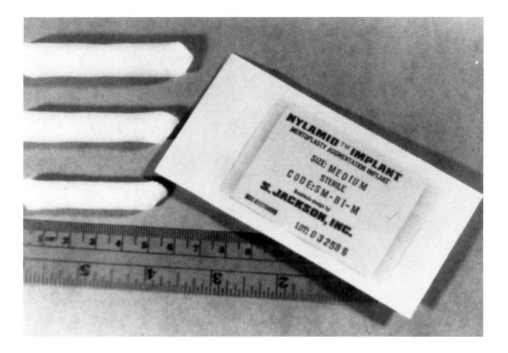

FIGURE 2.   Supramid™ is available in prerolled units for use in augmentation mentoplasty as shown here. It is also available as a suture material and as a flat sheet of mesh.

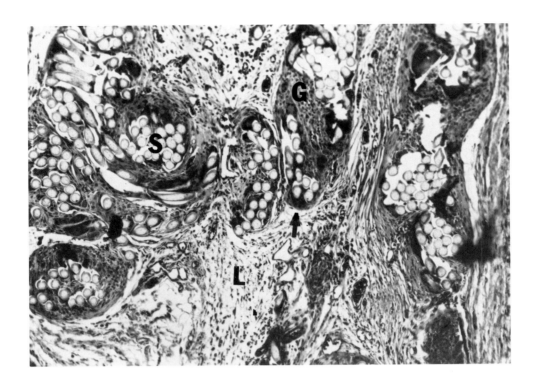

FIGURE 3.   Strands of Supramid® (S) are surrounded by dense granulomas (G) and foreign body giant cells (arrow). Between the strands there is loose granulation tissue (L). (Hematoxylin and eosin stain; magnification × 200) (Photograph   courtesy of Jeanne Adams, M.D.)

is also available as suture and in a mesh form (Ethicon, Inc.). Mersilene mesh is knitted by a process which interlinks each fiber junction. This provides for elasticity in all directions (Figure 4). Such construction also permits the mesh to be cut into any desired shape or size without unraveling. Animal studies have shown that implantation of Mersilene mesh elicits a minimum to slight inflammatory reaction which is transient. This is followed by the deposition of a thin fibrous layer of tissue which can grow through the interstices of the mesh thus incorporating the mesh into surrounding tissue (Figure 5). The mesh remains soft and pliable. The material is not absorbed nor is it subject to degradation or weakening by the action of tissue enzymes.

Clinically, we began using Mersilene mesh in 1985. We have found that it has persisted well without clinical indication of resorption.

III. ADVANTAGES OF MESH PRODUCTS

It might be stated that the ideal prosthetic material should be chemically inert, noncarcinogenic, capable of resisting mechanical stress, capable of being fabricated in the form required, sterilizable yet not physically modified by tissue fluids, or excite an inflammatory or foreign body reaction, or induce a state of allergy or hypersensitivity. While no alloplastic material meets all of these criteria, we believe that certain mesh products (especially Mersilene mesh) may fulfill many of them and, therefore, may be quite useful in facial augmentation.

The more permanent mesh products (Supramid and Mersilene) seemed to offer several advantages.

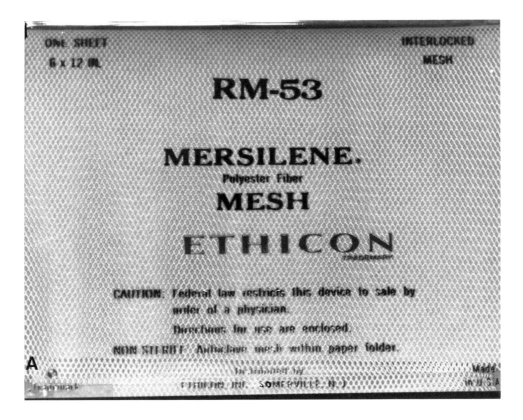

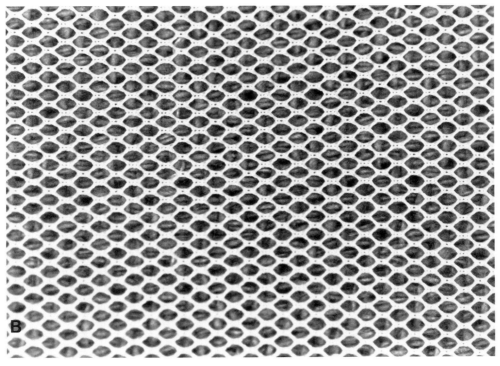

FIGURE 4.   Mersilene mesh is available in sheet form from Ethicon, Inc. (A). High power view of Mersilene™ mesh (B).

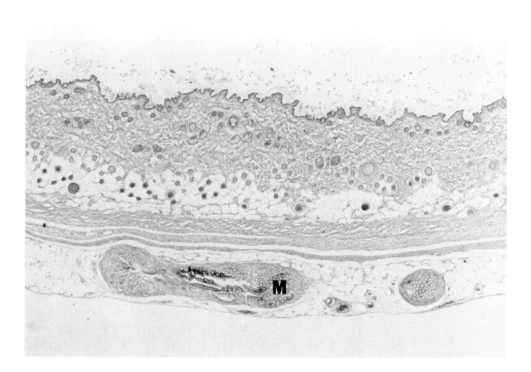

FIGURE 5A. Mersilene mesh (M) implanted in a surgically created abdominal-wall defect (2 × 2 cm segment of abdominal wall musculature removed) in a Long-Evans rat at 28 d following surgery. The individual mesh strands composed of multiple polyester filaments (M) are seen as discrete structures deep to the subcutaneous tissues in the panniculus muscle. Each strand is surrounded by a slight foreign body granuloma composed predominantly of macrophages and fibroblasts with less numerous macrophage giant cells. Note that in the rat model, collagen does not bridge between the strands of Mersilene mesh as it does in the human. (H & E stain; magnification × 50.)

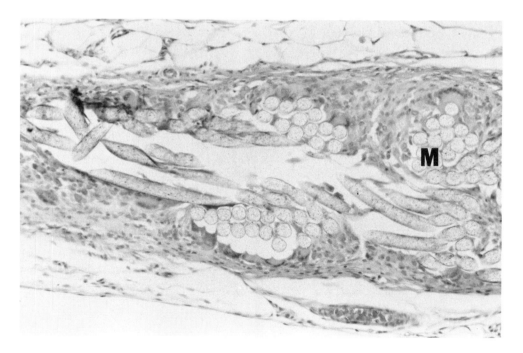

FIGURE 5B. A 250× view of the same section seen in Figure 5A. Results in examination of this tissue at 6 months show a slight decrease in the overall reaction.

1. Mesh is readily available. All mesh implants come in prepackaged sterile containers or containers that may be easily sterilized. These may be kept in inventory for use whenever the surgeon requires it. This is especially useful when large amounts of implant material are needed for augmentation or when augmentation is unexpectedly needed.
2. Mesh is relatively inexpensive. Compared to homograft cartilage, dura, fascia, etc., it is very reasonably priced.
3. There is no need for a second operative site. This can save operative time for the surgeon and it can save recovery time and postoperative pain for the patient. It is common knowledge that recuperation from a bone graft taken from the hip is extremely uncomfortable. Often, recovering from this part of the operation is much more difficult for the patient than recovering from the nasal or facial reconstruction in which the bone graft was used.
4. Mesh implants are very easy to work with. They are easily shaped with scalpel or scissors. They may be finely tailored to suit most any need.
5. Mesh implants have a very natural feel and give a very normal looking appearance. This can be particularly useful in high visibility areas such as the dorsum of the nose. Cartilage, no matter how carefully cut and shaped may give slight irregularities, ridges, and dents. Often these irregularities are not visible for a year or more following the original surgery. Mesh implants do not give this trouble. Mesh implants give a soft natural feel when touched either by the patient or by someone else.
6. Symmetry is easy to achieve. If placement is in a precisely shaped pocket, the roughness of the mesh will help prevent displacement. Fibrous tissue tends to grow into the spaces of the mesh, helping secure the implant and prevent its movement.
7. Mesh implants will absorb antibiotic solution into the spaces of the mesh. This helps lower the infection rate.
8. Mesh implants withstand trauma easily. They are not easily fractured or displaced after healing has been completed.
9. When properly used there is little incidence of infection or rejection. Care must be taken to handle the implant in a sterile fashion, as well as to impregnate the implant with a nonallergic antibiotic solution prior to insertion. If careful technique is observed, incidence of infection is low.

IV. DISADVANTAGES OF MESH PRODUCTS

The use of any alloplast may cause some concern among surgeons. Indeed, when considering any nasal reconstruction or augmentation, the benefits of the material to be used must be weighted against the possible risks and complications associated with that material. The surgeon must evaluate the pros and cons in his experience to decide on the best material.

Use of any alloplast will cause some host reaction to the material. Hopefully the material chosen should have a limited or mild reaction at best. The implantation of any foreign material may cause infection or rejection of the implanted material. Our experience with mesh products has been that, if an antibiotic solution is used to impregnate the implant, the chances of infection and subsequent rejection are small.

Since fibrous tissue tends to grow into the spaces of the mesh implant, its removal may be quite difficult. If the implant must be trimmed, it must be done with sharp dissection. Because of the fibrous tissue ingrowth, total removal of the implant is probably not possible.

V. CLINICAL APPLICATIONS

Mesh materials can be considered for any site requiring augmentation. Since the material does not have much support strength, it works best for areas which require onlay grafting for contour defects. Mesh materials are not particularly useful if rigid support is needed (such as in the area of the tip of the nose). However, mesh materials can be quite useful for augmenting areas such as the dorsum of the nose, the chin, the cheeks, and other facial defects.

In 1979, McCollough and Weil reported the successful use of Mersilene mesh for chin augmentation and for correction and repair of a case of Rhomberg's hemifacial atrophy.[10] They also reported success in recontouring the jawline of a patient who suffered a crush injury of the jaw. Mesh was used to reconstruct the contour at the angle of the mandible. Mersilene mesh can be used to recontour the forehead, to soften the supraorbital prominences found in some people (Figure 6).

Mesh products can be successfully used for chin augmentation. For many years we used Supramid mesh for mentoplasty. A variety of sizes of prerolled Supramid mesh implants are commercially available (Figure 2). Mersilene can be used similarly. It, however, does not come prerolled. It would have to be fashioned at the time of use.

Although we do not have any personal experience with cheek augmentation using mesh products, we believe mesh products could be successfully used in this application.

Our largest clinical experience has been the use of mesh implants to augment the nasal dorsum.[11-17] We feel that, in carefully chosen cases, mesh can be used along the nasal dorsum to achieve repair of a saddle deformity or other deformities along the dorsum of the nose. We will discuss our clinical experience later in this chapter.

We have discussed briefly the use of Vicryl mesh in an onlay technique to help cover irregularities along the dorsum of the nose at the conclusion of rhinoplasty. It is felt that the use of Vicryl, which is absorbed, causes a fibrous layer to form which helps hide cartilage and bony irregularities along the nasal dorsum.

A. TECHNIQUE

No matter which mesh product is chosen and no matter where it is placed, certain basic considerations in technique must be observed. Close attention to proper handling will decrease the chance of infection and rejection of the implant.

The implant itself should be handled only in a sterile manner. We try to avoid touching the implant to the skin even in areas inside the sterile operative field. We believe that this helps prevent the implant from picking up contaminants from the skin which might then be introduced into the implant site. This might cause infection.

Mesh implants should be soaked in an antibiotic solution prior to implantation. We have used liquid Gentamycin successfully for many years. In all likelihood, any broad spectrum liquid antibiotic would be useful and acceptable. The patient should not be allergic to the antibiotic solution selected.

The incision should be kept well away from the implant itself and the implant site. One should strive to create a precise pocket into which the implant is placed. This helps prevent movement and distortion of the implant. The rough nature of the mesh itself will help prevent movement and dislodgement, as well. After healing is well under way, fibrous tissue, which grows through the implant, will further secure it and prevent movement. The implant may be fashioned in any way—it may be tightly rolled, stacked, or folded. A suture may be placed through this rolled or stacked implant for stability. The implant may then be trimmed to the proper size and shape. It is very important to have complete soft-tissue coverage of the implant. A meticulous, careful, tight closure is mandatory. If there is incomplete coverage, infection almost certainly will result. This will necessitate removal of the implant.

When using mesh implants in the nose, it is important to isolate the pocket from the nasal chamber. In such cases, it is best not to separate upper lateral cartilages from the septum or use medial osteotomies. Both of these maneuvers open the pocket created along the dorsum of the nose with the nasal chamber, thus increasing chance for infection in the postoperative period.

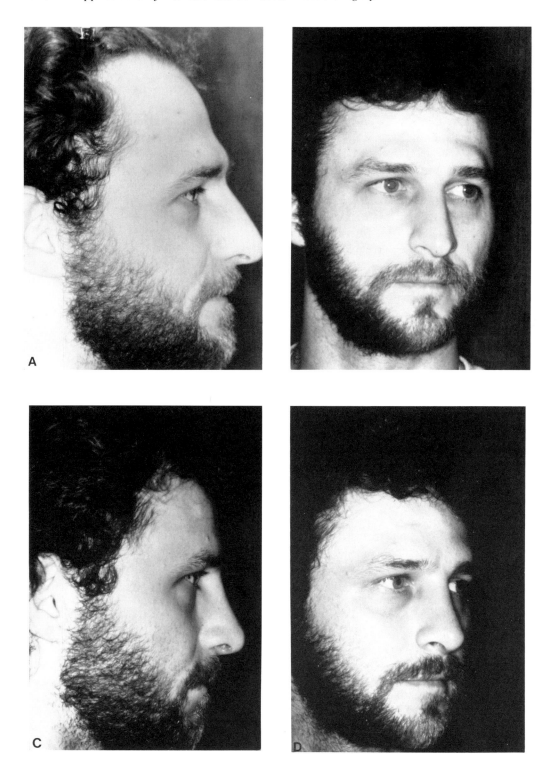

FIGURE 6A—D.   Implantation of Mersilene in the forehead through two separate mid-brow incisions to correct a congenital protrusion of the brow and supraorbital area. This was combined with rhinoplasty. Preoperative photos (A and B) and postoperative correction (C and D) attained with onlay grafting of Mersilene mesh.

TABLE 1
Mersilene Mesh in Nasal and Facial
Augmentation (1985 to Spring 1989)

113 Total cases
  93 Nasal dorsum
    8 Nasal tip and lobule
    1 Supratip area
    4 Nasolabial angle
    1 Premaxilla
    1 Jawline (jowl area)
    5 Chin
   4 Implants removed for infection
    2 Nasal tip
    2 Nasal dorsum

In addition to soaking the implant in an antibiotic solution, we administer intravenous antibiotics (a broad spectrum Cephalosporin) in the preop area. This allows for adequate blood levels at the time of the surgical procedure. Patients are maintained on an oral Cephalosporin for 10 d following the procedure.

When infection has occurred it has usually been in the immediate postoperative period. In the cases where antibiotic has not been successful in resolving the infection the implant has been removed. It has been easily removed because tissue ingrowth has not taken place as yet.

If exposure takes place, this may allow infection to begin secondarily. At early exposure an attempt may be made to close the offending area. We have found that this usually does not work very well. Removal of the implant is usually indicated.

Infection is usually characterized by redness over the implant and foul drainage into the nose. Careful examination usually reveals a small exposed piece of mesh and drainage. A culture can be taken and antibiotics begun. If drainage and smell persist for longer than 7 to 10 d, removal is usually indicated. After a suitable healing period (6 to 8 weeks) the implant can be replaced.

B. PERSONAL CLINICAL EXPERIENCE

Our interest in mesh products for nasal and chin augmentation dates back many years. The senior author (Beekhuis) reported his experience with Supramid mesh in the mid-seventies.[17] We have reported our experience with mesh products periodically from that time.[11-16] The initial experience with Supramid was encouraging. However, in the early eighties it appeared that the Supramid was resorbing. Patients who have received implants in both the nose and the chin were returning with the loss of the original correction. For this reason we looked for a suitable alternative to the Supramid mesh. We believe that we have found a suitable alternative in Mersilene mesh.

Our experience with Mersilene mesh began in 1985. Primarily, Mersilene mesh has been used for augmentation of the nasal dorsum. Five years later the material seems to be holding up well. We have not encountered problems with resorption. There have been few postoperative infections, signs of inflammation, or rejection.

Mersilene mesh has been used in 113 cases (through the spring of 1989). Primarily, it has been for augmentation of the nasal dorsum in postrhinoplasty or saddle nose deformity reconstructions. The early results seem quite gratifying. In small numbers of cases we began to use mesh in other places around the nose (see Table 1). Small pieces of mesh were used to plump the nasal labial angle when cartilage was not readily available. The same principle was applied to the nasal tip. Small ball-like pieces of implant were placed into the nasal tip to increase tip projection and definition.

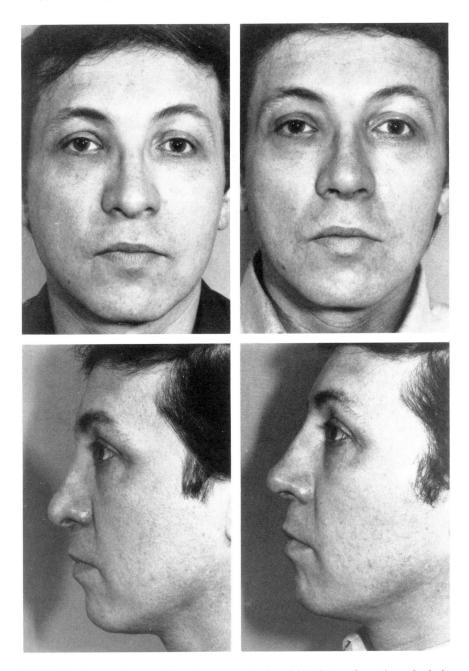

FIGURE 7.   Preoperative (on left) and postoperative (on right) photos of a patient who had a traumatic nasal deformity and previous rhinoplasty done approximately 2 years before to correct the problem. At the time of his original surgery, he underwent nasal polypectomy and developed a septal perforation. The current surgery consisted of placement of a silicone septal button and removal of polyps. Irradiated cartilage was used to support the nasal tip and Mersilene mesh was used along the nasal dorsum for augmentation. He did not wish augmentation mentoplasty which was suggested.

We have used mesh for chin augmentation. We have, however, almost exclusively changed to Silastic chin implants for chin augmentation. This is because we have enjoyed the wide variety of shapes and sizes available for mentoplasty procedures.

Almost universally the mesh implants used along the dorsum of the nose have been well tolerated (see Figures 7, 8, 9). There have been occasional infections which have required

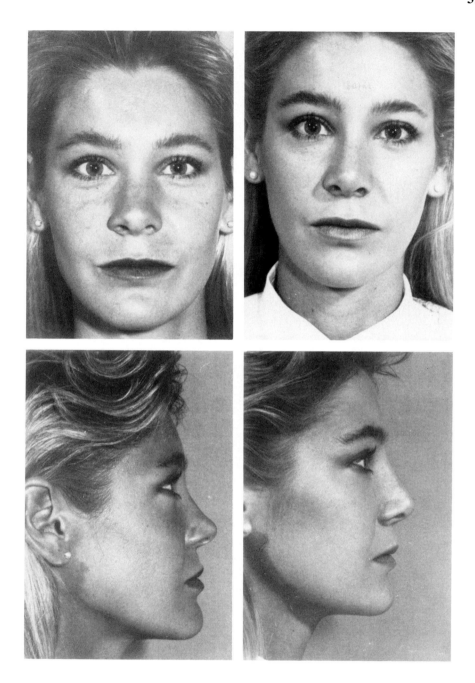

FIGURE 8. Preoperative (on left) and postoperative (on right) photos of a patient who had undergone two rhinoplasties many years previously. The patient had very little structural support in the septum. Mersilene mesh was used along the nasal dorsum and irradiated cartilage was used to support the nasal tip.

antibiotic treatment. Four of these infections were resolved with appropriate antibiotic care. Four were not resolved and the implants were removed because of the infection.

To the best of our knowledge the mesh implants along the dorsum of the nose have persisted without resorption and have remained satisfactory for 5 years.

Approximately a year and a half ago, feeling comfortable with the safety and persistence of Mersilene mesh, we began to use it in certain other areas (Table 1). In our experience

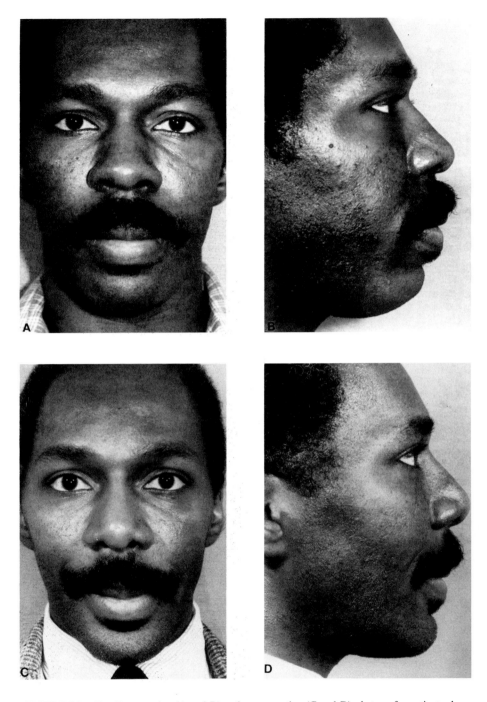

FIGURE 9A—D.   Preoperative (A and B) and postoperative (C and D) photos of a patient who underwent primary rhinoplasty surgery with augmentation of the nasal bridge using Mersilene™ mesh. The nasal lobule was narrowed and chin augmentation was accomplished with Silastic™ chin implant.

mesh grafts placed in the tip of the nose have not fared as well as those placed along the dorsum. Twenty-five percent of these have become infected or exposed and removal has been necessary. We can only speculate about reasons for this occurring. Perhaps areas of higher movement do not allow for good fixation. Placing a graft in the nasal tip requires an incision through the hair-bearing skin of the nasal vestibule. This may introduce infection, or in some other way create an unfavorable environment for subsequent stabilization and fixation of the implant. Implants used in other selective areas seem to be tolerated well, at least thus far.

Those implants which have been used in the chin have been very well tolerated.

VI. SUMMARY

Every procedure in surgery carries certain possible advantages and disadvantages. Each physician must weigh a multitude of factors including potential advantages and disadvantages before deciding how best to treat his patient. This certainly is true in choosing implant materials for facial augmentation. The authors have had long experience with the use of mesh implants to augment the nose and chin. The results have been quite gratifying except for the long term resorption of the Supramid mesh. Because of this, Mersilene mesh has been used and found to be more persistent. We believe it has the benefits of any mesh product and does not seem to have any unusual disadvantages. Although our main indication for using Mersilene mesh remains augmentation along the nasal dorsum, we feel that mesh products can be safely used to correct any facial defect as long as the principles of use are closely followed. At this point we can report no evidence of resorption of Mersilene mesh. Our overall complication and rejection rate has been low.

We feel that mesh products, especially Mersilene mesh, are safe and useful products for certain cases of facial and nasal augmentation.

REFERENCES

1. **Jenkins, S. D. et al.,** A comparison of prosthetic materials used to repair abdominal wall defects, *Surgery,* 94, 392, 1983.
2. **Maurer, P. K. et al.,** Vicryl (Polyglactine 910) mesh as a dural substitute, *J. Neurosurg.,* 63, 448, 1985.
3. **Glasgold, A. I.,** Personal communication.
4. **Gilmore, J.,** Personal communication.
5. **Adams, J.,** Grafts and implants in nasal and chin augmentation: a rational approach to material selection, in *Oto clinics of North America,* W. B. Saunders, Philadelphia, 1987, 913.
6. **Kronenthal, R. L.,** Intraocular degradation of nonabsorbable sutures, *Am. Intra-Ocular Implant Soc. J.,* 3, 222, 1977.
7. **Postlethwait, R. W.,** Long term comparative study of nonabsorbable sutures, *Ann. Surg.,* 171, 892, 1970.
8. **Brown, B. L., Neal, H. B., and Kern, S. B.,** Implants of superficial Proplast, Plasti-pore, and Silastic, *Arch. Otolaryngol.,* 105, 605, 1979.
9. **Beekhuis, G. J.,** Surgical correction of saddle nose deformity, *Trans. Am. Acad. Ophthalmol. Otolaryngol.,* 103, 461, 1977.
10. **McCollough, E. G. and Weil, C.,** Augmentation of facial defects using Mersilene mesh implants, *Otolaryngol. Head Neck Surg.,* 87, 515, 1979.
11. **Beekhuis, G. J.,** Alloplastic implants in facial plastic surgery: Use of Supramid mesh, in *Plastic and Reconstructive Surgery of the Head and Neck,* Ward, P. H. and Berman, W. E., Eds., C. V. Mosby, St. Louis, 1984, 129.
12. **Beekhuis, G. J.,** Augmentation mentoplasty using Polyamide mesh, *Laryngoscope,* 86, 1602, 1976.
13. **Beekhuis, G. J.,** Augmentation mentoplasty with Polyamide mesh: update, *Arch. Otolaryngol.,* 110, 364, 1984.
14. **Beekhuis, G. J.,** Polyamide mesh implants in revision rhinoplasty and the severely traumatized nose, *Laryngoscope,* 90, 339, 1980.
15. **Beekhuis, G. J.,** Polyamide mesh used in facial plastic surgery, *Arch. Otolaryngol.,* 106, 642, 1980.
16. **Beekhuis, G. J.,** Saddle nose deformity, in *Current Therapy in Otolaryngology—Head and Neck Surgery,* Gates, G. A., Ed., B. C. Decker, Trenton, 1982, 126.
17. **Beekhuis, G. J.,** Saddle nose deformity: etiology, prevention, and treatment; augmentation rhinoplasty with Polyamide, *Laryngoscope,* 84, 2, 1974.

Chapter 19

USE OF HYDROXYAPATITE, TRICALCIUMPHOSPHATE, AND GORE-TEX® IN FACIAL AUGMENTATION AND FACIAL RECONSTRUCTION

Claus Walter

TABLE OF CONTENTS

I. INTRODUCTION

Tissue loss is a consequence of normal aging, fat degeneration, and bony atrophy. In addition, other instances that result in tissue loss include excisional therapy for treatment of malignant cancer involving bony structures, as well as injuries resulting from automobile, bicycle, aviation travel, sports, and work related accidents. According to Hensch two to three million artificial prosthetic parts are implanted each year in the U.S. as a consequence of these injuries.[1]

Choosing the most suitable graft or implant material for tissue augmentation can be difficult as there are a number of good materials available, all having particular advantages and disadvantages. The surgeon must consider the characteristics of both the material (e.g., firmness, ease of contouring, degree of absorption, availability, biocompatability), and site of implantation.

Materials for implantation can be classified as being either biologic or synthetic. The biologic materials include autogenous tissues (e.g., cartilage, bone, fat), homografts (e.g., irradiated cartilage), and heterografts (e.g., cartilage, bone, collagen). Synthetic or alloplastic materials that have been used include silicone (fluid or solid silastic), Proplast®, Supramid®, hydroxyapatite and PTFE. During the past 10 years, we have almost exclusively used methylmethacrylate, hydroxyapatite and polytetrafluoroethylene (PTFE) for facial reconstruction.[2]

Selection of an implant is based upon several factors. The biomaterial used must be nontoxic to host tissues in cell culture screening tests or short-term animal implantation tests. In addition, it must not initiate an immune response nor cause infection. Finally, the match in physical properties between the host tissue and implant is a formidable scientific challenge. Development of biomaterials that have physical properties similar to host tissue, that are nonallergenic, nontoxic, and prevent bacteriological growth is the goal of materials research.[3]

Inert biomaterials are differentiated from reactive ones by virtue of the fibrous tissue capsule that surrounds an implant. Inert materials are associated with only a thin fibrous capsule while reactive materials are surrounded by a thick capsule. Progressive thickening and contraction of capsules surrounding silicone breast implants produce pain and necrosis of underlying tissues because of the material reactivity.

II. BIOCERAMIC IMPLANTS

A. BACKGROUND AND GENERAL INFORMATION

Hench[1] points out that interfacial problems associated with "inert" biomaterials have led to intensive research during the last decade directed at stabilizing the tissue-biomaterial interface. This requires surface depressions or pores that are large enough for cells to cross the interface. In this manner fibrous tissue connects the host tissue to the implant and increases the interfacial area between the two materials.

One consequence of the large interfacial surface area is the possibility of rapid corrosion and biodegradation of an implant. Bioceramics have potential for microstructural control of the interface without formation of potentially toxic corrosion products. Of other materials, only titanium possesses sufficient corrosion resistance to be considered for use as a porous implant.

Quantitative analysis of the growth of tissue into pores with different sizes shows that soft connective tissue will grow into pores greater than 50 μm in diameter and remain healthy over periods over at least several years. Bone will grow into pores bigger than 100 μm.[4]

According to Roth and co-workers,[5] hydroxyapatite and tricalciumphosphate with the same porosity but with different pore sizes were implanted into the metaphysis of the distal femur bones in rabbits up to 6 months. The hydroxyapatite ceramic was not resorbed whereas up to 85% of the tricalciumphosphate material was degraded after 6 months. The rate of implant substitution by bony ingrowth for tricalciumphosphate and hydroxyapatite depended upon pore size. The implant with the smaller pore size range (50 to 100 μm) showed a significantly higher rate of implant degradation and bony ingrowth than the implants with a larger pore size range (200 to 400 μm). Preexisting pore interconnections up to 20 μm in diameter between the smaller pores allow rapid ingrowth of vessels and cells involved in implant resorption and bone formation.

Certain conclusions can be drawn from the results of animal studies. The existence of pore interconnections rather than pore size determines the rate of bone ingrowth and in the case of tricalciumphosphate the rate of implant resorption. Tricalciumphosphate is biodegradable whereas practially no degradation takes place in hydroxyapatite. Bearing in mind these facts, one can choose the adequate ceramic material for the application such as bone substitution or drug delivery. Ceramics with smaller pore sizes are of future interest because rapid tissue ingrowth is in most situations an important advantage.[6]

Tricalciumphosphate and hydroxyapatite are powderous ground substances and can be converted into granules and blocks of different micropore sizes by a chemical/physical process (Fa. Friedrichsfeld, Mannhein, Fa. Ceros, and other companies).

Approximately 12 years ago we were confronted with the interesting experimental work and publications by De Groot and Osborn[7] who used hydroxyapatite and tricalciumphosphate in the facial region.

In conjunction with the ENT-Department of the University of Munich, Klinikum rechts der Isaar, over 300 implants in the head and neck field were used and observed. The producer (Fa. Friedrichsfeld, Mannhein, Fa. Ceros) supplied blocks and granules. Our clinical experience with these two implant materials based on X-ray analysis of implants indicate that hydroxyapatite is resorbed more slowly than tricalciumphosphate which is readily resorbed, but total replacement of the hydroxyapatite granules by newly formed bone tissue is not observed. Total replacement of hydroxyapatite or tricalciumphosphate by new bony ingrowth, as well as replacement of only the surface structures invaded by newly formed bone are not observed. However, this material retains its bulk and is fixed to the surrounding tissue by bony ingrowth allowing facial tissue augmentation or filling of cysts.

In the past, it was difficult to choose which of these two materials to use in facial augmentation. Although hydroxyapatite is brittle and therefore difficult to carve, it remains intact for longer periods when implanted. In addition, one has the choice of materials with small or large pore diameters. In comparison, tricalciumphosphate is easier to carve and work with; however, its higher absorption rate is a problem.

Recently, the Ceros Company has come up with the new combination of hydroxyapatite and tricalciumphosphate which combines both positive features; it is easy to carve and drill but offers the advantages of hydroxyapatite for longer lasting implant correction of facial defects.

B. CLINICAL STUDIES

We have used the above named materials (hydroxyapatite and tricalciumphosphate) all over the facial skeleton for augmentation over 8 years on more than 300 patients.

It was inserted into the forehead, and particularly the supraorbital rim, to augment bony tissue loss after trauma or other surgical interventions in maxillary canine fossa and the infraorbital rim. There is a wide use to build up the premaxilla, and especially in mandibular reconstruction, we found its use very successful.

Before the operation begins, the size of the implant needed is measured using a moulage of wax or a piece of silicone which is applied externally or into the pocket which is created for inserting the implant. The size of the moulage gives the surgeon a model to copy when cutting the block of hydroxyapatite or tricalciumphosphate (Figure 1).

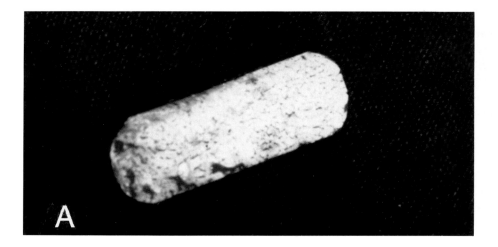

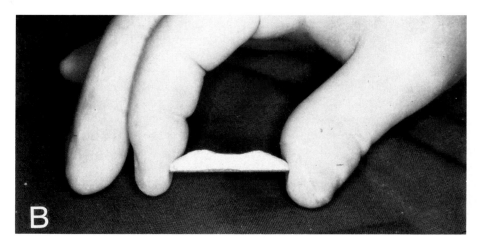

FIGURE 1.   Photographs showing a block of hydroxyapatite before (A) and after carving (B) to form a chin implant.

After using several approaches, we found that a diamond-dust plated, circular saw, similar to what dentists use, was a most useful device for carving the blocks. We used a motor-driven handpiece similar to that used in ear and maxillofacial surgery, and under constant cooling of the saw blade and cooling of the implant with water, we succeeded in avoiding excessive dust production and overheating of the saw. Tilting the instrument and the saw blade, we carved the implant into the desired shape, smoothed the sharp edges, and excavated the implant according to the facial bone contours.

As another safeguard against infection we placed the final product into a syringe of 10 or 20 cc filled with an antibiotic solution. By pulling on the piston of the syringe while closing the outlet, we created a vacuum. The applied vacuum pulled out the remaining air bubbles from the implant and allowed the antibiotic solution to enter the implant.

The pocket found in the host tissue should be of sufficient size to allow the implant to be inserted without great force and to avoid breaking the implant. It must be placed flat on the host surface because kinking of the implant may cause it to break.

While we had very good success in the augmentation of facial areas (Figures 2 and 3), the use of hydroxyapatite or tricalciumphosphate in nasal surgery was a bit disappointing. They cannot be used in the columella because there is no bony contact, resulting in more rapid absorption. In the nasal dorsum they were only useful over the bony portions because

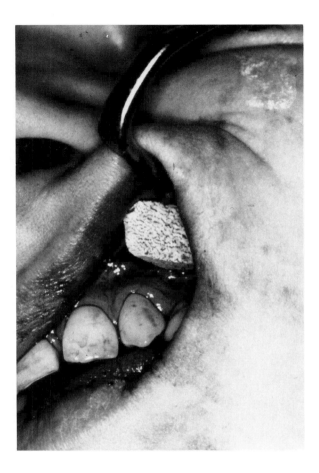

FIGURE 2.   Photograph of a block of tricalciumphosphate used for
nasolabial augmentation.

they could not withstand the constant motion when placed over the cartilaginous part of the nose.

In some of our cases additional augmentation or further carving, after the first intervention, allowed us to remove small portions of this implant. We found that the implant was so well embedded that we could chisel away and drill away parts of its surface for histological examination. We were able to use more of the implant by laying it on top of the well-embedded piece of hydroxyapatite.

In four cases in which the implant had to be partially removed, we found that there were only loose pieces with rather sharp edges which had broken off from the original piece.

Based on the very favorable long-lasting results obtained using hydroxyapatite and tricalciumphosphate, we can recommend their further use in all those cases in which there is a very well-defined bony bed. The newer combination of tricalciumphosphate and hydroxyapatite (Ceros) offers even further advantages by allowing screws to be drilled into it or use of circumferential wiring to secure the implant to the host bone. Using hydroxyapatite alone was not always possible. To assure a good long-lasting result the implant must be carved to have as large a bony contact as possible.

These implants fulfill almost ideally Hulbert's three postulations of ready availability, noncarcinogenic, and nonallergenic stimulation of bony invasion, and allowing tissue ingrowth on the surface, avoiding dead spaces or capsule formation.

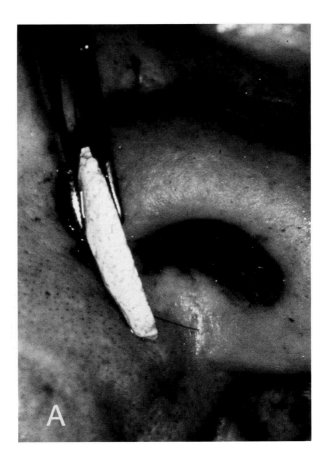

FIGURE 3.   Photograph showing approximate placement of a carved block of hydroxyapatite prior to implantation into the base of the nose to prevent nasal alar collapse and elevation of the floor of the nose (A) and post-op X-ray of implant (B) showing location (arrow).

III. GORE-TEX® SOFT-TISSUE IMPLANTS

A. BACKGROUND AND GENERAL INFORMATION

Use of polytetrafluoroethylene (PTFE) to replace large diameter vessels dates back to 1975 when the GORE-TEX® reinforced expanded PTFE vascular graft was introduced.[8] The high tensile strength, low deformation under load,[8] ability to incorporate tissue ingrowth, and the absence of a foreign body response[9] make expanded PTFE a suitable candidate for use in a variety of medical applications (Figure 4).

Some of these applications include use in hernia repair,[10-14] chest wall resection,[15] rectal prolapse,[16] augmentation of nasal dorsum,[17] and treatment of facial paralysis.[18,19] GORE-TEX® soft tissue patches are available in the U.S. from W. L. Gore & Associates, Inc., Flagstaff, AZ, 86002 and in Europe from W. L. Gore & Associates, Hermann-Oberth-Str. 22, D-8011, Putzbrunn, or its affiliates. These patches are available in varying sizes (5 × 10 cm, 10 × 5 cm, 15 × 20 cm, or 20 × 30 cm) in thicknesses of 1 and 2 mm and can be trimmed into appropriate size and shape for use in many facial cosmetic and reconstructive procedures.

B. CLINICAL USE

From January 1987 to February 1989, GORE-TEX® was implanted in 135 patients. The areas of implantation were as follows:

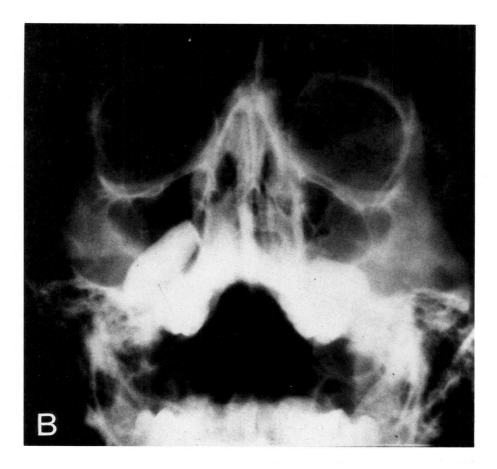

FIGURE 3B

	No. of procedures/patients
1. Nasolabial folds	66
2. Glabellar frown lines	22
3. Mandible - mentum	7
- body	5
4. Perioral, lip	7
5. Malar, zygomatic	13
6. Forehead (in conjunction with forehead lift)	5
7. Auricle and postauricular	1
8. Nasal dorsum	9

These implantations were performed under either local or general anesthesia and often in combination with other procedures which most commonly were facelifts, rhinoplasties, or total profile plasties.

The method of implantation varied according to the site of augmentation but basically it was either placed directly into a subcutaneous or subperiosteal pocket or inserted with a pull-through technique. This latter technique involves attaching a strip of GORE-TEX® to a suture and Keith needle. The needle and attached graft are pulled through a subcutaneous tunnel and once the needle is withdrawn from the skin, the suture is cut and removed, leaving the graft in place. This technique is useful to ensure smooth, even augmentation of long and narrow areas (nasolabial fold, glabellar frown lines). Specific methods of implantation of each site are described as follows.

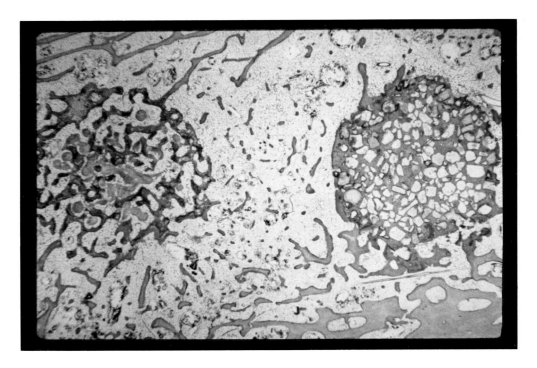

FIGURE 4. Light micrograph of GORE-TEX® soft tissue implant showing fibers and pores (arrow) that allow for cellular ingrowth. (Magnification × 50.)

Nasolabial folds—This area is augmented by making stab incisions along the floor of both nasal vestibules or less commonly at the alar margin at the superior end of the nasolabial fold. A narrow subcutaneous tunnel beneath the fold is then developed, and a thin 3 to 4 mm wide strip of GORE-TEX® is then placed usually with a pull through technique from a superior to inferior direction (Figures 5 and 6). Alternatively, several small pieces of GORE-TEX® may be placed directly into the tunnel. Either technique is supplemented with the placement of horizontal mattress sutures which are kept in place for two days as an attempt to add an everting force to the fold. Antibiotic caplets are placed into the wound if a nasal vestibular incision is used. Both incisions are closed primarily.

Glabellar frown line augmentation or filling up nasal defects—is performed through a stab incision at the inferior aspect of the frown line and after developing a subcutaneous tunnel, a thin strip of GORE-TEX® is advanced beneath the frown line with a pull through technique.

Chin augmentation—is usually performed via an intraoral incision through which several pieces of GORE-TEX® may be layered in a subperiosteal pocket.

Mandibular body augmentation—is achieved via a submental approach through which a subperiosteal pocket can be developed and a suitable sized implant placed with a pull through technique (Figure 7).

Lip augmentation—is performed by pulling the implant directly into the subcutaneous tissue without elevating a tunnel. This is achieved with a pull through technique via stab incision at the oral commissures (Figure 8).

Malar and zygomatic augmentation—is performed by direct placement of the implant via an intraoral or skin incision.

For implantation and augmentation during coronal forehead lifts, the GORE-TEX® can be placed as 1.5 to 2 cm strips across the pericranium of the glabellar and forehead areas. It is used in an attempt to smooth the defects caused by resection of the frontalis and corrugator muscles.

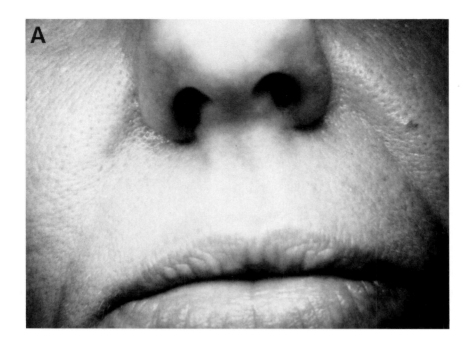

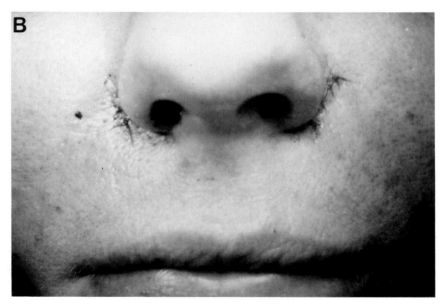

FIGURE 5. Photographs showing pre-op (A) and post-op views (B) of a patient treated with GORE-TEX® soft tissue patch for augmentation of the nasolabial region using an external approach.

Whenever the implant is placed through anything larger than a stab incision (e.g., forehead lift, malar augmentation), use of fibrin glue or a dissolvable suture is advisable to help maintain initial implant placement until soft tissue ingrowth occurs.

Aesthetic results with GORE-TEX® implantation and augmentation in patients treated so far have been comparable and in many ways better than results with the use of other biologic or synthetic materials. Advantages of GORE-TEX® are its ease of insertion, biocompatibility with minimal tissue reaction, and lack of absorption. It is a firm yet malleable material which allows the surgeon to accurately augment the specific defect. If revision is

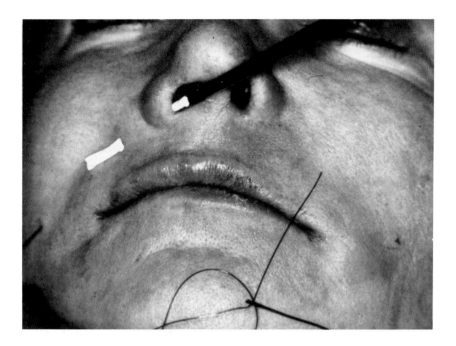

FIGURE 6.   Photograph showing a view of a patient treated with GORE-TEX® soft tissue patch for augmentation of the nasolabial region using an infranasal approach.

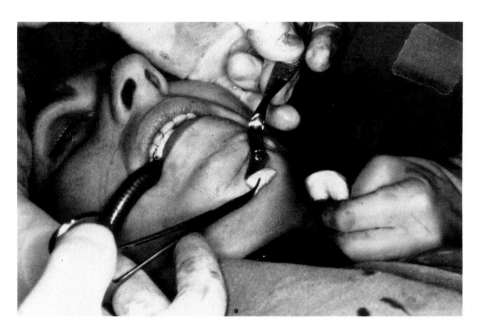

FIGURE 7.   Photograph showing approximate placement of GORE-TEX® soft tissue patch for mandibular augmentation.

needed early on in the postoperative period, the implant can be remodeled or revised with ease. Of the 135 patients receiving GORE-TEX® implants, only two developed infections resulting in extrusion of the implant. Following removal of the GORE-TEX® and local wound care and antibiotics both patients healed well with no significant cosmetic defect arising from the procedure.

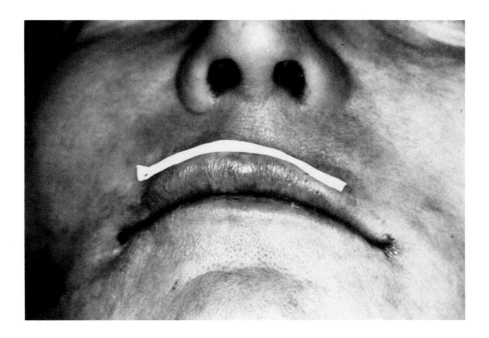

FIGURE 8.   Photograph showing approximate placement of GORE-TEX® soft tissue patch for lip augmentation.

In summary, GORE-TEX® has been successfully used for a variety of facial cosmetic and reconstructive problems as described. The ease of use, minimal morbidity and lack of absorption all make this material a very desirable option for tissue augmentation.

REFERENCES

1. **Hench, L. L.,** Biomaterials, *Science,* 208, 23, 1980.
2. **Berghaus, A., Axhausen,M., and Handrock, M.,** Porose Kunststoffe fur die Ohrmuschelplastik, *Laryngol. Rhinol. Otol.,* 62, 1983.
3. **Hulbert, S. F., Morrison, S. J., and Klawiterr, J. J.,** Tissue reaction to three ceramics of porous and non-porous structures, *J. Biomed. Mater. Res.,* 6, 347, 1972.
4. **Pizzoferrato, A.,** Biomaterials and clinical applications, *Proc. 6th Eur. Conf.,* Biomaterials, Bologna, Italy, September 1986.
5. **Roth, H., Muller, W., and Spiessl, B.,** Zur Behandlung grossvolumiger Knochendefekte im Kieferbereich mit Hydroxylapatite-Granulat, *Schweiz. Mschr. Zahnmed.,* 94, 222, 1984.
6. **Horch, H. H. and Koster, K.,** Resorbierbare Calciumphophatskeramik zur Fullung enoraler Knochendefekte—eine neue Methode der Behandlung grosser Zysten. Vortrag 29 Kongress der Deut. Ges. F. Mund-, Kiefer- u.d. Gesichtschir, Linz, 1979.
7. **DeGroot, K.,** Bioceramics consisting of calciumphosphate salts, *Biomaterials,* 1, 47, 1989; **Osborn, J. F.,** Implantawerkstoff Hydroxylapatile-Keramik, Grundiagen und Klinische Anwendung, Quintesseny-Verlay, Berlin, 1985.
8. **Boyce, B.,** Physical characteristics of expanded polytetrafluoroethylene grafts, in *Biologic and Synthetic Vascular Prostheses,* Stanley, J. C., Ed., Grune & Stratton, New York, 1982, 553.
9. **Silver, F. H. and Doillon, C. J.,** Cardiovascular implants, in *Biocompatibility: Interactions of Biological and Implantable Materials,* VCH Publishers, New York, 243, 1989.
10. **Bauer, J. J., Salky, B. A., Gelernt, I. M., and Kreel, I.,** Repair of large abdominal wall defects with expanded polytetrafluoroethylene (PTFE), *Ann. Surg.,* 206, 765, 1987.
11. **Hamer-Hodges, D. W. and Scott, N. B.,** Replacement of an abdominal wall defect using expanded PTFE sheet GORE-TEX®, *J. R. Coll. Surg. Edinburgh,* 30, 65, 1985.

12. **Murphy, J. L., Freeman, J. B., and Dionne, P. G.,** Comparison of Marlex and GORE-TEX® to repair abdominal wall defects in the rat, *Can. J. Surg.,* 32, 244, 1989.

13. **Smith, S., Gantt, N., Rowe, M. I., and Lloyd, D.,** Dura versus GORE-TEX® as an abdominal wall prosthesis in an open and closed infected model, *J. Pediatr. Surg.,* 24, 519, 1989.

14. **Wool, N. L., Straus, A. K., and Roseman, D. L.,** Clinical experience with the GORE-TEX® soft tissue patch in hernia repair: a preliminary report, *Proc. Inst. Med. Chicago,* 38, 33, 1985.

15. **Grosfeld, J. L. et al.,** Chest wall resection and reconstruction for malignant conditions in childhood, *J. Pediatr. Surg.,* 76, 803, 1989.

16. **McMahan, J. D. and Ripstein, C. B.,** Rectal prolapse: an update on the rectal sling procedure, *Am. Surg.,* 53, 37, 1987.

17. **Rothstein, S. G. and Jacobs, J. B.,** The use of GORE-TEX® implants in nasal augmentation operations, *EN Technol.,* September, 40, 1989.

18. **Daigeler, V. R. and Bohmert, H.,** Masseterplastik bei-fazialisparel, *Fortschr. Med.,* 15, 304, 1986.

19. **Levet, Y. and Jost, G.,** Utilisation du polytetrafluorethylene (GORE-TEX® E-PTFE soft tissue patch), *Ann. Oto Laryngol. (Paris),* 104, 65, 1987.

Index

INDEX

A

B

C

Columella strut, 120—122
Compact bone, see Bone, compact (Haversion)
Complement, 67—69
Conchal cartilage, see Cartilage, auricular
Connective tissue, 103
Connective tissue disease, see Adjuvant disease;
    Scleroderma, linear
Contamination, 93
Contour elevation, 226—227
Core proteins, 136—137
Cornea, 13
Corneocyte envelope, 9
Corneum, see Stratum corneum
Corrosion, 89
Cortical bone, see Bone, compact (Haversion)
Costal cartilage, see Cartilage, costal
Coup de sabre, see Scleroderma, linear
C-propeptide, see Chondrocalcin
Cranial bone, see Bone, cranial
Craniofacial bone, see Bone, craniofacial
Craniotomy, 202, 206
Creep experiment, 54
Creeping substitution, 170
Creutzfeldt-Jacob disease, 207
Cryofixation, 39, 41—42
CSF fistula closure, 201
Cytoactin, see Hexabrachion
Cytocrine secretion, 34

D

DBM, see Demineralized bone matrix
Decorin (DS-PGII), 14—15, 17
Decortication, 159—161
Decubitus ulcers, see Ulcers, decubitus
Deformation, 300
Demineralized bone, see Bone, demineralized
Demineralized bone matrix (DBM), 71
Dendritic cells, 34
Dental implants, 166
Dermatan sulfate, 12, 15, 35—36, 39, see also
    Glycosaminoglycans; Proteoglycans
Dermis, 8, 11—13, 35—38, 66, see also Skin
Dermo-epidermal junction, 33, 35
Dermographism, 233
Desmocollins, 9
Desmogleins, 9
Desmoplakins, 9, 12
Desmosomes, 8—9, 30
Diaphysis, 46, 48
Disinfection, 102
Disjunctum, see Stratum disjunctum
Donnan osmotic pressure, 53—54
Drift, 229, 235—236, see also Silicone, injectable-
    grade
DS-PGI, see Biglycan
DS-PGII, see Decorin
Dura mater, 103, 203—204, 207
Dyschromia, 234

E

Earlobes, 228
Ecchymosis, 233
Eccrine glands, 37
Ectoderm, 30—31, 34
Ectopic bone formation assay, 174
Edema, 233
Elastase, 140
Elastic cartilage, see Cartilage, elastic (hyaline)
Elastic fibers, 35, 44, 82—83
Elastic force, 138—139
Elastin, 11—12, 51—52
Elastin mRNA, 83
Electrochemical charge, 171—172
Electron Spectroscopy for Chemical Analysis
    (ESCA), 93—94
Embolism, 235
EMLA, 248
End bulbs of Krause, see Bulbs of Krause
Endochondral ossification, see Ossification
Endosteal surface, 46
Enophthalmos, 158
Epidermal growth factor (EGF), 10, 19, 70, 173
Epidermis, 8—10, 30—35, 81
Epidermolysis bullosa, 10
Epiphyseal growth plate, 47—48, 50
Epiphysis, 47
Epithelialization, 70
Erythema, 233—234
ESCA, see Electron Spectroscopy for Chemical
    Analysis
Ethmoid, 44
Eumelanin, 10
Excluded volume, 54
Extracellular matrix, 11—12, 19, 53, 83, see also
    Dermis
Extracellular matrix proteins (ECM), 95
Extrusion, implants, see Implants, extrusion
Eyelids, 198, 201, 227, 236

F

Facial reconstruction, see also individual entries
    alloplastic implants, 213—214
    bioceramic implants, 325
    biomaterial selection, 101
    fascia lata graft, 193—195
    irradiated cartilage, 148—149
    Mersilene, 317
    paralysis, 193
    serial puncture technique, 229—230
Fanning technique, 232
Fascia
    clinical applications, 190, 193—199
    facial reanimation, 193—195
    histology, 189, 191—192
    lata, anatomy, 188—189
Fascial sling, 193, 195, 197—199
Fat, injectable